ANESTHESIA AND THE LUNG 1992

DEVELOPMENTS IN
CRITICAL CARE MEDICINE AND ANESTHESIOLOGY

Volume 25

The titles published in this series are listed at the end of this volume.

ANESTHESIA AND THE LUNG 1992

edited by

T. H. STANLEY and R. J. SPERRY

Department of Anesthesiology,
The University of Utah Medical School
Salt Lake City, Utah, U.S.A.

SPRINGER SCIENCE+BUSINESS MEDIA, B.V.

Library of Congress Cataloging-in-Publication Data

Anesthesia and the lung 1992 / edited by T.H. Stanley and R.J. Sperry.
        p.   cm. -- (Developments in critical care, medicine and
anesthesiology ; v. 25)
      "Contains the refresher course manuscripts of the presentations of
the 37th Annual Postgraduate Course in Anesthesiology ... at Cliff
Conference Center in Snowbird, Utah, February 28-March 3, 1992"-
-Pref.
      ISBN 978-0-7923-1563-6   ISBN 978-94-011-2724-0 (eBook)
      DOI 10.1007/978-94-011-2724-0
      1. Lungs--Diseases--Complications and sequelae--Congresses.
2. Anesthetics--Pathophysiology--Congresses. 3. Lungs--Effect of
drugs on--Congresses. 4. Lungs--Pathophysiology--Congresses.
I. Stanley, Theodore H. (Theodore Henry), 1940-   . II. Sperry, R.
J. III. Postgraduate Course in Anesthesiology (37th : 1992 :
Snowbird, Utah) IV. Series: Developments in critical care medicine
and anaesthesiology ; 25.
      [DNLM: 1. Anesthesia--congresses. 2. Lung Diseases--therapy-
-congresses. 3. Lung Diseases--physiopathology--congresses.
4. Pulmonary Circulation--congresses.   W1 DE997VRL v. 25]
RD87.3.L85A54 1992
617.9'6041--dc20
DNLM/DLC
                                                            91-35394
ISBN 978-0-7923-1563-6

Table of Contents

PREFACE

Theodore H. Stanley, M.D.

Anesthesia and the Lung 1992 contains the Refresher Course manuscripts of the presentations of the 37th Annual Postgraduate Course in Anesthesiology which took place at the Cliff Conference Center in Snowbird, Utah, February 28 - March 3, 1992. The chapters reflect recent advances in the diagnosis, pre-, intra-, and postoperative anesthetic management of patients with lung disease, presenting for pulmonary and non-pulmonary surgery. They also deal with ventilation-perfusion issues, the lung as a metabolic organ, the effects of anesthesia on pulmonary mechanics and pulmonary blood flow. In addition, there are chapters that focus around hypoxia; regional differences in the lung; pulmonary surfactant; recent advances in the understanding of pulmonary edema; high altitude disease; anesthesia and the control of breathing; recent development in oximetry; instrumentation designed to measure pulmonary oxygen tension, PO_2 and PCO_2 transcutaneously; differential lung ventilation; reactive airways; septic shock; the adult respiratory distress syndrome and numerous aspects of ventilatory support. The purposes of the textbook are to 1) act as a reference for the anesthesiologists attending the meeting, and 2) serve as a vehicle to bring many of the latest concepts in anesthesiology to others within a short time of the formal presentation. Each chapter is a brief but sharply focused glimpse of the interests in anesthesia expressed at the conference. This book and its chapters should not be considered complete treatises on the subjects addressed but rather attempts to summarize the most salient points. This textbook is the tenth in a continuing series documenting the proceedings of the Postgraduate Course in Salt Lake City. We hope that this and the past and future volumes reflect the rapid and continuing evolution of anesthesiology in the late twentieth century.

LIST OF CONTRIBUTORS

Allen, S. J.
Department of Anesthesiology, Center for Microvascular and
Lymphatic Studies, University of Texas - Houston, Houston, TX
77225, U.S.A.

Benumof, J. L.
Anesthesia Research Laboratory, The University of California, San
Diego, La Jolla, CA 92093, U.S.A.

Bone, R. C.
Department of Internal Medicine, Rush-Presbyterian/St. Luke's
Medical Center, Chicago, IL 60612, U.S.A.

Corbeil, C.
Meakins-Christie Laboratories, McGill University, and Hôpital
Saint-Luc, Université de Montréal, Montreal, Quebec, Canada

Downs, J. B.
Department of Anesthesiology, The University of South Florida,
Tampa, FL 33612-4799, U.S.A.

Eissa, N. T., Meakins-Christie Laboratories, McGill University, and Hôpital
Saint-Luc, Université de Montréal, Montreal, Quebec, Canada

Frasch, H. F.
Department of Anesthesia, The University of Pennsylvania School
of Medicine, Philadelphia, PA 19104-4283, U.S.A.

Hornbein, Th. F.
Department of Anesthesiology, The University of Washington
School of Medicine, Seattle, WA 98195, U.S.A.

Lumb, A. B.
Division of Anaesthesia, Clinical Research Centre, Watford Road,
Harrow, Middlesex HA1 3UJ, U.K.

Marshall, C.
Department of Anesthesia, The University of Pennsylvania School
of Medicine, Philadelphia, PA 19104-4283, U.S.A.

Marshall, B. E.
Department of Anesthesia, The University of Pennsylvania School
of Medicine, Philadelphia, PA 19104-4283, U.S.A.

Milic-Emili, J.
    Meakins-Christie Laboratories, McGill University, Montreal,
    Quebec, H2X 2P2, Canada

Nunn, J. F.
    Division of Anaesthesia, Clinical Research Centre, Watford Road,
    Harrow, Middlesex HA1 3UJ, U.K.

V.M. Ranieri,
    University of Bari, Bari, 70100, Italy

Severinghaus, J. W.
    Anesthesia Research Center, The University of California, San
    Francisco, School of Medicine, San Francisco, CA 94143-0542, U.S.A.

West, J. B.
    Department of Medicine, Section of Physiology, The University of
    California, San Diego, School of Medicine, La Jolla, CA 92093,
    U.S.A.

Zapol, W. M.
    Department of Anaesthesia, Massachusetts General Hospital,
    Boston, MA, 02114, U.S.A.

Zimmerman, G. A.
    Division of Respiratory, Critical Care, and Occupational Medicine,
    Department of Internal Medicine, The University of Utah School of
    Medicine, Salt Lake City, UT 84132, U.S.A.

GRAVITY AND THE LUNG: LESSONS FROM SPACE

J. B. West

The normal lung is exquisitely sensitive to gravity, which causes regional differences in blood flow, ventilation, gas exchange, alveolar size, intrapleural pressure, and mechanical stress (1). These topographical differences of structure and function have many implications in the way in which disease processes develop. Recent work on pulmonary function in the absence of gravity, including measurements in Spacelab SLS-1 in June 1991, have clarified the effects of gravity on the lung.

BLOOD FLOW

Blood flow decreases up the upright human lung, reaching very low values at the apex. The inequality of blood flow is altered by change of posture; thus in the supine position, apical and basal blood flow are the same, but there is an increase in blood flow from the anterior to posterior (dependent) region of the lung. During upright exercise, both apical and basal blood flows increase, and the distribution becomes more uniform.

The regional differences in blood flow can be explained by the effects of the pulmonary arterial, venous, and alveolar pressures on the pulmonary capillaries. Basically, the gradient can be attributed to the hydrostatic pressures in the column of blood in the lung which are not balanced by similar pressures in the alveoli. In addition, lung volume plays a role because when the expansion of the lung is decreased, the extraalveolar vessels narrow, and this contributes to an increase in vascular resistance. The result is a region of reduced blood flow at the lung base.

1

T. H. Stanley and R. J. Sperry (eds.), Anesthesia and the Lung 1992, 1–7.
© 1992 Kluwer Academic Publishers.

It is known that increased acceleration exaggerates the normal regional inequality of blood flow. Extensive centrifuge studies of $+g_z$ acceleration (headward) and $+g_x$ (forward acceleration) have been carried out. Pilots are subjected to $+g_z$ accelerations during tight turns in high-performance aircraft, and astronauts lie supine in the spacecraft during lift-off ($+g_x$) because tolerance to acceleration is better in this position.

VENTILATION

Because the lung distorts under its own weight, the alveoli at the base of the upright lung are relatively compressed compared with the apical alveoli; and because poorly expanded lung is more compliant, ventilation increases down the upright human lung. Thus the changes in ventilation are in the same direction as those for blood flow, but the magnitude of the inequality of ventilation is less.

A striking change in the regional distribution of ventilation occurs at low lung volumes because the basal airways close, and for small inspirations from residual volume, no gas enters the basal regions. Therefore under theses conditions, the normal pattern of ventilation is reversed, with the apex being ventilated best.

Increase acceleration has been shown to exaggerate the normal regional differences in ventilation, as for blood flow. At high $+g_z$ levels (aircraft in a tight turn) an interesting dissociation of ventilation and blood flow can occur. Blood flow is confined to the base of the lung because of hydrostatic effects, whereas ventilation is confined to the upper regions because of basal airway closure. As a result there is little meeting of the two, and gas exchange is greatly impaired.

GAS EXCHANGE

Because gas exchange in any region of the lung is determined by the ventilation-perfusion ratio, the regional differences of blood flow and ventilation imply regional differences of gas exchange. For example, because the ventilation-perfusion ratio is relatively high at the apex of the lung, this region has a high PO_2, low PCO_2, and high pH. Furthermore, the uptake of oxygen and elimination of carbon dioxide by the upper regions of the lung are relatively small because of the reduced blood flow and ventilation to that region. On exercise, when the pulmonary artery pressure rises and the distribution of blood flow becomes more uniform, the upper regions of the lung take on larger proportions of total gas exchange.

ALVEOLAR SIZE

Because the lung distorts under its own weight, the basal alveoli are less well expanded than the apical alveoli. In anesthetized dogs frozen in the head-up position, the apical alveoli are four times larger by volume than those at the base. However, when the animals were frozen in the supine position, the size of the apical and basal alveoli were the same, confirming that gravity was responsible of the differences. These differences in alveoli size are closely related to the regional differences in ventilation described above.

INTRAPLEURAL PRESSURES

The weight of the lung is supported, to a large extent, by the rib cage and diaphragm. As a result of the downward-acting weight force, the pressure near the bottom of the lung must be greater than the pressure near the top. This means that the intrapleural pressure is less negative at the bottom of the lung than at the top. Regional differences in intrapleural pressure were first demonstrated in head-up anesthetized dogs and subsequently in many other animals. Early evidence in humans was obtained by measuring esophageal pressure at different levels.

PARENCHYMAL STRESSES

Just as the relative overexpansion of the lung at the apex is associated with very low intrapleural pressures, it also causes large mechanical parenchymal stresses. Because of technical difficulties, these have not been measured directly, but the pattern of stress distribution has been analyzed by finite element techniques. The higher stresses near the apex may explain the pattern of development of centrilobular emphysema, spontaneous pneumothorax, and other diseases.

EFFECTS OF SHORT PERIODS OF WEIGHTLESSNESS ON TOPOGRAPHICAL DIFFERENCES

All the regional differences of structure and function referred to above are caused by gravity. The weight of the column of blood in the lung is responsible for the regional differences of blood flow, whereas the distortion of the lung itself by its own weight causes the regional differences in ventilation, alveolar size, intrapleural pressure, and parenchymal stress. Therefore, presumably the regional differences will be greatly reduced by weightlessness, though there are reasons to think that they might not be completely abolished.

In 1978 we carried out studies on a Learjet aircraft flying parabolic arcs (2) which give 20-25 seconds of weightlessness. The measurements were made with prototype equipment being developed for the experiment on Spacelab SLS-1, and data were obtained from four normal subjects during 112 weightless periods.

The inequality of ventilation was measured from single-breath nitrogen washouts which were performed with a test inspiration containing an initial bolus of argon at residual volume. Striking alterations in the pattern were seen during weightlessness compared with the measurements obtained at 1g flying straight and level. The cardiogenic oscillations on the alveolar plateau were greatly diminished at 0g, and there was a striking reduction of terminal rises for both nitrogen and argon. The cardiogenic oscillations are caused by preferential emptying of the lung bases due to movement of the beating heart, whereas the terminal rises of nitrogen and argon are the result of basal airway closure. These measurements provided strong evidence that under weightless conditions, the topographical differences of lung expansion and ventilation were dramatically reduced.

An interesting feature of these studies is that the nitrogen tracings for 0g showed larger cardiogenic oscillations and terminal rises (though these were both small) than did the argon tracings. The probable reason for this is the compression of the base of the lung caused by a period of increased g forces prior to the weightless parabolic arc, along with the fact that the lung takes a few seconds to recover from this distortion. The point is mentioned here partly to bring out a limitation of parabolic profile maneuvers in that these are preceded and succeeded by periods of increased gravitational loading. This factor, along with the short duration of the microgravity, limits the value of this type of measurement. However, flying Keplerian arcs is the only way to generate the microgravity state for more than 2 or 3 sec (free fall) in the absence of orbital flight.

At the time that these measurements were made, there was disagreement on whether the topographical inequality of ventilation was caused by distortion of the lung by its own weight, or whether it was due to distortion of the chest wall by gravity. To answer this questions, chest radiographs were taken in both the 1g and 0g states, and the shape of the rib cage and diaphragm was traced (3). These results showed that there was very little change, although during microgravity there was a tendency for the diaphragm to be higher and for the rib cage to be slightly wider.

Information was also obtained on the topographical distribution of pulmonary blood flow in these experiments. For these measurements, the subject first hyperventilated for about 5 sec, and then he held his breath at total lung capacity for approximately 15 sec. Subsequently, expired PO_2 and PCO_2 were measured with the mass spectrometer during a steady flow exhalation to residual volume. The size of the cardiogenic oscillations on the alveolar plateau was determined by how rapidly the PO_2 and PCO_2 had changed during the breathhold period, and this was a measure of blood flow per unit lung volume. We found that the cardiogenic oscillations were exaggerated by increased acceleration, but they were almost abolished under weightless conditions. Again, this was strong evidence that the topographical inequality of blood flow is grossly reduced in the microgravity environment.

PULMONARY FUNCTION DURING EXTENDED SPACEFLIGHT AS MEASURED SPACELAB SLS-1

Spacelab is a cylindrical laboratory about 7 meters long and 4 meters in diameter which is carried into low earth orbit by the Space Shuttle. The first spacelab dedicated to life sciences flew in June 1991, and one of the 20 experiments on board was our experiment to measure the effects of weightlessness on pulmonary function. The measurements included resting gas exchange, distribution of ventilation and blood flow in the lung, diffusing capacity for carbon monoxide during air and oxygen breathing, lung volumes, cardiac output by rebreathing, and forced expiration. This was by far the most extensive investigation of pulmonary function in space to date.

Although at the time of writing this, the flight landed less than a month ago, it is already clear that there are some surprises. The single breath nitrogen washout, with an argon bolus included at the beginning of inspiration, showed obvious cardiogenic oscillations in both nitrogen and argon during the test expiration. This presumably means that there is some residual topographical inequality of ventilation in the lung during extended periods of weightlessness. A similar result was found during the short-term parabolic profile flights in the Learjet flights but there the 20-27 sec period of weightlessness was preceded by a period of increased g forces as the aircraft pulled up in preparation for its maneuver and we could never be sure that we were seeing the pure effects of weightlessness.

Another interesting finding from Spacelab SLS-1 was that the test of inequality of blood flow which was the same as used in the Learjet experiments also showed obvious cardiogenic oscillations. Again this presumably means that there is some remaining topographical inequality of blood flow in the lung when all the gravitational forces have been removed. Finally, we looked for evidence of inequality of ventilation-perfusion ratios by measuring the changes in the respiratory exchange ratio during a long expiration. Again, to our surprise there was clear evidence of ventilation-perfusion inequality.

It will take many months to complete the analysis of the extensive series of measurements obtained on Spacelab SLS-1. However it is already clear that we have much stimulating and provocative data on the effect of gravity on pulmonary structure and function.

ACKNOWLEDGEMENTS

This work was supported by NASA Grant NAG-2-616.

REFERENCES

1. West JB: Regional Differences in the Lung. New York, Academic Press, 1977
2. Michels DB, West JB: Distribution of pulmonary ventilation and perfusion during short periods of weightlessness. J Appl Physiol 45: 987-8, 1978
3. Michaels DB, Friedman PJ, West JB: Radiographic comparison of human lung shape during normal gravity and weightlessness. J Appl Physiol 47: 851-7, 1979

CONTROL OF THE PULMONARY CIRCULATION

B. E. Marshall, C. Marshall and H. F. Frasch

INTRODUCTION

The first essay, in this series of three, discussed the influence of anesthesia on pulmonary gas exchange and the role of ventilation/perfusion ratios in determining the outcome. Hypoxic pulmonary vasoconstriction was shown to be of critical importance. The second essay introduced a model of the pulmonary circulation that permits analysis of complex interactions to reveal the individual influences. Implicit to both these discussions was the concept that HPV contributes to regulation of ventilation/perfusion ratios ($\dot{V}A/\dot{Q}C$) and that $\dot{V}A/\dot{Q}C$ distribution is an important determinant of steady state pulmonary hemodynamics. The purpose of this discussion is to introduce the beginnings of the resolution of this long standing pulmonary research problem.

HEMODYNAMIC EFFECT OF $\dot{V}A/\dot{Q}C$ DISTRIBUTIONS

Measurement of $\dot{V}A/\dot{Q}C$

The multiple inert gas technique developed by Wagner and West (1) permits the assignment of flow and ventilation to the lung in 50 compartments with $\dot{V}A/\dot{Q}C$ varying from zero to infinity. These compartments have no *a priori* anatomic localization and the ordinate (Fig. 1) represents the total flow or ventilation to each compartment. The sum of all the flows is the cardiac output. This approach also yields the alveolar oxygen and carbon dioxide tensions for each compartment which together with the blood flow and the mixed venous gas tension permit calculation of the final mixed arterial gas tension. For any combination of mean and log standard deviation of $\dot{V}A/\dot{Q}C$ ratios, cardiac output, oxygen

9

T. H. Stanley and R. J. Sperry (eds.), Anesthesia and the Lung 1992, 9–18.
© 1992 Kluwer Academic Publishers.

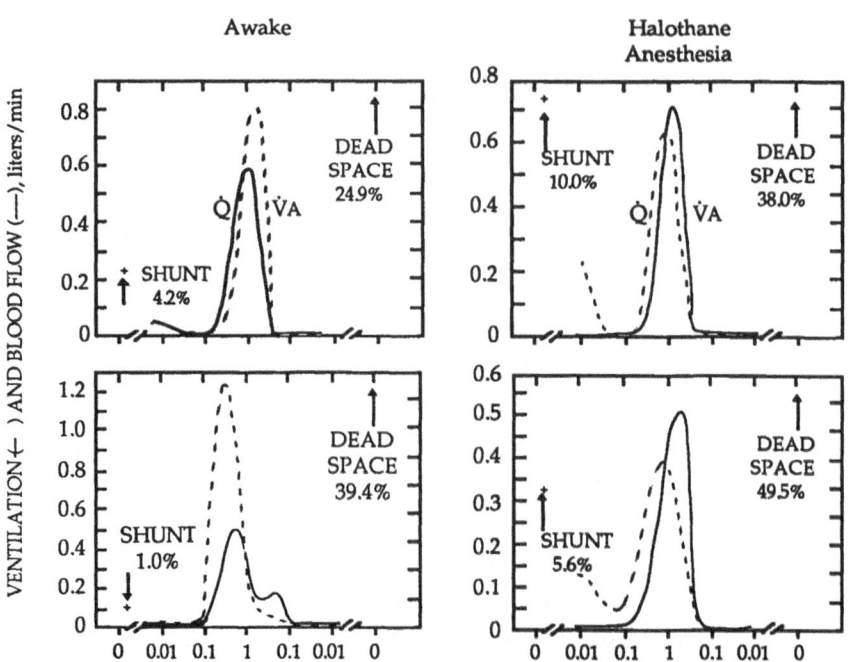

Figure 1. Multiple-Inert Case Measurement of Ventilation-Perfusion Distribution in Humans. (Left) Results from two awake individuals (Right) Results from the same two subjects during halothane anesthesia. The effects of the anesthetic are to increase shunt and dead space, and ventilation-perfusion distribution data have an increased spread particularly evident in the low $\dot{V}A/\dot{Q}C$ regions. (Redrawn from Dueck R et al: Altered distribution of pulmonary ventilation and blood flow following induction of inhalational anesthesia. Anesthesiology 52:113-25, 1980).

consumption, inspired oxygen and blood hemoglobin and pH, the resulting gas exchange can be predicted. Furthermore utilizing the relationships introduced in the first essay, because the mixed venous oxygen tension is common to all compartments and the alveolar oxygen tension is calculated as above therefore the stimulus oxygen tension (PSO_2) for HPV can be defined for each compartment together with its pH (Fig. 2).

Derivation of the Pressure/Flow Relations

For each compartment the pressure/flow plot can be calculated utilizing the information obtained from the $\dot{V}A/\dot{Q}C$ analysis (Fig. 3) to obtain

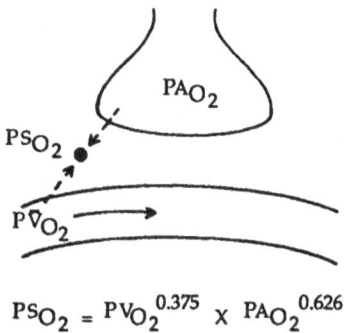

$$PSO_2 = PV_{O_2}^{0.375} \times PA_{O_2}^{0.626}$$

Figure 2 . The stimulus oxygen tension (PSO_2) is illustrated as a discrete site in the wall of the precapillary arteriole influenced by both the alveolar (P_aO_2) and mixed venous (PvO_2) oxygen tensions.

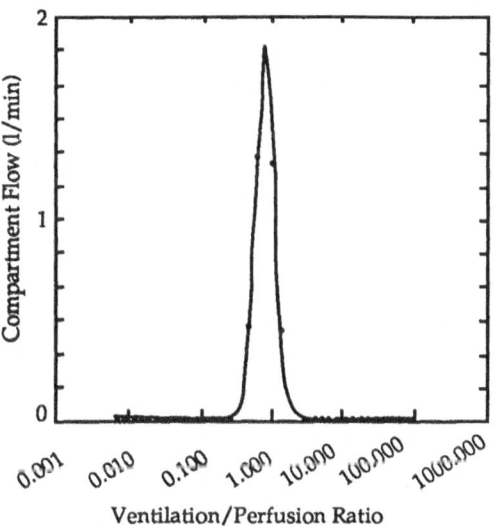

Figure 3. Calculation of effect of $\dot{V}A/\dot{Q}C$ ratio on pressure flow relations to illustrate calculation the 50 compartment lung is modelled with perfusion to only 9 compartments, normally distributed and with no shunt. From these data the PSO_2 for each compartment is derived.

Table 1. Derivation of the hypoxic stimulus (PSO$_2$) for nine components from the $\dot{V}A/\dot{Q}C$ distribution

$\dot{V}$ l/m	$\dot{Q}$ l/m	$\dot{V}/\dot{Q}$	P$_{\bar{v}}$O$_2$ mmHg	PAO$_2$ mmHg	PACO$_2$ mmHg	PSO$_2$ mmHg
0.002	0.006	0.291	40	60.4	44.2	51.2
0.029	0.076	0.375	40	68.7	43.7	55.3
0.218	0.452	0.483	40	79.2	42.9	50.2
0.816	1.311	0.623	40	90.3	41.8	65.2
1.491	1.857	0.803	40	100.4	40.4	69.5
1.330	1.285	1.035	40	109.1	38.7	73.0
0.579	0.434	1.334	40	116.3	36.7	75.9
0.123	0.072	1.720	40	122.2	34.5	78.2
0.013	0.006	2.217	40	127.1	32.0	80.0

the PSO$_2$ (Table 1) and applying the generalized model outlined in the second essay (3). In brief the left atrial pressure is the starting point for each calculation and working backwards across the pulmonary circulation the pulmonary artery pressure is calculated that would be necessary to conduct the flow across the generation of vessels in the particular circumstance of passive and active forces that apply. These calculations provide a complete pressure/relative flow curve for each compartment (Fig. 4). Solutions of these curves are then derived for a particular pulmonary artery pressure and the total cardiac output is calculated that would have been present in the absence of HPV. The calculation is repeated interactively until the solution converges on unique values that match the sum of the relative flows to the normoxic cardiac output. This is the dashed line in Figure 4.

The result is, therefore, a prediction of pulmonary artery pressure and pulmonary vascular conductance (resistance) that accompany a particular $\dot{V}A/\dot{Q}C$ distribution. With this tool it is, therefore, possible to examine systematically, and for the first time, the role of HPV in the regulation of $\dot{V}A/\dot{Q}C$ and the significance of these effects on steady state pulmonary hemodynamics.

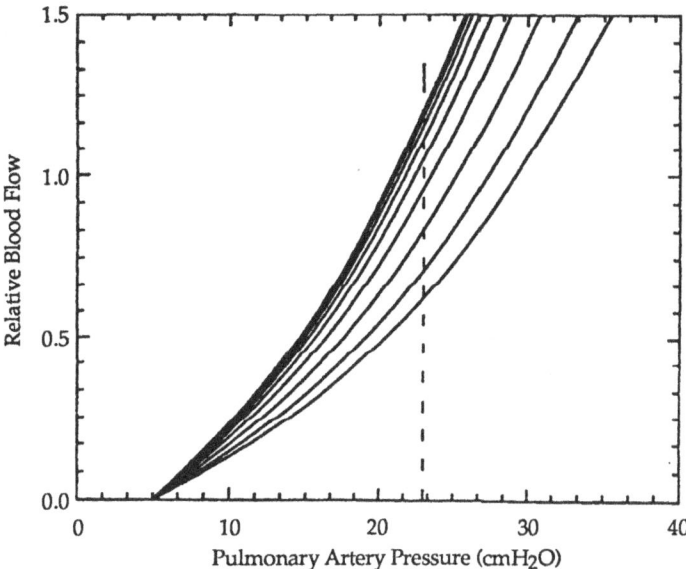

Figure 4. Calculation of effect of V̇A/Q̇C rate on pressure/flow relation. From the PSO₂ derived in Fig. 3 the pressure/flow curve for each of the nine compartments is calculated together with a curve (the thick line) when the HPV is present. The dashed vertical line indicates the unique solution that satisfies the total flow (sources of all seven compartments with flow) and a particular pulmonary artery pressure. See text for discussion.

Regulation of V̇A/Q̇C by HPV

Chronic bronchitis is a condition in which impairment of gas exchanges is prominent and is due to the broadened distribution of the V̇A/Q̇C ratios as documented by several clinical studies (2). These patients also demonstrate increased pulmonary vascular resistance. The questions to be examined are, therefore, to what extent does HPV improve oxygenation by reducing the V̇A/Q̇C abnormality and at the same time by how much is the pulmonary vascular resistance increased. Intuitively both these questions are qualitatively correct but until now no convincing quantitation has been advanced.

The data for inert gas analysis of patients with chronic bronchitis were analyzed as above to provide the pulmonary vascular resistance and arterial oxygen tension (Fig. 5). The model was then modified so that the

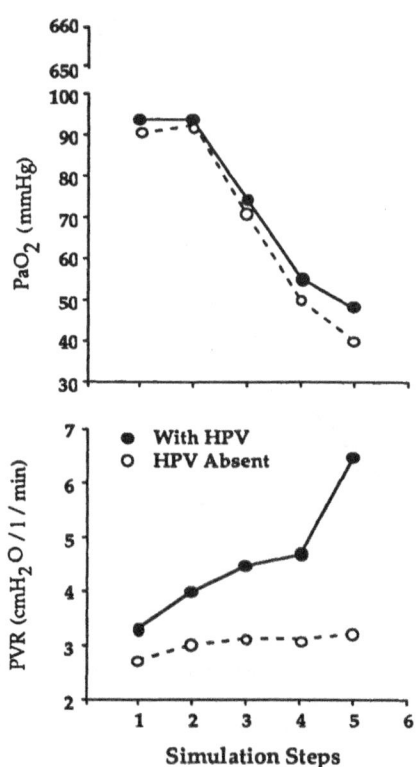

Figure 5. Role of HPV in the pathophysiology of chronic bronchitis. The P_aO_2 and PVR of a normal subject (Step 1) the same subject. With chronic bronchitis (Step 5) breathing air. Step 1 normal lung, mean $\dot{V}A/\dot{Q}C$ = 8, Log Sd = 0.3; Step 2 with 25% of lung vascular bed lost; Step 3 and mean $\dot{V}A/\dot{Q}C$ = 0.6; Step 4 and Log SD - 1.1; Step 5 and cardiac output reduced by 25%. Step 6 in the influence of 100% O_2 breathing on Step 5. (Pulmonary shunt is assumed to be zero for the purpose of demonstrating the HPV to $\dot{V}A/\dot{Q}C$ interaction).

derivations were recalculated in steps corresponding to the pathophysiologic characteristics of this disease. Step one was, therefore, the normal
subject free of disease, step 2 a reduction of the cardiac output by 25%, step
3 plus a reduced mean $\dot{V}A/\dot{Q}C$, step 4 plus an increased log standard
deviation for the mean $\dot{V}A/\dot{Q}C$ distribution (no shunt was included), step
5 plus a reduced cardiac output which corresponds to the fully developed
disease. The calculations reveal that the arterial oxygen tension is
progressively reduced and the pulmonary vascular resistance increased at
each step. However, the calculations were then repeated in the absence of
HPV and the result is surprising in that the effect on the arterial

oxygenation is real but quite small, while that on vascular resistance is impressively large. This result is, therefore, the theoretical support for the conclusion of the first essay that inhibition of HPV by anesthetic agents has only a modest effect on the hypoxemia that results from overall $\dot{V}A/\dot{Q}C$ maldistribution, where its effect on the hypoxemia that results from shunt or very low $\dot{V}A/\dot{Q}C$ regimen is more pronounced. In contrast the very substantial increase in pulmonary vascular resistance is consistent with the tendency of such patients to ultimately succumb to right heart failure.

$\dot{V}A/\dot{Q}C$ Changes with One Lung Hypoxia

A study by Domino, et al. (4) measured the $\dot{V}A/\dot{Q}C$ distribution in each lung before and after one of the lungs was subjected to hypoxia. The data revealed changes in the blood flow distribution such that $\dot{V}A/\dot{Q}C$ in the normoxic lung improved while that in the hypoxic lung did not. The authors kindly supplied us with the original data and the computer model was characterized with the data from the animals when both lungs were normoxic and then the model was changed only to make one lung hypoxic. The influence of this condition on the resulting $\dot{V}A/\dot{Q}C$ distribution in each lung and on the gas exchange were then calculated and compared to the experimental result. The computer experiment and the animal experiment coincide remarkably (Table 2) indicating that the observed result is that expected from the normal physiologic response and no new hypotheses are required to explain the result. This conclusion is of some significance because it was not possible in the original paper to elucidate the various interactions.

Estimation of Differential Lung Blood Flow by Carbon Dioxide Excretion

Because the blood flow to the lung is the source of carbon dioxide excretion, it is possible to estimate the functional blood flow to each lung by measuring the fraction of the total carbon dioxide that is excreted by each lung. This technique has been established and used for many years and more recently has been adopted for the same purpose when one lung

Table 2. Effect of left lower lobe hypoxia on $\dot{V}A/\dot{Q}$ distribution in both lungs. Comparison of experimental data and computer modelling

		Experiment	Model
	Q_T	3.14	3.14
	Q_R	2.80	2.76
	Q_L	0.34	0.38
	Q_R	1.44	1.41
	Q_L	1.93	1.66
	$LOGSD_R$	0.56	0.6
$\dot{V}/\dot{Q}$	$LOGSD_L$	0.89	0.85
	$P_{\bar{v}}O_2$	50	48
	$P_{\bar{v}}CO_2$	40	38
	P_aO_2	303	446
	$PACO_2$	33	30

is hypoxic. However, unilateral hypoxia introduces several complicating factors. In the usual experimental situation the ventilation is maintained constant to the hypoxic lung while HPV reduces the blood flow. The result is that the carbon dioxide excretion is overestimated and the profound alkalosis that develops in the hypoxic lung leads to inhibition of HPV and an oscillation of the blood flow change (5). However, if carbon dioxide is added to the hypoxic lung so as to maintain the alveolar carbon dioxide tension constant two theoretical difficulties are apparent. The first is the Haldane effect, whereby desaturated hemoglobin retains carbon dioxide, so that the carbon dioxide excretion from the hypoxic lung is underestimated. The second is the possibility that hypoxia may so exaggerate the influence of a maldistribution of $\dot{V}A/\dot{Q}C$ as to impair carbon dioxide excretion. Experimental data in dogs have shown that the Haldane effect can account for a 25% reduction in carbon dioxide excretion when one lung is exposed to 3% oxygen and the end-tidal carbon dioxide tension is maintained constant. The result demonstrated wide variability (Fig. 6).

A modelling experiment was, therefore, undertaken to investigate these effects. The results demonstrate that the Haldane effect is large and predictable and that the influences of hypoxia on the $\dot{V}A/\dot{Q}C$ distribution of carbon dioxide excretion is very small. However, these analyses demonstrated the exquisite sensitivity of the preparation to these conditions. Thus very small changes in added inspired carbon dioxide or in ventila-

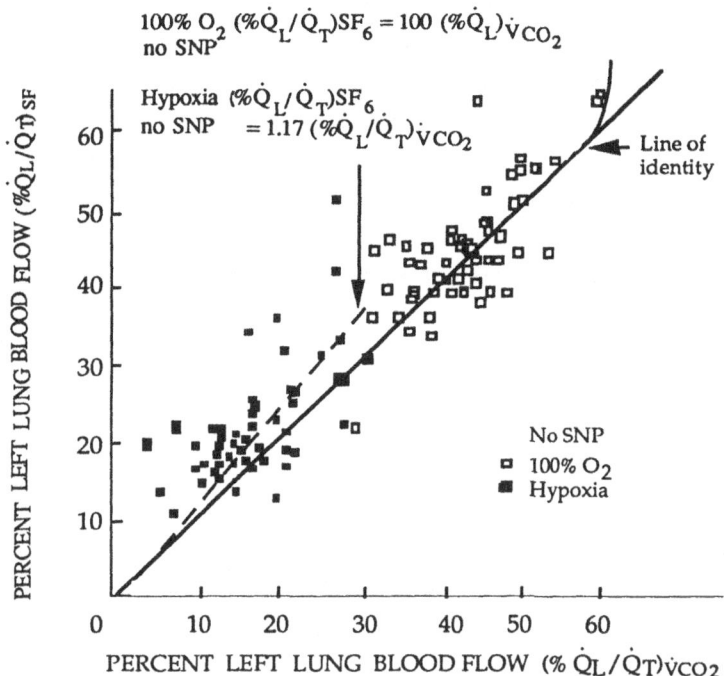

Figure 6. Comparison of blood flow distribution to left lung of dogs measured with sulfur hexafluride (SF) and carbon oxide excretion. The dashed line fitted to the values measured during hypoxia is shifted from the line of identity (solid line and open squares) because of the haldane effect. See text for discussion of variability (personal communication, L. Chen).

tion result in large changes in carbon dioxide excretion and this appears to account for the variability observed experimentally. The conclusion, therefore, is that these techniques must be applied with great care.

CONCLUSION

A new method is described to combine the computer model of the $\dot{V}A/\dot{Q}C$ distribution with the steady state hemodynamic model. The power of this technique is illustrated by analysis of some previously intractable questions. Concerning the influence of anesthesia on gas exchange and pulmonary hemodynamics, the more complete analysis confirms the conclusion regarding the experimental work of the previous

two essays. Namely that HPV has profound importance during all distur-
bances of $\dot{V}A/\dot{Q}C$. For areas of shunt and very low $\dot{V}A/\dot{Q}C$, HPV is the
mechanism responsible for reducing hypoxemia, and anesthetic agents, by
inhibiting HPV, are not infrequently associated with arterial hypoxemia.
For patients with diseases increasing the distribution of $\dot{V}A/\dot{Q}C$ ratios the
influence of HPV is to provide only a modest improvement of arterial
oxygenation while at the same time considerably increasing the pulmonary vascular resistance and, therefore, the right heart work. Perhaps
this is one of the reasons that some patients with severe preoperative
pulmonary impairment improve clinically when subjected to general
anesthesia.

Acknowledgement

This work was supported in part by NIGMS Grant Number
RO19M29628 for NIH.

REFERENCES

1. West JB, Wagner PD: Pulmonary Gas Exchange. Bioengineering
   Aspects of the Lung. West JB (ed.). New York, Marcel Dekker, 1977,
   pp 361-458
2. Dueck R, Young I, Clausen J, et al: Altered distribution of pulmonary
   ventilation and blood flow following induction of inhalational anesthesia. Anesthesiology 52:113-25, 1980
3. Marshall BE, Marshall C: A model for hypoxic pulmonary vasoconstriction. J Appl Physiol 64:68-77, 1988
4. Domino KB, Hlastrala MP, Eisenstein BL, et al: Effect of regional
   alveolar hypoxia on gas exchange in dog. J Appl Physiol 67:730-5, 1989
5. Benumof JL, Mathers JM, Wahrenbrock EA: Cyclic hypoxic pulmonary vasoconstriction induced by concomitant carbon dioxide
   changes. J Appl Physiol 41:466-9, 1976

A PRIMER ON PULMONARY CELL BIOLOGY: LUNG CELLS AND THEIR FUNCTIONS

G. A. Zimmerman

CELL BIOLOGY OF ALVEOLI AND AIRWAYS

The lung contains over 40 different cell types. Each has a variety of structural and metabolic functions that may be altered by disease states. The potential functions of some of these cells have been studied in detail (1,2), while the activities of other cell types are little known. In this discussion we will emphasize several specific cells that are important in a variety of syndromes of lung injury. For practical purposes the cells of the pulmonary parenchyma can be divided into a few groups.

A. Cells of the Alveolar-capillary Membrane

The "alveolar-capillary membrane" has as its major function *gas exchange*, and is lined on both sides by specialized cells. Approximately 95% of the alveolar surface is covered by *Alveolar Type I cells*, which are thin, attenuated cells with a very large surface area relative to their volume, and with relatively few organelles. The narrow barrier formed by the cytoplasm of these cells facilitates the diffusion of gases across the alveolar surface. At the same time they form tight junctions with other alveolar Type I cells that make them essentially impermeable to water and low molecular wight substances that may be present in the interstitium. Thus they serve *transport* (gases, and some other substances), *"barrier"* (some fluids and solutes), and *structural* roles.

The *pulmonary capillary endothelial cell* is the other major cell type of the alveolar capillary unit. The endothelial cell also has a very large surface area relative to its volume, which is an important feature for O_2

19

T. H. Stanley and R. J. Sperry (eds.), Anesthesia and the Lung 1992, 19–29.
© 1992 *Kluwer Academic Publishers.*

and CO_2 exchange. The pulmonary endothelial cells allow the passage of water and small molecular weight molecules into the interstitium, and thus the endothelium is somewhat more "permeable" than the alveolar surface. In this regard the pulmonary endothelium performs a function that is common to capillaries in general: the transport of fluids and solutes to adjacent extravascular cells. In addition, pulmonary endothelial cells metabolize a variety of biologically-active compounds. As an example, bradykinin is degraded and angiotensin I is converted to angiotensin II by an enzyme bound to the luminal surface of the endothelial cells (angiotensin converting enzyme, kininase II).

As mentioned, the major "business" of the alveolar capillary membrane is gas exchange. The large surface area covered by the Type I cells and endothelial cells (greater than 100 M2 for each), and the thin cytoplasmic barrier of each cell, facilitate this function. The barrier for the diffusion of O_2 from the alveolar gas to the plasma in the capillaries is only 0.5-1.0 µM, even though it is composed of a) cytoplasm of the Type I cells, b) cytoplasm of the endothelial cells, and c) the basement membranes of both cell types. However, the large surface covered by each cell, and their attenuated, delicate cytoplasmic processes, appear to also predispose them to injury by toxic agents carried in the alveolar gas or the plasma. Injury to the cells of the alveolar capillary membrane can interfere with O_2 and CO_2 exchange. One common manifestation of injury to cells of the alveolar capillary membrane is *pulmonary edema*. Acute pulmonary vascular injury often results in increased permeability of the endothelium of the microvessels to water and large molecular weight substances (such as proteins), resulting in *"increased permeability" pulmonary edema*. There is also evidence that pulmonary edema can result from increased permeability of the alveolar surface formed by the Type I cells. In either event, gas exchange will be impaired by the accumulation of edema fluid in the alveoli or in the interstitial space. Increased permeability pulmonary edema is one important feature of adult respiratory distress syndrome (ARDS), which can result from fulminant injury to alveolar endothelial cells, Type I epithelial cells, or both.

Impaired gas exchange can also result from other manifestations of cellular injury besides edema, such as swelling of the endothelial cells or Type I cells, replacement of the Type I cells with Type II cells (which are thicker than Type I cells—see the next paragraph), infiltration of the inter-stitial space with inflammatory cells, fibroblasts, or fibrous tissue, or actual destruction of capillaries with loss of part of the vascular surface. These are just a few examples of how injury to Type I cells and endothelial cells can impair the vital *gas exchange function* of the lung.

The *alveolar Type II cells* are more numerous than the Type I cells, but the Type II cells cover only 3 to 5% of the alveolar surface. Therefore, they have a much smaller surface-to-volume ratio than the Type I cells. In addition, they have many intracellular organelles and are specialized to produce phospholipids and protein components of the alveolar lining material known as *surfactant*. Surfactant is secreted onto the alveolar sur-face in a regulated fashion. Since surfactant diminishes alveolar surface tension and prevents alveolar collapse, Type II cells are critically impor-tant in the maintenance of normal gas exchange, although their role is less direct than that of the Type I cells and endothelial cells. Infant Respiratory Distress Syndrome ("Hyaline Membrane Disease") is a human disease in which immaturity of the Type II cells in premature infants prevents sur-factant secretion. This results in alveolar collapse and severe hypoxemia and hypercarbia. Type II cells have other functions besides surfactant secretion, including the ability to divide and to differentiate into Type I cells. This is an important activity since Type I cells are not able to divide; thus Type II cells appear to repopulate the alveolar surface after limited injury.

The *alveolar macrophage* will be discussed later.

B. Specialized Airway Cells

The airway epithelium contains *secretory cells* and *ciliated epithelial cells* that are specialized to participate in the process of *mucociliary clearance* (see section, Lung Defense: Mechanical and Cellular Mechanisms). This highly regulated process is one of the major dense mechanisms for the handling of inhaled particulate materials that may be injurious to the lung. *Nonciliated bronchiolar epithelial cells*, also termed *Clara cells*, are found primarily in the bronchioles and appear to have a variety of functions, including secretion of some components of the extracellular surface lining layer of the bronchioles and alveoli, and the metabolism of exogenous substances. Furthermore, the Clara cells may be the chief cells that repopulate the bronchiolar epithelium after injury. They may also differentiate into other specialized epithelial cells.

C. Interstitial Cells

The basement membranes of the alveolar epithelial and endothelial cells define the boundaries of the alveolar interstitial region. This area, which contains a connective tissue matrix composed of elastin, Types I and III collagen, proteoglycans, and fibronectin, represents about 50% of the tissue volume of the normal lung. Its major cell type is the pulmonary interstitial *fibroblast*, which is likely a *group* of cell types with somewhat similar morphology but different biochemical and functional activities. The most important activities of the fibroblast-like cells are thought to be the synthesis of matrix components and remodeling of the interstitial matrix. They probably perform many other important functions. As an example, there is evidence that some highly specialized fibroblasts may contract, thereby influencing capillary caliber and alveolar volume.

D. Inflammatory and Immune Cells.

The normal pulmonary parenchyma contains many *macrophages* and *lymphocytes* that are found both on the alveolar surface and within the interstitium. *Polymorphonuclear leukocytes* (PMNs) are *not* frequently found in the normal human lung, but they can be rapidly recruited from the blood and are important in lung defense against bacteria and other agents. Each of these three cell types is a critical component of the lung defense system, and is an important *effector cell* in inflammatory lung injury (see chapter, "Mechanisms of Lung Injury--An Overview").

Alveolar macrophages make up the majority of the resident inflammatory/immune cells in the normal lung. They can be retrieved from the alveoli by lavage. The normal role of the alveolar macrophage is to defend the lower respiratory tract by phagocytizing bacteria and particulate matter. Some bacteria can be directly ingested by alveolar macrophages, but for virulent encapsulated bacteria this process usually requires opsonins such as the C3b component of complement, or specific antibodies; the alveolar macrophages have surface receptors for C3b and the FC region of IgG that are important in this process. In response to appropriate stimulation the normally quiescent alveolar macrophages undergo a complex process termed *activation*, resulting in the ability to synthesize and release a variety of mediators that can initiate or amplify inflammatory events.

Ninety percent of the leukocytes in the normal lung are alveolar macrophages; most of the rest are *lymphocytes*. Lymphocytes are found free on the alveolar surface, scattered throughout the interstitium, and concentrated in specialized regions in the submucosa of proximal airways (called *bronchus-associated lymphoid tissue*). The relative proportions of the various lymphocyte subtypes recovered from the normal human lung by lavage is similar to that found in the blood. The cells are able to respond to mitogens, secrete lymphokines, and produce immunoglobulins when they are activated.

The *polymorphonuclear leukocyte (PMN)*, although not found as a resident cell in the normal lung parenchyma, is an extremely important effector cell in lung inflammation. When appropriately *activated* (after stimulation by chemotactic factors, for instance), it has a variety of biologic potentials that allow it to participate in lung defense and in inflammatory lung injury (Table 1).

In addition to the alveolar macrophages, lymphocytes, and PMNs, the *lung mast* cell is an important cellular mediator of certain immune reactions, notably those involving antibody-mediated airway reactions (such as asthma, anaphylaxis, and others). Mast cells are found in subepithelial regions of the airways and in perivascular compartments. Thus either airborne or blood-borne antigens trigger the release of mast cell products, mediated by IgE binding to the mast cell surface. IgE-stimulated mast cells isolated from human lung fragments release a variety of chemical mediators, notably histamine, prostaglandin D, a chemotactic factor for *eosinophils* (another important cell in some immune responses of the lung), and leukotriene components of (LTC_4, LTD_4, and LTE_4) a complex mediator termed "slow reacting substance of anaphylaxis" (SRS-A). The release of SRS-A from human lung mast cells appears to require interaction with interstitial mononuclear cells; this feature illustrates the concept that the activity of lung effector cells may be influenced by other cell types.

Table 1. Biologic activities of activated polymorphonuclear leukocytes.

I. *Biologic Activities*

    1. Adherence to endothelial surfaces
    2. Aggregation
    3. Chemotaxis
    4. Phagocytosis
    5. Production of biologically-active
        products

II. *Products*

    1. Oxygen Metabolites

       A. Superoxide anion
       B. Hydrogen peroxide; hypo-
          chlorous acid
       C. Hydroxyl radical
       D. Singlet O_2

2. Arachidonic Acid Metabolites

       A. Leukotriene B4
       B. 5 HETE
       C. Smaller amounts of PGE_2,
          thromboxane A_2

3. Platelet Activating Factor
4. Granular Enzymes

       A. Acid hydrolases (B-gluc-
          uronidase, cathepsins B and
          D, others)
       B. Neutral proteases (elastase,
          collagenase, cathepsin G,
          Proteinase 3)
       C. Myeloperoxidase

5. Defensins and Granulins

E. Blood and Blood Cells

The lung has the largest capillary bed in the human body and is the only organ besides the heart to receive the entire cardiac output. The circulating blood cells represent a reservoir that can contribute to the intraparenchymal pool of lung effector cells. As mentioned, the *PMN* is a example of an intravascular cell that is recruited to the alveoli and interstitium in response to appropriate stimuli. Additional examples of circulating blood cells that contribute to pulmonary responses include *monocytes*, which are the precursors for most alveolar macrophages, and *platelets*, which may participate in a variety of syndromes of pulmonary vascular damage.

In addition to cells, the circulating blood may provide humoral substances that are important in pulmonary responses. Examples include components of the complement system that may "feed the fire" of acute lung inflammation, and alpha-1-antiprotease, an inhibitor of proteolytic enzymes that may cause alveolar destruction in some forms of emphysema.

LUNG DEFENSE: MECHANICAL AND CELLULAR MECHANISMS

The volume of gas transported from the environment to the alveoli in a single 24-hour period is enormous (5600 liters, assuming an alveolar minute ventilation of 4 l/min) and is contaminated by a variety of potentially toxic agents. One way for lung damage to occur is for the normal lung defense mechanisms that handle the toxic materials in the inhaled gas to fail, allowing the toxic agents to reach or remain in the lower respiratory tract (see chapter, "Mechanisms of Lung Injury—An Overview"). The defense mechanisms of the lung fall into 3 general categories, including *mechanical, phagocytic,* and *humoral* factors.

A. Mechanical Factors

Laryngeal and epiglottic reflexes are important in keeping solids and large volumes of toxic liquids and gases from reaching the tracheobronchial tree. Thus reflex laryngospasm may result from the inhalation of noxious gases, regurgitation of gastric acid, etc.

Most airborne particles greater than 10 μM in diameter are trapped in the nose, nasopharynx, and pharynx where they impact on the mucosal surfaces as the inspired gas flows through this anatomic "maze." They are then swallowed. Particles, including microorganisms, smaller than 10 μM may gain access to the lower respiratory tract where they settle onto mucosal surfaces of the bronchi, bronchioles, and alveoli; maximal alveolar deposition occurs with particles 1 to 2 μM in diameter. One factor involved in their clearance is a forceful and coordinated *cough.* In addition, removal of the particles requires a functional *mucociliary apparatus.* The specialized airway *secretory epithelial cells* produce a complex mucus lining material in the conducting airways that includes sol and gel layers. This liquid sheet is propelled upward to the pharynx by the coordinated beating of cilia of the *ciliated epithelial cells.* The process is under complex neural and humoral control. *Cystic fibrosis* is a disease resulting from a heritable defect in the regulation of water and solute content of airway fluid. It results in thick, viscid mucous and impaired mucociliary clearance, leading to recurrent bacterial infection and airway destruction.

Mucociliary transport can also be disrupted or depressed by a variety of acquired insults, many of them iatrogenic (Table 2).

Table 2. Factors that impair mucociliary transport.

Congenital:	1. Cystic Fibrosis
	2. Other inherited defects (example: Kartaganer's Syndrome)
Acquired:	1. Decreased airway humidity
	2. Endotracheal intubation
	3. Aspirated gastric acid
	4. Cigarette smoke
	5. Air pollutants
	6. Hyperoxia
	7. Viral respiratory tract infections
	8. Abdominal and thoracic incisions
	9. Inhalational anesthetics
	10. Other drugs: local anesthetics, narcotics, etc.

B. Phagocytic Mechanisms

The *alveolar macrophage* is the phagocyte that is most important in ingesting particles, including bacteria, that reach the alveolar surface. After phagocytosis, the macrophages are transported up the trachea (via the mucociliary apparatus) and out of the lung, or they may move into the interstitium to the lymphatics. If they enter the lymphatic system, there is evidence that they can be transported to regional lymph nodes and present ingested antigens for immune recognition and processing.

Depending on the nature of the particle, the macrophages may also degrade the phagocytized material without leaving the alveoli. This is a major defense mechanism against many bacteria, such as staphylococci. Phagocytosis and killing of microorganisms by alveolar macrophages may be enhanced by *non-specific opsonins* (example: complement component C3b) and by *specific immunity*. In the case of many bacteria, immunity is expressed as a specific antibody directed against the organism that enhances opsonization and phagocytosis (although some bacteria can be ingested without specific opsonizing antibody). The lipid fraction of the alveolar lining material ("surfactant") also facilitates the killing of some bacteria, such as staphylococci and pneumococci. The *rate of killing* of different microorganisms by alveolar macrophages varies; as an example, the killing of staphylococci and pneumococci is much faster than the killing of Klebsiella species.

A second group of organisms, termed *intracellular pathogens*, survive easily in quiescent macrophages after phagocytosis, and may actually multiply. Examples include M. *Tuberculosis*, some fungi, and *Legionella pneumophilia*. Specific immunity against these organisms involves the *activation* of the macrophages, mediated via sensitized subpopulations of lymphocytes. This process is required for the generation of biochemical products required by the macrophages to kill the organisms (see "lung Cells and Their Functions"). A defect in macrophage killing of intracellular pathogens may be an important cause of severe lung infection in the *acquired immunodeficiency syndrome*.

Alveolar macrophages may ingest inorganic materials such as silica and asbestos particles, particulates in cigarette smoke, etc. Under some conditions these particulates can stimulate the macrophage to become activated and to continuously release mediators that can promote alveolitis and alveolar injury. Death of the macrophage with release of enzymes and mediators can also occur. This sequence of events is thought to be important in the human lung diseases *silicosis* and *asbestosis,* and may mediate some of the pathologic responses associated with infection with intracellular pathogens such as *Mycobacterium Tuberculosis*. This is an example of how a process that is vital for *lung defense* (i.e. the phagocytosis of particulate matter and activation of the phagocyte) may become a process that effects *lung injury* when its regulation is altered by a pathologic stimulus (the undigestible particle).

Polymorphonuclear leukocytes become important alveolar phagocytes when the inoculum of bacteria (and perhaps other types of particulates) is so great that the alveolar macrophage's capacity to ingest and kill them is surpassed, or when biologic characteristics of the bacterium stimulate rapid recruitment of PMNs from the blood to the alveoli. The latter mechanism appears to be important in the early clearance of *Streptococcus pneumoniae*, which cause rapid recruitment of PMNs to the alveoli of experimental animals.

C. Humoral Factors

The role of specific antibody (usually of the *IgG class*) against bacteria in facilitating phagocytosis and killing of bacteria by alveolar macrophages and PMNs has been mentioned. Specific antibodies of the IgG class may also be important in the neutralization of viruses and toxins. IgG is found in lavage fluid from normal human lungs.

Another limb of the antibody system may be especially important in the lung. *Plasma cells* in the submucosa of the tracheobronchial tree produce *IgA*, which is secreted onto the mucosal surface. The *"secretory IgA"* has a number of roles in lung defense, including inhibition of viral infection of epithelial cells, decreasing mucosal adherence of certain bacteria (streptococci), and serving as a nonspecific opsonin for particles and some microorganisms. Secretory IgA is also found on the mucosal surfaces of the nasopharynx and in the gastrointestinal tract. Isolated IgA deficiency is one of the most common of the genetic immunodeficiency syndromes, and is characterized by recurrent bacterial infections of the sinuses and lungs.

Lung explants can produce components of the *complement system*. In addition, lung monocytes, macrophages, and plasma in pulmonary vessels may serve as sources of complement components. Activation of the complement "cascade", by either the classic or alternative pathways, produces C3b, mentioned previously as an important nonspecific opsonin, and C5a, which is chemotactic for PMNs. Other complement components are produced as well and may be important for the defense against certain microorganisms. Activation of the complement system can occur in response to live bacteria, bacterial lipopolysaccharides, and cell wall components of certain microorganisms, as well as in response to antigen-antibody complexes, products of tissue injury, and other stimuli.

Lung cells also produce other humoral mediators, termed *chemotactic factors*, that may be important in the recruitment and activation of circulating phagocytes (see, Mechanisms of Lung Injury-an overview). As previously mentioned, C5a is a chemotactic factor, as is its desarginated form, C5a desarg (C5a desarg is produced when the terminal arginine is cleaved from C5a by a plasma carboxypeptidase. C5a and C5a desarg are commonly termed "C5a fragments"). Other chemotactic factors that are important in the lung include bacterial peptides, leukotriene B4, platelet activating factor, and interleukin 8.

REFERENCES

1. Gail DB, Lenfant JM: Cells of the lung: Biology and clinical implications. Am Rev Resp Dis 127:366-87, 1983
2. Crystal RG, West JB, Barnes PJ, Cherniack NS, Weibel ER. The Lung. Scientific Foundations. New York, Raven Press, 1991
3. Harada RN, Repine JE. Pulmonary host defense mechanisms. *Chest* 87:247-52, 1985
4. Kaltreider HB. Immune defenses of the lung. In Respiratory Infections (Sande MA, Hudson LD, Root RK, eds.) New York, Churchill Livingston, 1986, p 47-70

PULMONARY CIRCULATION DURING ANESTHESIA

B. E. Marshall and C. Marshall

INTRODUCTION

The anatomic arrangement and composition of the lung has evolved so as to allow gas exchange across a large and exquisitely thin membrane at the blood/gas interface (1). The entire cardiac output must be accommodated at low pulmonary vascular pressures and this imposes a design constraint that is common to all mammals. The low pressure is necessary to avoid the development of edema. The plasma oncotic pressure is normally about 35 cm H_2O and, according to the relationships governing fluid flow enunciated by Starling a century ago, this is also the upper limit for the normal pulmonary artery pressure. Patients with pulmonary artery pressure consistently above 35 cm H_2O are diagnosed as having pulmonary hypertension (2). Interestingly in all these species the vital capacity of the lung is achieved with transpulmonary pressures of 35 cm H_2O, and barotrauma occurs in otherwise normal lungs ventilated with pressures in excess of this. The pulmonary circulation is therefore a system of elastic tubes in parallel the dimensions of which are governed passively by intravascular and extravascular forces and by vasoactivity.

The purpose of this discussion is to review the factors influencing pressures and flows in the pulmonary circulation.

PULMONARY PRESSURE/FLOW RELATIONS

If pressure and flow are measured simultaneously as pulmonary artery pressure (PAP) is increased from zero, the relationship is curvilinear (Fig. 1).

T. H. Stanley and R. J. Sperry (eds.), *Anesthesia and the Lung 1992*. 31–43.
© 1992 *Kluwer Academic Publishers*.

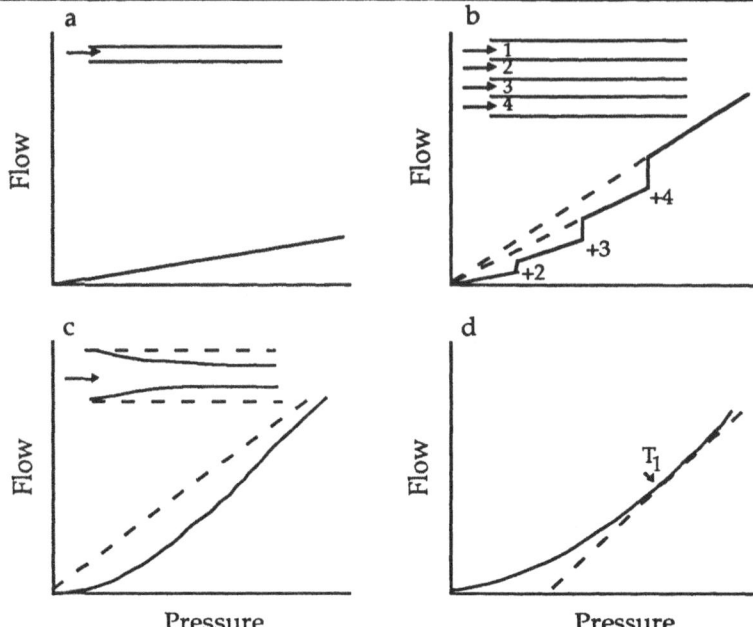

Figure 1. Pressure and flow in tubes (Panel a) As pressure is increased across a single rigid tube, the flow increases in a linear manner, and the conductance is a single value represented by the slope of the line. (Panel b) Recruitment: From the origin, pressure is increased across a single rigid tube as in panel a, but subsequently second (+2), third (+3), and fourth (+4) tubes are added. At each addition, the flow exhibits a step increase, and because the new pressure-flow line can be extended back through the origin, the new slope established after each step is the true conductance, representing precisely the number of tubes that are present. If, however, many more tubes are added in smaller increments, the step becomes smoothed to a curved line that becomes sigmoid when no further tubes are added, as in panel c. (Panel c) Distensibility: An elastic tube is depicted, with its walls at the start represented by the solid lines, while the maximum diameter is indicated by the dashed lines. As pressure is increased, the flow increases; however, because the wall stretches with each increment of pressure, the conductance also increases, and the pressure-flow relation is a smooth curve. The curvature is sigmoid because, at high pressures, the elastic tube will begin to resemble a rigid tube as its diameter approaches the limit. (Panel d) The problem of interpreting conductance from the smooth curve resulting in recruitment or distensibility in panel b or c is illustrated here. At the point indicated by T_1, the true conductance is best calculated from the slope of a straight line passing from T_1 through the origin; therefore, a unique conductance value exists for every point on the pressure-flow curve. The slope of a tangent to the curve drawn at this point reflects both the conductance and the change in conductance and will always be greater than or equal to the value of the intercept of this tangent with the pressure ordinate. Note that the sigmoid curve is not usually recognizable with in vivo data because the range of flows is usually limited.

The basis for the curvilinear relation has been the source of considerable controversy. Originally it was ascribed entirely to the recruitment, or opening, of previously closed vessels (Fig. 1b) and even today it is not uncommon for a straight line to be drawn through a graph of experimentally determined pressure and flow points and extrapolated to the pressure axis at zero flow (Fig. 1d). This pressure has been called by various names (i.e., critical opening pressure, starling resistor pressure, downstream pressure, etc.) all implying that it is a measure of a pressure limit which once exceeded the flow corresponds to the opening of all vessels as if they were rigid tubes. Each vessel was thought to have an individual opening pressure and the curvature represented the distribution of such pressures. However there is no obvious physical reason for a critical opening pressure; fluid entering fluid lined vessels do not encounter the surface tension barriers present when attempting to re-expand collapsed alveoli. In truth most pulmonary vessels require positive compression forces before becoming collapsed (3) or in the case of capillaries open or close with minute pressure changes (4).

These considerations have led many workers to reduce or abandon the role of recruitment and to emphasize the importance of distension. The pulmonary vessels are all elastic and therefore as the pressure increases so the diameter of the vessels increase again resulting in a curvilinear pressure/flow relationship (Fig. 1c).

It is important to understand that the calculation of conductance (flow divided by perfusion pressure), or its reciprocal, resistance, is a simple and useful expression of the state of the vasculature. The perfusion pressure is obtained by subtracting the output pressure (left atrial pressure LAP) from the input pressure (PAP) and thus the conductance calculated is directly analogous to the slope of a straight pressure/flow line that would be obtained for a rigid tube (Fig. 1a). Because the pressure/flow relation is curved the conductance changes with pressure and furthermore the tangent to the curve is not the same as the conductance (Fig. 2) because the tangent includes both a conductance and the change in conductance, it has been called an incremental conductance.

As a corollary of this all vessels distend elastically to some diameter, beyond which the compliance rapidly decreases. Further distension requires greater pressure and when all vessels are in this state then the pulmonary circulation behaves more like a system of rigid tubes and the pressure/flow relation is almost linear.

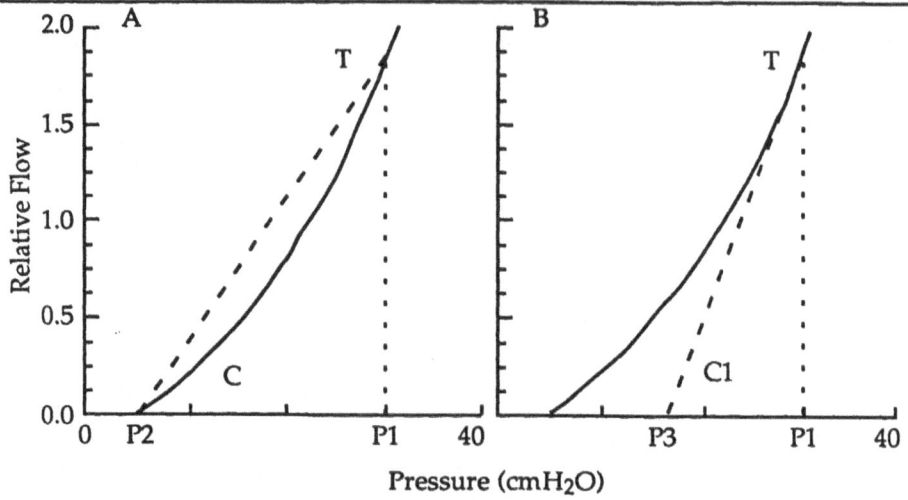

Figure 2. The difference between the conductance (C) and the incremental conductance (1c). A simultaneous measurement of pressure and flow identifies the point T. In panel A the conductance is calculated as the slope (C) of a straight line connecting T with the outflow pressure (P2). This line then corresponds to the pressure/flow behavior of a rigid tube the radius (r) of which is identical to that exiting at point T. The conductance is useful but because of the curvature, unique to each point. In Panel B the slope CI is for the line tangent to the curve at point T. This slope is called the incremental conductance and differs from the conductance because; $CI-c=2Q.r/hE$ where h&E are the wall thickness and elasticity respectively. The intercept of this line extrapolated to the pressures axis (P3) has no special physiology significance.

The interaction of forces is well illustrated during exercise where not only are large increases in cardiac output accompanied by large increases in conductances of vascular distend but this distension is so augmented by the increased respiratory efforts that the mean pulmonary artery pressure may not change at all. A principal deficit in pathologic pulmonary hypertension is the reduction of this ability to accommodate large flow changes, when the vascular distensibility has been reduced (Fig. 3).

ANALYSIS OF THE VARIABLES

A Model for the Pulmonary Circulation

With so many interacting variables it has been difficult to interpret many research studies in which an experimental manipulation alters several parameters simultaneously. A comprehensive model was

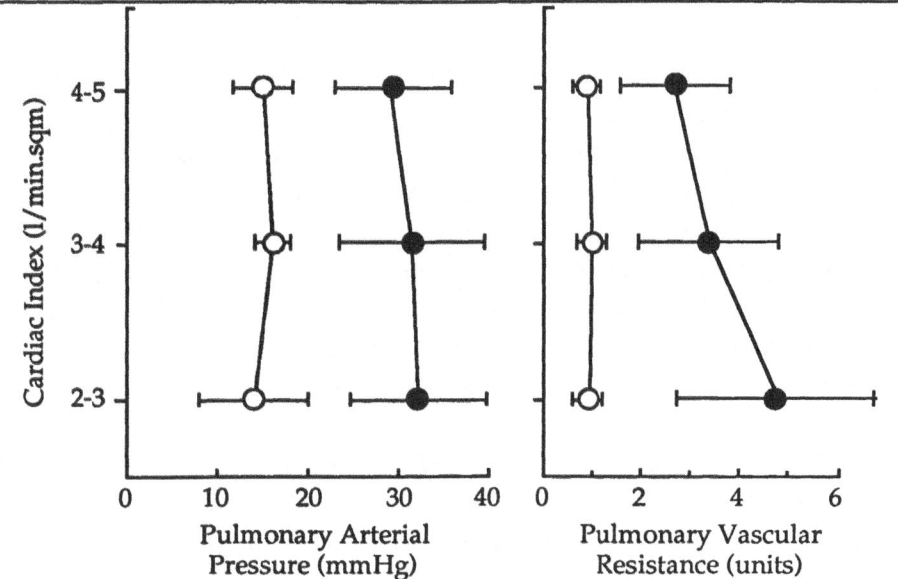

Figure 3. Comparison of normal subjects and patients with ARDS when cardiac output increased by isoproterenol infusion (55). In normal subjects (O), the pulmonary artery pressure and pulmonary vascular resistance are little altered by a twofold increase of flow. In patients with ARDS ●, pulmonary hypertension is present, but the dilation induced by the increasing dose of isoproterenol reduces the vascular resistance. These data show that pulmonary vascular tone is normally low and that much of the increase with ARDS is due to active vasoconstriction.

therefore developed that is of general application and incorporates the many variables in a quantitative manner. The basis for such a model was the work of Fung and his colleagues (6) which provided detailed measurements of the dimension and properties of all the pulmonary vessels of a cat. This model was then generalized and expanded to include the compliance limits and vasoactive components (7).

In brief with the number, length, diameter and compliance properties of all the vessels characterized, the pressure in the pulmonary artery can be calculated by working backwards from the left atrial pressure and the flow. By repeating the calculations as flow is systematically increased the complete pressure/flow curve can be described uniquely. The model incorporates the influence of airway pressure, pleural pressure, left atrial pressure, hypoxic pulmonary vasoconstriction, pH, PCO_2, temperature, hemoglobin, posture, and anesthetic and other drugs and can therefore be utilized to predict and analyze the results of experimental vs. clinical manipulations for any number of compartments.

Hypoxic Pulmonary Vasoconstriction (HPV)

HPV is a property of the pulmonary vascular smooth muscle cells
(8) and endothelium is not required (9). The stimulus is the oxygen tension
in the vicinity of these muscle cells and for the small pulmonary
arteries (≤500μmm in diameter) both the alveolar and the mixed venous
oxygen tension contribute to the stimulus (PSO_2). From the modelling
perspective the PSO_2 causes a constriction resulting in a smaller diameter,
for vessels involved, starting at zero flow. At each flow the pressure is
increased compared to the non-hypoxic lung and the pressure/flow curve
is shifted to the right in accordance with the dose/response relation for
hypoxia.

For a two compartment model, if one lung is hypoxic and the other
normoxic their specific pressure/flow curves are calculated. The unique
distribution of blood flow is then arrived at iteratively to satisfy the
requirements for the correct total blood flow and a common pulmonary
artery pressure. Such a calculation during one-lung ventilation then
allows the analysis of each of the contributing variables to be evaluated
quantitatively and independently (Table 1).

A further influence of HPV has also been demonstrated recently to
result from changes in arterial oxygen tension. The walls of all the
pulmonary arteries with diameters greater than about 500 micrometers are
supplied with vasa vasorum, not from their lumens which contain mixed
venous blood, but from branches of the bronchial arteries containing
systemic arterial blood. Reduction of the arterial oxygen tension causes a
progressive HPV response in the larger pulmonary arteries down to a tension
of about 40 mmHg. Further reduction of oxygen tension results in a
reversal of the constrictor response (Fig. 4)(10). This bimodal behavior
appears to explain the variable HPV responses that have been reported
when global hypoxia is present and may be of considerable clinical
importance in chronic and acute lung disease and perhaps lung
transplantation.

Table 1. Simulation of non-dependent left lung blood flow and P_aO_2 with anesthesia for thoracic surgery.

Step	1	2	3	4	5	6	7
Posture	Supine	Lateral	Lateral	Lateral	Lateral	Lateral	Lateral
Vent	Two	Two	Two	One	One	One	One
Thoracot.	No	No	Yes	Yes	Yes	Yes	Yes
Anesth MAC	0	0	0	0	1.5	1.5	1.5
Constr. fract.							
Left	1	1	1	0.7	0.7	0.7	0.7
Right	1	1	1	1	1	1	1
PALV (CMH2C)							
Left	2.5	2.5	2.5	0	0	5	0
Right	2.5	2.5	2.5	2.5	2.5	2.5	10
P_pL (cmH2O)							
Left	-2	-5	0	0	0	5	0
Right	-2	0	+2	+2	+2	+2	10
Pap (cmH2O)	18.5	14.4	18.8	20.7	20.0	20.9	22.3
Left lung flow (% total)	45.0	33.8	35.1	21.1	26.7	19.7	33.8
P_aO_2	400	400	400	150	115	170	85

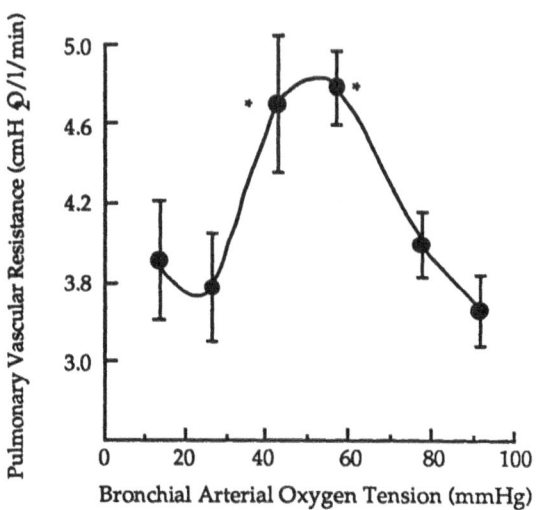

Figure 4. The influence of bronchial arterial oxygen tension on pulmonary vascular resistance. The oxygen tension was varied in an external oxygenator circuit and the bronchial artery cannulated and perfused while the lungs were ventilated with air and all other known variables maintained constant. The changes in pulmonary vascular resistance are at least bimodal. It is suggested that hypoxemia of the large vessel walls initially induces HPV but that profound hypoxemia (≤40 mmHg) results in sufficient generation of vasodilator materials in the systemic bronchial vessels that HPV is decreased progressively (5).

Importance of Pressure

It has long been known that the effectiveness of HPV is reduced when pulmonary vascular pressures (11) are increased but the basis for this has not been elucidated. Measurements in isolated perfused rat lung have allowed disassociation of the left atrial and pulmonary artery pressure effects. Simulation of these circumstances in the computer model reproduces quite closely the experimental observations (Fig. 5) and demonstrates that the hypoxic response is reduced progressively by increased left atrial pressure but changes in a bimodal fashion with increasing pulmonary artery pressure. This behavior results because the entire pulmonary vascular bed is elastic and because all vessels have a reduced compliance at a limited diameter and because vessels constricted by hypoxia require a higher distending pressure to achieve their limiting diameter. At one extreme, if left atrial pressure could be increased

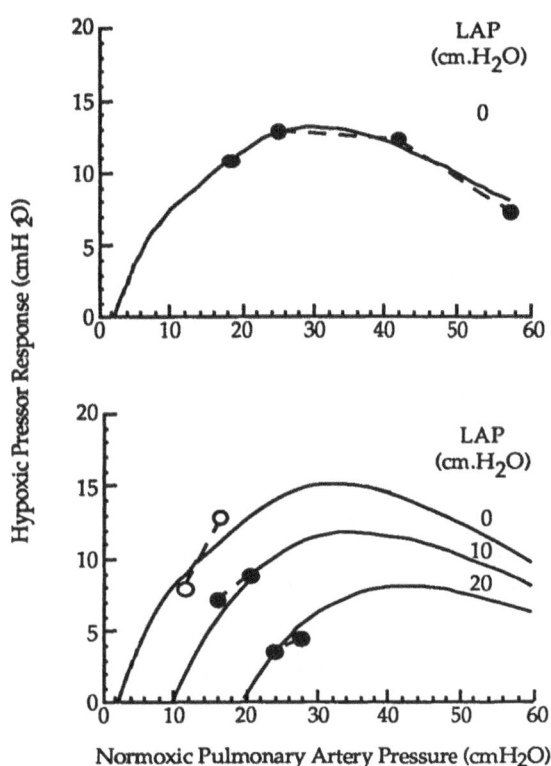

Figure 5. Effects of Vascular Pressures on the hypoxic pressor response in isolated perfused rat lungs. In the upper part the pulmonary artery pressure was increased by increasing the flow while the left atrial pressure was maintained at zero. The circles are the mean experimental results and the solid line is derived for the computer model. In the lower part the experimental observation consists of measurements of pulmonary artery pressure at two flow levels while the left atrial pressure was increased (0, 10 and 20 cm H_2O). The circles are the experimental observations and the solid lines results of the computer model. The hypoxic response is monotonically decreased as left atrial pressure increases but the affect of increasing pulmonary artery pressure is bimodal.

sufficiently (without causing edema) then all vessels, whether constricted or not, would have reached their limiting diameters and the HPV response would be undetectable. At the other extreme with left atrial pressure at zero, small flows do not distend the vessels so that constriction has little influence and HPV response is small; as flow increases the intravascular pressure increases and the HPV response becomes maximal in the range when most vessels have not yet reached a limiting diameter.

The precise clinical application of these observations has yet to be determined.

PULMONARY EMBOLISM

Many of these concepts are illustrated by consideration of the pathophysiologic effects of pulmonary embolism. An experiment (12) reported that in normal dogs increasing the left atrial pressure resulted in a substantial increase of pulmonary artery pressure but following pulmonary embolization the same increase of left atrial pressure resulted in a much smaller increase of pulmonary arterial pressure. The authors assumed that the pressure/flow relation in each case was linear and extrapolated to the pressure axis. The intercept pressure derived was found to be markedly increased after embolization and it was concluded that "embolic pulmonary hypertension produces an effective waterfall." It is difficult to identify any reasonable pathophysiologic basis for this conclusion although it is an inevitable result of regarding the pulmonary circuit as rigid tubes and the curvature as due to recruitment.

The same data can be reexamined using the principals outlined above. When a portion of the lung is subjected to embolization, the blood flow to those areas is abolished (or reduced) and the blood flow to the remaining lung is increased. In addition the embolization leads to the release of vasoconstrictor materials. A plot of relative flow versus pulmonary artery pressure therefore shows that even when the total cardiac output remains constant, following embolization, the pulmonary artery pressure is increased (Fig. 6). Furthermore if for each point a tangent to the curve is estimated and pressure intercept is derived their values are similar to those reported, but now they are revealed to depend only on geometry and to have no specific physiologic insights. The reasons for the decreased transmission of left atrial pressure changes following embolization are the following. First if no constriction has occurred a qualitatively similar but smaller effect would have been observed because the venous end of the circulation will always have a lower conductance with low left atrial pressure than with high and the difference decreases as the flow increases. If left atrial pressure is increased progressively the pulmonary artery pressure changes reflects more and more closely the left atrial

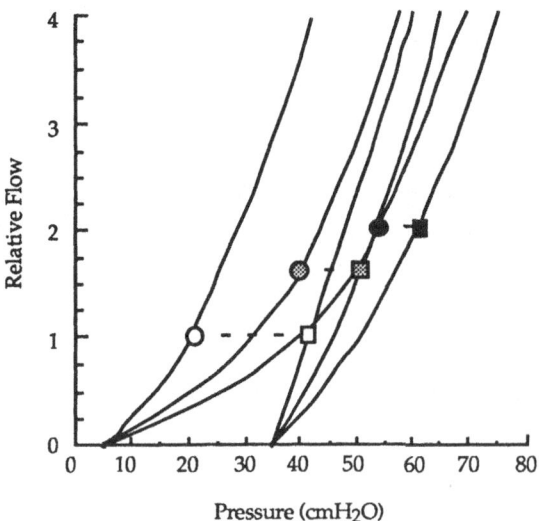

Pressure (cmH₂O)

Figure 6. Pulmonary Embolism reduces the pulmonary arterial pressure change with increased left atrial pressure. The data points are estimated from observation in dogs (12) and the solid lines are the corresponding pressure flow lines generated from the computer model. The open circle is the control observation with normal left atrial pressure indicated by the 5 cm H₂O origin for the pressure flow curve and open square is following the increase of left atrial pressure to 35 cm H₂O. The horizontal dashed line is the pulmonary artery pressure change and is approximately 20 cm H₂O for these points. When a large quantity of embolic is infused (solid symbols) the flow to the remaining perfused lung is increased and vasoconstriction occurs. For the model this state was approximated by constricting the small arteries to shift the curve to the right and by estimating an almost two-fold increase in flow to the perfused lung. The horizontal difference between the pressure/flow curves (O) to solid data points) before and after increasing to left atrial pressure is clearly reduced. For a lesser degree of embolization (hatched points) the effect is intermediate. For interpretation and discussion see text.

pressure changes. However when constriction occurs the curvature of the pressure/flow relation is enhanced in proportion with the degree of constriction at low left atrial pressure, but this enhanced curvature is progressively diminished as the left atrial pressure is increased coinciding with the fraction of the pulmonary vessels that have reached their limiting diameters. From this arrangement it is evident that increasing the left atrial pressure from normal to moderately increased levels will be associated with a diminished reflection in the pulmonary artery pressure that will be exaggerated when the relative flow increases as in the reported study. However it is also predicted that as the left atrial pressure is increased further transmission to the pulmonary artery pressure change will be more closely affected even in the presence of vasoconstriction stimuli.

CONCLUSION

The pulmonary circulation is influenced by many variables. The present analysis has revealed that some concepts originally introduced to simplify the understanding of these variables have not been effective. A model based on biodynamic and anatomic problems of the lung is discussed and used to illustrate the importance of considering the curved pressure/flow relationship when interpreting steady state observations of the pulmonary circulation.

Acknowledgment

This work was supported in part by NIGMS Grant Number R01 GM 29628 from NIH.

REFERENCES

1. Weibel ER: The Pathway for Oxygen. Cambridge, Harvard University Press, 1984
2. Marshall BE, Marshall C: Pulmonary hypertension. The Lung: Scientific Foundation. Crystal RG, West JB, Cherniak H, Weibel R (eds.). New York, Raven Press, pp. 1177-89, 1991
3. Yen RT, Foppiano L: Elasticity of small pulmonary veins in the cat. J. Biomech Eng 103:38-42
4. Warrell DA, Evans JW, Clarke RO, et al: Pattern of filling of the pulmonary capillary bed. J Appl Physiol 32:346-56, 1972
5. Zapol WM, Snider MT: Pulmonary hypertension in severe acute respiratory failure. N Engl J Med 296:476-80, 1976
6. Fung YC: Biodynamics. New York, Springer Verlag, p. 290-369, 1984
7. Marshall BE, Marshall C: A model for hypoxic pulmonary vasoconstriction in the pulmonary circulation. J Appl Physiol 64:68-77, 1988
8. Murray TK, Chen L, Marshall BE, et al: Hypoxic contraction of cultured pulmonary vascular smooth muscle cells. Am J Resp Cell & Mol. Biol 3:457-65, 1990
9. Marshall C, Marshall BE: Endothelial cells are not required for the HPV response in isolated pulmonary arteries. Anesthesiology 73:A1141, 1990

10. Marshall BE, Marshall C, Magno M, et al: The influence of bronchial artery oxygen tension on pulmonary vascular resistance. J Appl Physiol 405-15, 1991
11. Benumof JL, Wathrenbrock EA: Blunted hypoxic pulmonary vasoconstriction by increased lung vascular pressures. J Appl Physiol 38:846-50, 1975
12. Hasinoff I, Ducas J, Schick U, et al: Pulmonary vascular pressure-flow characteristics in canine pulmonary embolism. J Appl Physiol 68:462-7, 1990

PULMONARY EDEMA CAUSED BY STRESS FAILURE
OF CAPILLARIES

J. B. West

A cardinal feature of the human lung is that alveolar gas and blood are separated by an extremely thin membrane. This is essential because the respiratory gases pass through it by passive diffusion, and the diffusion resistance is proportional to the thickness of the membrane. However despite the extreme thinness of the blood-gas barrier, maintenance of its integrity is essential for efficient gas exchange. Mechanical failure will cause alveolar edema or even frank alveolar hemorrhage. We, therefore, decided to investigate the strength of the blood-gas barrier by raising the pressure inside pulmonary capillaries and looking for evidence of ultra-structural changes in their walls.

Another reason for our work was some recent intriguing data obtained in high altitude pulmonary edema. There is now very strong evidence that the occurrence of high altitude pulmonary edema is strongly correlated with the increase in pulmonary artery pressure caused by hypoxic pulmonary vasoconstriction (1). This strongly suggests a hydro-static basis for the edema although it is not immediately clear how the increased pressure is seen by the capillaries. Presumably the constriction of the small pulmonary arteries caused by the alveolar hypoxia is uneven, as first suggested by Hultgren (2) and, as a result, those capillaries that are not protected from the increased pulmonary artery pressure are exposed to an increased transmural pressure. As a result of the increased pressure, one would expect to see a low protein edema consistent with Starling's law. However Schoene and his colleagues (3) have shown that the protein content of the edema fluid is extremely high, often exceeding that in patients with severe adult respiratory distress syndrome. Thus the edema is of the high protein, high permeability type, and the problem we faced

T. H. Stanley and R. J. Sperry (eds.), Anesthesia and the Lung 1992, 45–51.
© 1992 *Kluwer Academic Publishers.*

was how to reconcile the high permeability type of edema with the presumed hydrostatic basis. It was these observations that stimulated us to look at the ultrastructural changes in pulmonary capillaries when these were exposed to high transmural pressures.

The measurements were done in anesthetized rabbits in which the pulmonary artery and the left atrium were cannulated so that the lung could be perfused with the rabbit's own blood. After only one minute of perfusion, the red cells were rapidly washed out with a saline/dextran mixture, and this was followed by buffered glutaraldehyde to prepare electron micrographs. Since we used a small arterial-venous pressure difference of only 5 cm water, the capillary pressure could be calculated to within 2.5 cm water. Knowing the alveolar pressure of 5 cm water, we could calculate the capillary transmural pressure, and studies were made at pressures of 12.5, 32.5, 52.5 and 72.5 cm water.

We made two interesting observations. The first was that at the high pressures, the capillaries bulged prominently into the alveolar spaces. This was not unexpected because Glazier et al. (4) had showed the same thing using an entirely different preparation in which dog lungs were rapidly frozen by inundating them with liquid freon gas. The other observation was surprising. We found that at capillary transmural pressures exceeding 52.5 cm water (about 40 mmHg) disruption of the capillary endothelium, alveoli epithelium or both were seen in some locations (5). The cells often appeared to be pulled apart along their intact basement membrane, though we also frequently saw instances where the basement membrane was also broken. These changes were consistently seen in preparations where the capillary transmural pressure was 40 mmHg or higher. Occasionally the disruptions were seen at lower pressures. We attributed the changes to the high mechanical stresses to which the capillary walls were exposed.

An analysis was made of the three principal forces acting on the capillary wall. The first is the circumferential or hoop tension caused by the transmural pressure, and determined by the Laplace law. The second force is the surface tension of the alveolar lining layer because, since the capillaries bulge into the alveolar spaces, this surface tension supports the capillary walls and tends to prevent stress failure. The third force is the tension of the tissue elements in the alveolar wall associated with lung inflation. This may contribute to the circumferential tension of the alveolar wall depending on the geometry.

The capillary wall stress can be calculated for typical conditions at failure. The transmural pressure is 40 mmHg, capillary radius 5 microns, and capillary wall thickness on the thin side is about 0.3 microns (6). Gehr et al. (6) reported that in the human lung, the harmonic main thickness of the blood-gas barrier is about 0.6 microns, but over approximately half of its area, that is the "bulging" or thin side of the capillary, the thickness is only 0.2-0.4 microns. Using these figures, the calculated wall stress is about 8×10^5 dyn/cm^2 (8×10^4 N/m^2). This is an extremely high stress being approximately the same as the wall stress of the normal aorta which is predominantly composed of collagen and elastin. By contrast, the thin side of the blood-gas barrier has approximately half of its thickness made up of the single layers of capillary endothelial and alveolar epithelial cells, the other half being composed of the extra-cellular matrix.

We have given a good deal of thought to what is responsible for the strength of this part of the blood-gas barrier. There are several pieces of evidence suggesting that the strength can be attributed to the collagen-IV of the basement membranes. First, we often see intact basement membranes in capillaries in which the capillary endothelium or alveolar epithelium or both have been disrupted. This in itself suggests that the basement membranes are the strongest component. Another piece of evidence comes from the work of Welling and Grantham (7) who took isolated renal tubules from rabbit kidneys and exposed them to increasing transmural pressures by inflating through a micropipette. They found that the mechanical properties of the tubules were the same irrespective of whether the epithelium was present of not. In other words, the mechanical properties of the isolated tubules in extension, were essentially determined by the basement membranes since this was the only structure remaining when the epithelium was removed. A third piece of evidence is that in systemic capillaries, the thickness of the basement membrane is known to increase down the body as the hydrostatic pressure in the systemic capillaries rises (8). Also, we know that in patients with mitral stenosis where the capillary pressure is raised over long periods, the basement membrane is thickened (9). These observations suggest that the basement membranes have a stress-bearing role.

Basement membranes contain collagen-IV, laminin, heparin sulfate proteoglycans and entactin/nidogen. The main structural component is believed to be collagen-IV which has an interesting structure (10). Two molecules join at the C-terminal end, and four molecules come together at the N-terminal end, to give a "chicken-wire" structure which apparently confers both porosity and great strength. Indeed the tensile strength of basement membranes approaches that of collagen-I (11), the structure responsible for the great strength of tendons such as the Achilles tendon.

There is evidence that the collagen-IV is not uniformly distributed throughout the extra-cellular matrix of the pulmonary blood-gas barrier. Vaccaro and Brody (12) have shown that the extra-cellular matrix has a central laminar densa with a lamina rara on either side. There is evidence that most of the collagen-IV is located in the laminar densa which has a thickness of only about 50 nm. This is presumably the principal structure responsible for the great strength of the normal blood-gas barrier. Thus, nature's solution to designing a very thin, but strong blood-gas barrier, is to have a very thin sheet of extremely strong collagen-IV within the extra-cellular matrix.

We have seen that the capillaries in the rabbit lung fail when the capillary transmural pressure exceeds about 40 mmHg. Is this such an unphysiologically high pressure that it is of little practical importance. The answer seems to be no because there is evidence that normal subjects during heavy exercise developed pulmonary capillary pressures exceeding 30 mmHg. For example, studies of humans exercising in the upright position, show that at an oxygen consumption of 3.7 l/min, mean pulmonary pressure was about 37 mmHg, and mean pulmonary artery wedge pressure about 21 mmHg (13). There is experimental evidence that the capillary pressure is about half way between arterial and venous pressures (14), and taking the wedge pressure as equal to venous pressure, this gives us a capillary pressure at mid lung of about 29 mmHg. Since the bottom of the lung is some 10 cm lower, this gives a mean capillary pressure there of about 36 mmHg. No claim is made for great accuracy here but the carry-home message is that the capillary pressure in the human lung during heavy exercise must exceed 30 mmHg. Of course, we cannot assume that the strength of the capillaries in the rabbit and human are the same, but nevertheless the results suggest that the safety factor is not very large.

What are the physiological consequences of stress failure? As the capillary transmural pressure is raised, fluid will move out into the interstitial space and perhaps the alveolar space, according to Starling's law. In addition, there may be some separation of the capillary endothelial cells with the movement of large molecules into the interstitial space, a phenomenon known as pore-stretching (15). At even higher pressures, disruption of the capillary endothelium and/or alveolar epithelium will occur with the development of a high permeability type of pulmonary edema.

What diseases can be attributed to stress failure of pulmonary capillaries. We have already referred to high altitude pulmonary edema which seems to be a good candidate, although the characteristic ultrastructure lesion has not yet been described. However, in neurogenic pulmonary edema, it is now known that pulmonary vascular pressures are high, presumably as a result of massive catecholamine release, and that the protein content of the alveolar fluid is also high indicating a high permeability type of edema. Furthermore, ultrastructural studies have actually demonstrated disruption of the capillary endothelium and alveoli epithelium (16) which is precisely the appearances we see in stress failure.

In high altitude pulmonary edema and neurogenic pulmonary edema, the capillary transmural pressure rises relatively slowly over a period of hours or days. What happens if the pressure rises very abruptly? We think this may be the cause of exercise-induced pulmonary hemorrhage which is well known to occur in galloping race horses (17). Indeed tracheal washings of thoroughbreds in training show that all of them have hemosiderin laden macrophages indicating that they have bled. Bleeding into the lung has also been described in racing greyhounds. Indeed there have been one or two case reports suggesting that the same thing happens in some humans following violent exercise.

Finally, stress failure can be expected when either the capillary transmural pressure is abnormally high, or the strength of the extracellular matrix is abnormally low. The later probably occurs in Goodpasture's Syndrome where the collagen-IV is cleaved by auto antibodies which specifically attack this molecule. The result is bleeding both into the lung and the kidney, the two microcirculations most at risk from a raised capillary pressure. It is also conceivable that the break down of alveolar walls seen in alpha 1 antitrypsin deficiency where the collagen is attacked by neutrophil elastase could be considered stress failure though this takes place over years rather than days or seconds.

As indicated earlier, the safety factor for stress failure seems to be relatively small. Initially this finding surprised us greatly because it seemed strange that the lungs should have evolved in this way. However we now realize that a small safety factor is inevitable in the design of the lung. The blood-gas barrier treads a knife edge between being thin enough for adequate passive diffusion of respiratory gases across it, and being strong enough to withstand the wall stress of the capillary during maximal exercise. We know that the barrier cannot be any thicker because measurements show that in elite human athletics, oxygen transfer maybe diffusion-limited at very high work levels. Therefore, the thinness of the barrier confers a clear evolutionary advantage. This thinness means that necessarily the amount of type IV collagen is severely limited. This appears to be the fundamental bioengineering dilemma of the lung. Indeed the fact that the blood-gas barrier needs to be extremely strong as well as exceedingly thin poses a unique design requirement which has not previously been recognized.

ACKNOWLEDGEMENTS

This work was supported by NIH program project HL17331-16.

REFERENCES

1. Oelz O, Ritter M, Jenni R, Maggiorini M, Waber U, Vock P, Bartsch P: Nifedipine for high altitude pulmonary oedema. Lancet 2:1241-44, 1989
2. Hultgren HN: High altitude pulmonary edema. In Biomedicine Problems of High Terrestrial Altitude, AH Hegnauer (ed.). New York, Springer-Verlag, 1969, pp 131-41
3. Schoene RB, Hackett PH, Henderson WR, Sage EH, Chow M, Roach RC, Mills WJ, Martin TR: High-altitude pulmonary edema. Characteristics of lung lavage fluid. JAMA 256:63-9, 1986
4. Glazier JB, Hughes JMB, Maloney JE, West JB: Measurements of capillary dimensions and blood volume in rapidly frozen lungs. J Appl Physiol 26:65-76, 1969
5. West JB, Tsukimoto K, Mathieu-Costello O, Prediletto R: Stress failure in pulmonary capillaries. J Appl Physiol 70: 1731-42, 1991

6. Gehr P, Bachofen M, Weibel ER. The normal human lung: ultrastructure and morphometric estimation of diffusion capacity. Respir Physiol 32:121-140, 1978

7. Welling LW Grantham JJ: Physical properties of isolated perfused renal tubules and tubular basement membranes. J Clin Invest 51:1063-75, 1972

8. Williamson JR, Vogler NJ, Kilo C: Regional variations in the width of basement membrane of muscle capillaries in man and giraffe. Am J Path 63:359-67, 1971

9. Haworth SG, Hall SM Patel M: Peripheral vascular and airway abnormalities in adolescents with rheumatic mitral stenosis. Int J Cardiol 18:405-16, 1988

10. Timple R, Wiedemann H, Delden VV, Furthmayr H, Kuhn K: A network model for the organization of type IV collagen molecules in basement membranes. Eur J Biochem 120:203-11, 1981

11. Stromberg DD, Wiederhielm CA: Viscoelastic description of collagenous tissue in simple elongation. J Appl Physiol 26:857-62, 1969

12. Vaccaro CA, Brody JS: Structural features of alveolar wall basement membrane in the adult rat lung. J Cell Biol 91:427-37, 1981

13. Wagner PD, Gale GE, Moon RE, Torre-Bueno JR, Stolp BW, Saltzman HA. Pulmonary gas exchange in humans exercising at sea level and simulated altitude. J Appl Physiol 61:260-270, 1986

14. Bhattacharya J, Nanjo S, Staub NC: Micropuncture measurement of lung microvascular pressure during 5-HT infusion. J Appl Physiol 52:634-37, 1982

15. Wasserman K, Loeb L, Mayerson HS: Capillary permeability to macromolecules. Circ Res 3:594-603, 1955

16. Minnear, FL, Connell RS: Increased permeability of the capillary-alveolar barriers in neurogenic pulmonary edema (NPE). Microvasc Res 22:345-66, 1981

17. O'Callaghan MW, Pascoe JR, Tyler WS, Mason DK: Exercise-induced pulmonary hemorrhage in the horse: results of a detailed clinical, post-mortem and imaging study. VIII. Conclusions and implications. Equine Vet J 19:428-34, 1987

MECHANISMS OF LUNG INJURY: AN OVERVIEW

G. A. Zimmerman

One of the most rapidly evolving areas related to respiratory patho-physiology and disease involves the mechanisms of lung injury. Until a few years ago, pulmonary pathophysiology was dominated by questions that involved the mechanisms by which gas flow and blood flow in the lung occur, how these two flows are regulated and matched, and how they are altered by disease. These questions were addressed by studies that involved the whole organ (the lung) and usually the whole organism. Such issues continue to be important, and the questions are not completely answered. However, in recent years much investigation has focused on the role of specific lung cells and their products in the functions of the normal lung, and on how cellular functions are altered in disease states. Information on the cell biology of lung disease is accumulating at a rapid rate, and is influencing the management of clinical lung problems. The emphasis on the cell biology and biochemistry of the lung has not replaced the traditional approach (based on gas and blood flow at the whole organ level) but it is definitely altering our understanding and view of these processes. Physicians in general, as well as lung specialists, will need a basic understanding of lung cell biology and cellular mechanisms of lung injury in the future in order to understand and rationally apply new therapies. This chapter will provide an overview of cellular mechanisms of lung injury. Many of the mechanisms, such as those involved in pulmonary inflammatory processes, are similar to mechanisms that are important in the pathophysiology of other organs and are not unique to the lung. They do, however, mediate alterations in functions of the lung that are unique.

T. H. Stanley and R. J. Sperry (eds.), Anesthesia and the Lung 1992, 53–67.
© 1992 *Kluwer Academic Publishers.*

The material in this chapter is not encyclopedic, but will emphasize mechanisms that are currently thought to be important in a variety of different disease processes.

OUTLINE OF CHAPTER

A. *Failure of normal lung defenses*
B. *Direct injury by inhaled toxins: O_2 toxicity as an example*
C. *Enzyme-mediated destruction of alveolar walls: the concept of "protease-antiprotease imbalance"*
D. *Injury caused by cellular and humoral mediators of inflammation*
  1. *Inflammatory effector cells*
  2. *Humoral mediators of inflammation*
  3. *Examples of animal models: PMNs, chemotactic factors, other mediators*
  4. *Examples of human diseases that appear to involve inflammatory cells and mediators*
E. *Lung repair*

FAILURE OF NORMAL LUNG DEFENSES

Pulmonary infections occur because of a failure of one or more of the lung defense mechanisms. The nature and severity of the lung injury that results will depend in part on: 1) the state of ancillary or "backup" defenses and the host's ability to contain the infection as well as repair the damage, 2) biologic features of the organism (factors that contribute to its "virulence"), 3) the nature of the lung inflammatory response, and 4) therapeutic interventions. As an example, a single episode of pneumococcal pneumonia may occur in an otherwise normal adult because *an unusually large inoculum* of pneumococci (of a subtype that the host has *no specific antibody against*) remains in the alveoli because *mucociliary clearance* and *alveolar macrophage* function have been depressed by a preceding *viral infection*. The patient rapidly clears the infection by recruiting circulating PMNs that phagocytize and kill the pneumococci; this process is facilitated when the physician decreases the bacterial growth rate by administering penicillin. The patient has no subsequent episodes of pneumonia because his defense systems return to normal after the viral infection and he develops specific antibody to the pneumococcus species. On the other hand, a chronic alcoholic with pyorrhea has repeated episodes of bacterial pneumonia, and ultimately develops necrotizing pneumonia and a lung abscess because of: a) increased numbers of anaerobic bacteria in his mouth due to poor dentition, and colonization of his oral mucosa with aerobic gram negative rods because of poor general health (*Klebsiella* and *E. Coli*, which are not part of the usual mouth flora of healthy subjects); b) recurrent aspiration of large inocula of bacteria in oropharyngeal secretions while intoxicated; c) chronic impairment of mucociliary clearance due to cigarette smoking and recurrent aspiration; and d) impaired PMN function (and possibly alveolar macrophage function) due to the effects of alcohol and chronic malnutrition.

DIRECT INJURY TO LUNG PARENCHYMAL CELLS BY INHALED TOXINS; O_2 TOXICITY

Some materials are directly toxic to lung parenchymal cells if they gain access to the lower respiratory tract. Certain *gases* are particularly toxic to lung cells, including ammonia, chlorine, nitrogen dioxide, and oxygen in high concentrations. Highly soluble gases such as ammonia and chlorine cause major injury to cells of the proximal tracheobronchial epithelium with little of the gas usually reaching the alveoli, whereas less soluble gases such as O_2 and N_2O penetrate more deeply to the alveoli.

It is ironic that too much O_2, as well as too little, can cause organ damage and death, but oxygen-induced injury to the lung (*"oxygen toxicity"*) is an important pathogenetic mechanism. Clinical O_2 toxicity becomes increasingly more frequent at inspired O_2 concentrations greater than 50%. Under the appropriate conditions O_2 avidly accepts electrons, causing oxidation of the electron donor molecule and reduction of the O_2 molecule. The primary site of reduction of molecular O2 is at the terminal cytochrome (cytochrome a/a3) of the mitochondrial electron transport chain, which handles most of the O_2 metabolized in the generation of energy from foodstuffs. Electrons can also be "leaked" to O_2 in the electron transport chain at points prior to cytochrome a/a3. The mechanisms by which this occurs appear to be nonsaturable and first order with respect to the O_2 concentration; therefore, the rate at which oxygen products (that result from the reduction of the molecule by the "leaking" electrons) are produced is directly proportional to the PO_2 at the site of production. While all cells have to deal with this phenomenon, lung cells are particularly susceptible because they are exposed to the highest O_2 tensions of any of the cells in the organism. Thus when the inspired O_2 tension is increased from 21% toward 100%, the rate at which reduced O_2 products are generated in lung cells is also increased dramatically. Generation of oxygen radicals by lung cells can also be induced by ionizing radiation and by certain drugs (Table 1).

Table 1: Mechanisms of alveolar cell injury by active oxygen metabolites ("O_2 radicals")

1. Generation of O_2 radicals by alveolar Type I cells and endothelial cells stimulated by *hyperoxia*	O_2 toxicity of the lung
2. Generation of O_2 radicals by lung cells, induced by *ionizing radiation*	Lung injury induced by radiation therapy for mediastinal or lung tumors
3. Generation of O_2 radicals by lung cells, induced by *drugs*	Lung injury caused by *bleomycin* (cancer chemotherapy), *nitrofurantoin* (antibiotic), *paraquat* (herbicide that may contaminate marijuana smoke)
4. Generation of O_2 radicals by *activated leukocytes* (neutrophils, alveolar macrophages)	Injury of alveolar epithelial cells in hypersensitivity pneumonitis, asbestosis, others; injury to endothelial cells in ARDS, others; inactivation of alpha-1-antiprotease in cigarette smoking, leading to emphysema

The reduction of oxygen by electrons results in the generation of one or more *active O_2 metabolites* (also termed "toxic O_2 species" and "O_2-derived free radicals"). These active metabolites occur when the 1, 2, or 3 electron reduction of molecular O_2 yields *superoxide anion* (O_2-), *hydrogen peroxide* (H_2O_2), and *hydroxyl radical* ($OH\cdot$). In addition, the 4 electron reduction of O_2 can result in an active intermediate termed "singlet O_2" under the appropriate conditions. The order of reactivity appears to be $OH\cdot$, singlet $O_2 > H_2O_2 > O_2-$. Each appears to be capable of causing tissue damage and cytotoxicity. There is evidence that O_2 metabolites, especially H_2O_2, can directly injure pulmonary endothelial cells (the lung cell that appears to be most sensitive to O_2-induced injury), alveolar Type I cells, and others.

In addition to directly damaging lung cells, O_2 radicals may stimulate alveolar macrophages to release a factor that is chemotactic for PMNs. The resulting inflammatory response may amplify the direct lung cell injury, since activated PMNs themselves are a potent source of active O_2 metabolites.

When activated by pathologic stimuli, such as immune complexes or chemotactic factors, both alveolar macrophages and PMNs can release active O_2 metabolites. This is a mechanism by which these oxygen radicals can be generated and can cause tissue injury in the absence of high concentrations of molecular O_2.

It appears to be impossible for cells to avoid the production of active O_2 metabolites, even under normal conditions. Therefore, they possess mechanisms by which these metabolites can be scavenged and converted to non-toxic molecules. *Superoxide dismutase* is an enzyme that catalyzes the dismutation of O_2- to H_2O_2 and O_2; H_2O_2 can be metabolized by *catalase* or one of a family of *peroxidases* (especially *glutathione peroxidase*). Successful elimination of $O2$- and H_2O_2 appears to prevent the formation of OH^- and singlet O_2. *Erythrocytes* have been shown to be potential scavengers for toxic oxygen radicals that may be generated by PMNs and other cells in some forms of lung injury. Oxygen toxicity and cell injury mediated by active O_2 metabolites result when the generation of $O2$ radicals exceeds the capacity of the scavenging systems, or when the activity of the scavenging systems are depressed.

Other materials besides gases can directly injure lung cells (2). *Liquid chemicals*, such as hydrochloric acid present in stomach fluids, can directly injure airway epithelial cells, alveolar Type I cells, and endothelial cells, and can cause an explosive secondary inflammatory response. The aspiration of gastric contents is a common cause of chemical tracheobronchitis and pneumonitis in patients whose protective laryngeal reflexes are depressed (such as a patient with depressed consciousness due to a drug overdose or general anesthesia). *Inorganic particles*, such as silica and chrysolite particles, are directly toxic to cell membranes. In addition, ingestion of silica particles by alveolar macrophages can result in intracellular lysosomal rupture causing death of the macrophage, release of macrophage enzymes and mediators, and release of the silica particles to be ingested again and continue the cycle (see section on alveolar macrophages in the chapter titled, "A Primer on Pulmonary Cell Biology"). A similar response may occur with other particulates. Some *drugs* that are administered for therapeutic purposes may have cytotoxic effects on lung cells.

ENZYME-MEDIATED DESTRUCTION OF ALVEOLAR WALLS: "PROTEASE-ANTIPROTEASE IMBALANCE"

One of the earliest theories of lung injury based on biochemical and cellular mechanisms involved the concept of "protease-antiprotease imbalance." Emphysema results from destruction of alveolar connective tissue matrix. It is irreparable. Clinical observations indicated that some patients with early-onset familial emphysema had a heritable defect in *alpha-1-protease inhibitor* (a1PI; a1- antitrypsin). This enzyme inhibits the activity of elastase and to a lesser extent other proteases, such as collagenase and trypsin. Experimental studies then demonstrated that the intrapulmonary instillation of elastolytic proteases caused *destruction* of alveolar walls in animals; the histologic pattern was similar to human emphysema. These findings suggested that when there was a deficiency of the protease inhibitor (a1PI), the "unopposed" action of proteases could destroy elastin and other components of the connective tissue framework of the pulmonary interstitium, resulting in *emphysema*. Currently, the proteases are thought to be released from inflammatory effector cells. The exact cell type is unknown, but PMNs, resident alveolar macrophages, and mononuclear cells in transit between the blood and alveolar spaces have been implicated. Each is capable of releasing enzymes with elastinolytic activity under the appropriate conditions. Alpha-1-PI from human plasma can effectively inhibit elastases from PMNs and monocytes. Thus it is possible that *a genetic deficiency* of a1PI could result in *unopposed protease activity* and alveolar destruction.

Although familial emphysema is an instructive and important disease, most cases of emphysema are acquired and result from cigarette smoking. A second potential mechanism for decreased effective a1PI concentrations is the oxidative inactivation of the protease inhibitor by chemical or cell-derived oxidants. *Active oxygen radicals*, released from alveolar macrophages or PMNs, can oxidize a methionine residue in the elastase-binding site of a1PI. This decreases the affinity of the inhibitor for the elastase and causes it to be inactive. Furthermore, cigarette smoke can oxidize a1PI *in vitro*, suggesting that smoking can inactivate the antiprotease. The activity of a1PI in bronchopulmonary lavage fluid of smokers has been reported to be decreased compared to nonsmokers.

These observations indicate that there is experimental basis for the protease-antiprotease theory, although it is yet to be conclusively proven. The evidence is strong enough, however, so that clinical trials of the effect of infusion of a1PI into humans with genetic deficiency of the protease inhibitor are now in progress. In spite of this, it is likely that the factors that regulate lung connective tissue metabolism are more complex than can be explained simply by the relative concentrations of proteases and antiproteases in the fluid phase. Recent studies indicate that proteases expressed on the surface of human alveolar macrophages are protected from protease inhibitors, and can degrade elastin even in the presence of the inhibitor when the macrophages are in contact with a connective tissue matrix.

LUNG INJURY CAUSED BY INFLAMMATORY CELLS AND HUMORAL MEDIATORS OF INFLAMMATION

It is currently thought that many types of lung injury result from a markedly enhanced, or unregulated, response of one or more inflammatory/immune effector cells. Humoral mediators that activate inflammatory effector cells, and that may have additional biologic effects, are likely to be important in these pathologic responses. A general schema for this type of mechanism is as follows (Fig. 1): a pathologic stimulus directly activates a population of inflammatory effector cells, or causes the synthesis and/or release of one or more humoral mediators that activate the effector cells. This causes increased numbers of activated effector cells in the alveoli ("*alveolitis*"). The effector cells generate products that injure one or more lung target cells, causing tissue damage. Frequently, products of the effector cell also have the ability to recruit and activate additional inflammatory cells of the same or a different class, amplifying the inflammatory injury. This general mechanism is similar to that proposed for inflammatory injury to other organs (consider inflammatory joint injury in rheumatoid arthritis, acute hepatitis, glomerulonephritis, etc.). Aspects of inflammatory tissue injury specifically related to the lung will be outlined in the next part of this discussion.

Pathologic Stimulus → Activated Effector Cells → Alveolitis

(Immune Complexes, etc)

↓

Release of Humoral Mediators → Activated Effector Cells → Alveolitis

(Chemotactic Factors, etc)

Figure 1

---

1) Inflammatory Effector Cells of the Lung

The major effector cells that are thought to be important in inflammatory lung injury are the resident alveolar macrophages, lymphocytes, and PMNs recruited from the circulating blood (see chapter, A Primer on Pulmonary Cell Biology). Other circulating cells, such as monocytes and platelets, are also likely to be important in specific syndromes of inflammatory injury. Particularly important mechanisms of lung cell injury caused by the inflammatory cells include the release of *active O_2 metabolites* by PMNs and alveolar macrophages, and the release of *proteases* by these cells.

It is currently thought that the type of cell that predominates in a given syndrome of inflammatory lung injury is determined in part by the nature of the pathologic stimulus. An additional general theory is that the nature and extent of lung injury that results is influenced by the *cell type(s)* that are involved, the *number* of effector cells, and their state of *activation*. Finally, it is thought that *alveolar destruction* (emphysema) or *fibrosis* can occur as a result of *alveolitis*.

It should be noted that most of this section on inflammatory injury is specifically directed to mechanisms of damage to the *alveolar-capillary unit*. However, many of the mechanisms may also be important in *airway* inflammation as well.

2) *Humoral Mediators of Inflammation*

The lung is a particularly rich source of humoral agents that may be active in the initiation or amplification of inflammatory responses. Several of these "inflammatory mediators" are discussed in References 5 and 6. Some of the mediators are synthesized and stored in lung cells, and are released in response to an appropriate stimulus; others, such as arachidonic acid metabolites, are not stored in cells but are synthesized *de novo* in response to stimulation.

A group of mediators that may be particularly important in pulmonary inflammatory responses are loosely termed "*chemotactic factors*" (5,6). Chemotactic factors are generally defined as biochemical compounds that stimulate the directed migration of cells. The compounds belong to a variety of chemical classes, and frequently have relative specificity for the cells that they stimulate. As an example, sensitized lung lymphocytes produce a factor that is chemotactic for monocytes; elastin degradation products are also chemotactic for monocytes but have little ability to stimulate the motility of alveolar macrophages or PMNs.

Chemotactic factors for PMNs are thought to be very important mediators of acute lung inflammatory responses (6). The most important chemotactic factors for PMNs in lung inflammation are thought to be: the activated peptide fragments derived from the 5th component of complement (C5 fragments, including *C5a* and its desarginated form, *C5a desarg*), oligopeptide *bacterial chemotactic factors*, the arachidonic acid metabolite *leukotriene B4* (LTB$_4$), and "*alveolar macrophage-derived chemotactic factor.*" The latter factor was recently shown to be a polypeptide, IL-8. *Platelet-Activating Factor*, an unusual phospholipids that can stimulate both platelets and leukocytes, may also be important. C5a, LTD$_4$ and Platelet-Activating Factor can each be generated by human lung cells under the appropriate condition. Each can stimulate PMNs to adhere to endothelial surfaces, aggregate, generate active oxygen metabolites, and release granular enzymes—thus they can *activate* the leukocytes in addition to stimulating directed motility.

Models of lung injury mediated by *C5 fragments* have received a great deal of attention. The intratracheal instillation of C5, C5a, or C5a desarg in experimental animals produces a dose-dependent inflammatory response characterized by edema due to increased permeability of the alveolar capillary unit, fibrin deposition, and a PMN infiltrate. This is thought to be a model for lung inflammation resulting from the *intraalveolar release* of C5 fragments. The intraalveolar release of chemotactic factors of other classes may have similar effects.

Activated C5 fragments may also be generated in the *circulating blood* in response to endotoxemia, shock, and tissue injury. In experimental models the intravascular injection or generation of C5 fragments causes PMNs to become hyperadherent to one another (forming aggregates) and to pulmonary endothelial cells. The activated PMNs are "sequestered" in the lung capillary bed, an event that is associated with increased pulmonary capillary permeability and the accumulation of pulmonary edema. The increased capillary permeability appears to be due in part to injury of the endothelial cells by activated O_2 metabolites, especially H_2O_2, released from the stimulated PMNs. In experimental animals, the lung injury can be decreased by making the animals granulocytopenic prior to intravascular complement activation, demonstrating a requirement for PMNs. Human PMNs, activated by C5a, can cause the death of cultured human endothelial cells *in vitro*. These observations have suggested that the intravascular generation of complement fragments may cause granulocyte-mediated pulmonary capillary injury in humans.

In this section (and in the two sections to follow) we have emphasized the potential role of *C5a fragments*, as humoral chemotactic factors and mediators of inflammation, and *PMNs*, as the effector cells that respond most dramatically to C5a, in acute lung inflammatory responses. Examples of how C5a generated in the alveoli, or in the blood, could cause PMN-mediated lung injury have been given. Although we have focused on this particular mechanism, other cellular and humoral mediators are likely to be equally important in specific syndromes of lung injury, and several mediators may act in concert to modulate acute and chronic inflammatory states (see below). It is also important to note that several mechanisms exist that regulate the biologic activities of chemotactic factors (such as enzymes that cleave the molecules, etc) and that regulate the responses of effector cells to them. Thus lung injury caused by PMNs (or other effector cells) to these agents most likely involves a breakdown in one or more *control mechanisms*, as well as a *stimulus* for the release of chemotactic factors and the activation of the effector cells.

3) Examples of Experimental Models of Acute Inflammatory Lung Injury Involving PMNs and Chemotactic Factors that May Be Relevant to Human Disease

In the preceding section we mentioned that the intratracheal instillation of C5 fragments in experimental animals can result in alveolitis, and that infusion of C5 fragments can cause pulmonary vascular injury. This sort of model demonstrates the potential for C5 fragments, and other chemotactic factors, to mediate inflammatory injury. However, we have indicated that activated C5 fragments and other mediators are not continuously released from cells in the lung, but require some sort of a stimulus for their generation. Are there experimental models involving the generation of mediators and the recruitment of PMNs that may be relevant to human diseases?

a) <u>Immune Complex Alveolitis.</u> Experimental lung injury mediated by *immune complexes* is thought to be representative of certain types of clinical lung disease. In several animal models the ability of IgG immune complexes to cause lung injury is *dependent* on the presence of PMNs and complement; the lung injury is thought to be due to the generation of C5a, other mediators, and the recruitment and activation of the neutrophils (5). When immune complexes are instilled into the alveoli of experimental animals, alveolar macrophages appear to phagocytize the antigen-antibody complexes. They become activated, and generate C5a, an alveolar *macrophage-derived chemotactic factor* for PMNs, and potentially other classes of mediators. Neutrophils, recruited and activated by the chemotactic factors, release O_2 free radicals and proteases that injure the Type I cells and alter the interstitial connective tissue elements. Oxygen metabolites released from the activated alveolar macrophages may also cause cellular injury. If the immune complexes are eliminated, the generation of chemotactic factors is decreased and inflammation subsides. If the *stimulus* (immune complexes) is continuously delivered to the lung, *chronic inflammation* and *fibrosis* of the alveolar wall results. This animal model is thought to be similar to some forms of human lung disease that may be mediated by immune complexes such as *hypersensitivity pneumonitis* and *idiopathic pulmonary fibrosis*.

b) <u>Experimental Endotoxemia and Intravascular Complement Activation.</u> The infusion of live gram negative bacteria, or endotoxin isolated from gram negative bacteria, causes diffuse pulmonary microvascular injury in sheep. Endotoxin-induced pulmonary vascular injury in sheep is thought to be similar to diffuse pulmonary microvascular injury that occurs as a complication of bacteremia in human (see "ARDS", to be discussed later). The pulmonary capillary injury is characterized by increased permeability of the capillaries to water and protein, resulting in pulmonary edema. The increased permeability is thought to occur because of the activation and sequestration of PMNs in the lung capillaries, mediated by circulating C5a fragments that are formed when the endotoxin activates plasma complement components (see the previous discussion of circulating C5 fragments). This hypothesis is supported by the observations that activated PMNs cause increased capillary permeability by releasing active O_2 metabolites in other animal models, and that the endotoxin-induced pulmonary vascular injury is markedly diminished if the animal is made granulocytopenic before infusion of the endotoxin.

Sheep infused with endotoxin also develop pulmonary hypertension, impaired hypoxic pulmonary vasoconstriction, and decreased compliance of the lung. While these changes may in part be due to endothelial cell injury and the effects of the resulting edema, there is evidence that some of the abnormalities result from release of mediators from C5a-stimulated PMNs. Humoral mediators may also be released from cells such as platelets and injured lung parenchymal cells. Such mediators include thromboxane A2 and certain leukotrienes, agents with potent biologic effects in the lung. This information illustrates the concept that the interaction of effector cells and humoral mediators (in this case C5 fragments and PMNs) can result in *physiologic abnormalities* of the lung (pulmonary hypertension, decreased compliance, etc.) as well as cell injury.

4) Examples of Some Human Disease Processes that Appear to Involve Activated Inflammatory Cells

a) Idiopathic pulmonary fibrosis (IPF) is a human lung disease that is thought to be due to interaction of one or more unidentified *antigens* (viruses, organic dusts, etc) with *immunoglobulins* (produced by *lung B lymphocytes*) to form *immune complexes* (4). The immune complexes activate *alveolar macrophages* and cause them to release chemotactic factors for *PMNs*, resulting in an *alveolitis* characterized by increased numbers of these two cells. Bronchoalveolar lavage fluid from patients with IPF contains increased numbers of macrophages and PMNs (and to a lesser extent eosinophils and lymphocytes) when compared to fluid from normals. Release of oxidants and proteases from the activated PMNs and alveolar macrophages causes injury to lung parenchymal cells and interstitial connective tissue, eventually resulting in lung *fibrosis*. The activated alveolar macrophage is thought to be especially important in the process of fibrosis, because there is evidence that it can influence the local accumulation and replication of fibroblasts (2).

b) The adult respiratory distress syndrome (ARDS) is a syndrome of *acute diffuse alveolar capillary membrane injury* that results in lung edema due to increased permeability in its early stages. Pulmonary hypertension occurs in many patients as the syndrome progresses. In some patients, there is also pulmonary microvascular occlusion, with PMN aggregates and platelet-fibrin thrombi, and actual destruction of lung capillaries. Later stages of the syndrome may be complicated by pulmonary fibrosis. ARDS is a common complication of *gram negative bacteremia*, where circulating mediators injure alveolar capillary endothelial cells (see next paragraph). It can also result from injury to Type I cells (for example, by aspiration of gastric contents). The mortality is greater than 50% on average.

ARDS secondary to gram negative bacteremia is a classic example of blood-bourne injury to the alveolar-capillary membrane. Endotoxin and C5a may be key mediators (see Section 3b on previous page). It is currently believed that initiation or amplification of the syndrome in some patients involves *activated PMNs* and circulating or locally-produced humoral *inflammatory mediators*. Evidence for this includes the following: 1) increased numbers of PMNs are found in the microvessels and alveoli of patients with ARDS (determined by lung biopsy, bronchoalveolar lavage, and lung scanning after injection of autologous radiolabeled PMNs); 2) the plasma from many patients with established ARDS, and from patients at risk for ARDS, appears to contain a mediator that can activate PMNs and has antigenic and biologic characteristics of C5a; 3) PMNs collected from the pulmonary arterial blood of some patients with ARDS appear to be activated since they respond in an enhanced fashion to chemotactic stimuli, and generate increased quantities of O2 metabolites in response to stimulation.

While these data suggest that PMNs and C5a fragments may be involved in the pathogenesis of the syndrome, several things indicate that this is not the whole story. For example, many patients with intravascular complement activation and circulating C5a fragments *do not* develop ARDS; similarly, activated granulocytes circulate in some patients who do not develop the syndrome. This suggests that an additional feature, such as a breakdown in one or more of the mechanisms that control the responses of activated granulocytes or their interaction with the pulmonary endothelium, may be required for initiation of the syndrome. Furthermore, other mediators may also be involved. *Endotoxin* can itself injure endothelial cells, and it also stimulates the generation of *tumor necrosis factor* and *Interleukin* 1. These cytokins can initiate PMN-mediated endothelial injury and may also directly induce endothelial injury.

LUNG REPAIR

The mechanisms involved in the repair of alveolar structures are poorly defined. Alveolar Type I cells are not able to replicate. After lethal injury (caused by toxic O2 metabolites, etc) destroys some of these lining cells, the alveolar surface is repopulated by Type II cells (assuming that the Type II cells have not been irreversibly injured). The Type II cells then differentiate into Type I cells if the injury is limited. Epithelial cells that migrate from the distal bronchioles may also participate in the reparative process.

It is not known if alveolar endothelial cells can replicate. However, chemotactic factors for endothelial cells have been identified, and a growth factors that stimulate endothelial replication are produced by human platelets and other cells. These observations suggest that endothelial cells from uninjured areas may be attracted to sites of vascular injury and stimulated to divide.

Repopulation of the alveolus by Type II cells and endothelial cells is thought to require an *intact basement membrane* that serves as a surface for the adherence, differentiation, and "maturation" of new cells.

If the extent of injury is such that the alveolar lining cells cannot immediately repair, *fibrosis* is thought to result. Under some conditions mild fibrosis may be reversible. If the connective tissue matrix of the interstitium has been irreparably damaged, destruction of the alveolar walls (*emphysema*) rather than fibrosis results. Emphysema is not reversible, as we currently understand it.

REFERENCES

1. McCord, JM. Oxygen radicals and lung injury; the state of the art. Chest (Suppl):35S-37S, 1983
2. Cambell EJ, Senior RM. Cell injury and repair. Clin Chest Med 2:357-75, 1981
3. Chapman HA, et al. Degradation of fibrin and elastin by intact human alveolar macrophages in vitro. J Clin Invest 73:806-15, 1984
4. Crystal RG, et al: Interstitial lung diseases of unknown cause. Disorders characterized by chronic inflammation of the lower respiratory tract. Parts I and II. N Eng J Med 1984; 310:154-65, 235-44
5. Fantone JC, et al: Chemotactic mediators in neutrophil-dependent lung injury. Annu Rev Physiol 44:283-93, 1982
6. Reynolds NY: Lung inflammation: Normal host defense or a complication of some diseases? Annu Rev Med 38:295-23, 1987
7. Crystal RG, West JB, Barnes PJ, Cherniack NS, Weiber ER. The Lung. Scientific Foundations. New York, Raven Press, 1991

HEMODYNAMIC DETERMINANTS OF PULMONARY EDEMA AND PLEURAL EFFUSIONS

S. J. Allen

PULMONARY EDEMA

Clinical Manifestations

Pulmonary edema is a pathologic process in which the water content of the pulmonary interstitium is greater than normal. But what does this mean to the patient? Small amounts of edema in the lungs may cause little in the way of signs or symptoms. However, as pulmonary edema increases, lung function is impaired in two ways. First, the increased amount of fluid in the lung parenchyma *increases the stiffness* (decreases the compliance) of the lungs. This produces a restrictive type defect in pulmonary function testing. The typical ventilatory pattern of patients with restrictive defects is fast and shallow. Thus, tachypnea may be the first sign of pulmonary edema. In patients with marginal pulmonary reserve, the increased work of breathing may be sufficient to produce respiratory failure.

A second problem arises when edema *fluid leaks into the alveoli* (alveolar flooding) and interferes with gas exchange. Essentially, flooded alveoli cannot be effectively ventilated. In the left atrium, blood which perfuses unventilated alveoli (shunt) mixes with blood which is fully saturated and lowers the overall arterial partial pressure of oxygen. When the fraction of desaturated blood rises high enough, hypoxemia develops. In ventilation/perfusion studies, pulmonary edema produces an "all-or-none" phenomenon. That is, perfused lungs units either have appropriate ventilation or no ventilation. There are few areas which demonstrate low $\dot{V}/\dot{Q}$'s.

T. H. Stanley and R. J. Sperry (eds.), Anesthesia and the Lung 1992, 69–82.

Fluid accumulating in the bronchioles results in airway narrowing which may produce rales. Expiratory rales (cardiac asthma) are sometimes present in patients with pulmonary edema secondary to congestive heart failure. The recent finding that these expiratory wheezes can be reduced with bronchodilators has been a surprise. There are apparently other mechanisms at work in cardiac asthma besides just the presence of edema fluid. Edema fluid in the airway may contribute to the frothy secretions characteristic of pulmonary edema. These pathophysiologic processes account for the typical clinical presentation of respiratory distress and cyanosis.

Radiologic Manifestations

As water has a higher radiodensity than air, pulmonary edema presents as increased densities on the chest X-ray. Pulmonary edema may be detected on chest X-ray before it is clinically apparent. Familiarity with the various changes associated with pulmonary edema, which are listed in Table 1, can help to differentiate the process from atelectasis, pneumonia, and chronic lung disease.

Table 1. Radiographic signs of pulmonary edema.

Increased vascular markings

Blurred vessels edges

Increased cardiac silhouette

Kerley A lines (long, mid lung field)

Kerley B lines (short, periphery)

Peribronchial cuffing

'Bat wing' or butterfly appearance

Pleural effusions

Unilateral is unusual

Acinar shadows (patchy areas of consolidation which coalesce over time)

Air bronchograms

Physiology

There are several etiologies of pulmonary edema, all which alter normal lung fluid balance. Under normal conditions, a small amount of fluid is constantly leaving the pulmonary capillaries and then removed by the lymphatics. The primary factors which determine the rate at which fluid leaves the capillaries are the capillary pressure and permeability. Once fluid has left the capillaries, edema will not form as long as the lymphatics can carry the fluid away. The rate of lymph flow can increase to accommodate increases in the rate at which fluid leaves the capillaries. However, once fluid leaves the capillaries faster than the lymphatics can remove it, fluid accumulates and pulmonary edema occurs. The principle which determines the rate at which fluid leaves the capillary is described by Starling's Equation.

$$J_v = K_f[(P_{cap}-P_{int})-\sigma(\pi_{cap}-\pi_{int})]$$

where

J_v = rate of fluid leaving capillary
K_f = filtration coefficient
P_{cap} & Π_{cap} = capillary hydrostatic and protein osmotic pressure, respectively
P_{int} & Π_{cap} = interstitial hydrostatic and protein osmotic pressure, respectively.
σ = reflection coefficient

Figure 1. Starling Equation.

or more simply

Fluid out = capillary pressure — osmotic pressure gradient

Figure 2. Simplified Starling Equation.

The Starling Equation demonstrates that *capillary pressure* (P_{cap}) is the most important factor determining edema formation, regardless of the etiology. The effect of increases in permeability is to magnify the effect of any increase in capillary pressure. Unfortunately, we do not have a readily available technique for determining capillary pressure. What we can measure is *pulmonary capillary wedge pressure* (PCWP, also called pulmonary artery occlusion pressure {PAOP}) which is an estimate of left atrial pressure, not capillary pressure. Under normal conditions, the gradient between the pulmonary artery and left atrial pressure is small (10-12 mmHg) and capillary pressure is very close to PCWP (Fig. 3). Capillary pressure and PCWP increase together in diseases such as left ventricular failure, mitral stenosis and fluid overload. However, in the presence of pulmonary hypertension, true capillary pressure may be much higher than PCWP. Thus, there may be an increased hydrostatic force driving fluid into the pulmonary interstitium in the presence of a low PCWP. A common situation in which this may occur clinically is ARDS. In animals in which we gave endotoxin, the administration of nitroprusside, in doses sufficient to reduce the resultant pulmonary hypertension, decreased the amount of pulmonary edema even though left atrial pressure was not decreased (Table 2) (1).

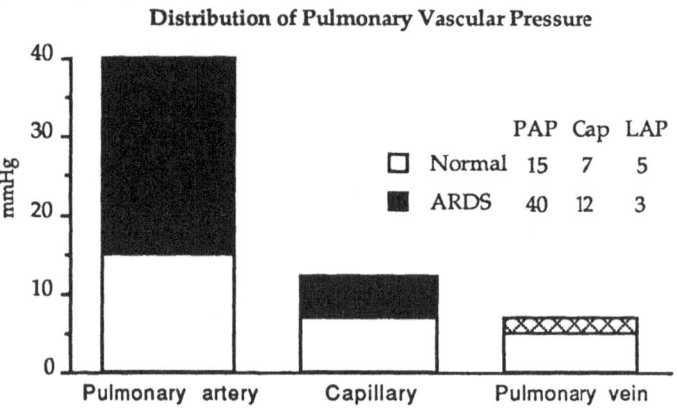

Figure 3. Decrease in vascular pressures across the pulmonary circulation in normal patients and in ARDS. Note in ARDS that despite a decrease in pulmonary venous pressure (or pulmonary capillary wedge pressure), capillary pressure is increased.

Table 2. Effect of sodium nitroprusside on pulmonary edema following endotoxin.

	PAP (mmHg)	LAP (mmHg)	EVF
Endotoxic	27.3	4.1	4.7
Endotoxin + SNP	20.9	4.1	3.9*

*P < 0.05, from Ref#1

In a patient study, Gattinoni et al found that the amount of pulmonary edema directly correlated with the pulmonary artery pressure (Fig. 4), but not with PCWP (2). These studies imply that some of the increased pressure in the pulmonary arteries is being transmitted to the level of the capillaries but not to the pulmonary veins and left atrium. Thus, pulmonary hypertension may increase the amount of fluid leaving the capillary even when PCWP is normal. Capillary pressure is even more important to maintain low in situations where permeability is increased. Smaller increases in capillary pressure produce edema which accumulate at a faster rate when permeability is increased (3).

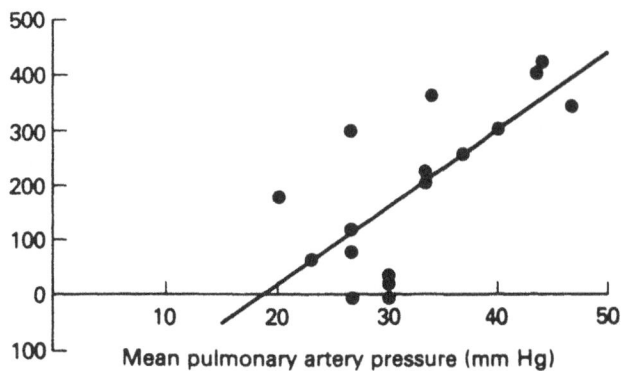

Figure 4. Effect of pulmonary hypertension on lung water in patients with ARDS. The vertical axis is the amount of excess lung water detected by CT. These data suggest that pulmonary hypertension contributes to pulmonary edema. No significant relation was found between excess lung water and PCWP. Ref. #2.

Lymph Flow

Even if the rate at which fluid leaves the capillaries increases, pulmonary edema does not occur as long as the lymphatics can remove the fluid at the same rate. Any factor which slows lymph flow can enhance the formation of pulmonary edema. For example, the lung lymphatics ultimately drain into the central venous system. Increased central venous pressure (CVP) decreases lymph flow rate. In a model of congestive heart failure, pulmonary edema was markedly exacerbated solely by increases in superior vena caval pressure (Fig. 5) (4). Similarly, in a model of increased permeability (endotoxin infusion), even increasing CVP by only 7 mmHg significantly increased the amount of pulmonary edema (Fig. 6) (5). Thus, increased CVP enhances pulmonary edema formation (caused by either increased left atrial pressure or increased permeability) by decreasing edema fluid removal. This is of particular concern to the critically ill population as many therapeutic maneuvers tend to increase CVP, such as positive pressure ventilation, vasoactive drugs, and fluid infusions. One option would be to lower CVP although this is not always feasible without producing hemodynamic compromise. An alternative is to divert the lymphatics so that they can flow against a lower outflow pressure. Thoracic duct drainage, which has been used in the past for immunosuppression and management of ascites and pancreatitis, allows the clinician the opportunity to optimize thoracic duct flow and thus, enhance edema fluid removal. Recently we subjected sheep to hydrostatic pulmonary edema and PEEP which increases CVP. Thoracic duct drainage resulted in significantly less edema and pleural effusions as shown in Figure 7 (6).

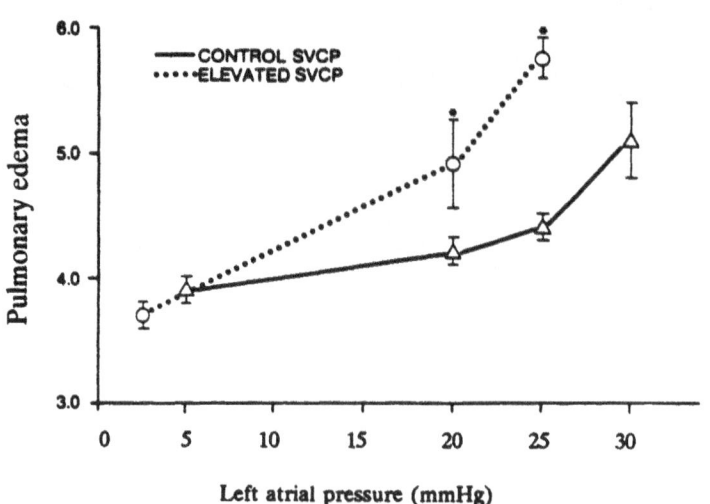

Figure 5. This graph demonstrates that increased venous pressure, opposing lymph drainage, exacerbates pulmonary edema formation (EVF). The triangles represent the amount of edema formed after three hours of left atrial pressure elevation (LAP). The open circles represent sheep in which superior vena caval pressure (SVCP) was also increased to 20 mmHg. * = P < 0.05. Ref. #4.

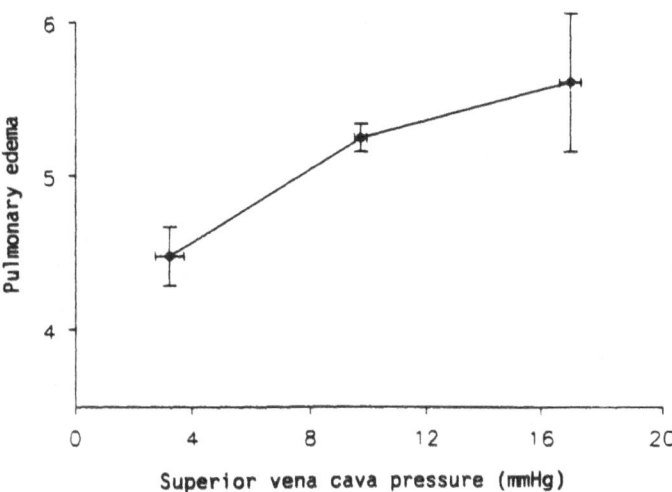

Figure 6. Effect of increase in superior vena caval pressure (SVCP) on pulmonary edema caused by endotoxemia. Increases in SVCP to 10 and 17 mmHg significantly (P<0.05) increased the amount of edema. Ref. #5.

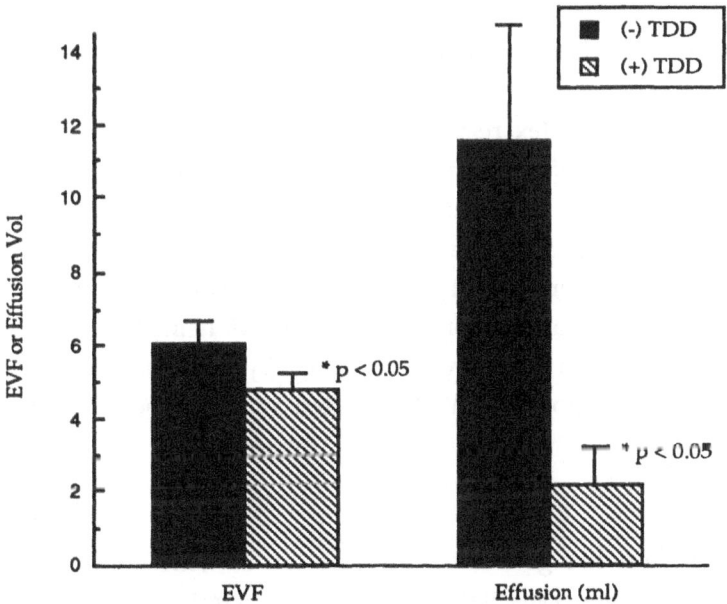

Figure 7. Effect of thoracic duct drainage on pulmonary edema (EVF) and pleural effusion volume in animals receiving PEEP. Ref. #6.

SPECIFIC ETIOLOGIES OF PULMONARY EDEMA

Congestive Heart Failure

Cardiac dysfunction results in pulmonary edema when left atrial and pulmonary capillary pressures rise and increase the rate at which fluid is pushed out of the capillaries. Because of the reserve of the lymphatics, left atrial pressure can typically be elevated by 15 mmHg above normal before pulmonary edema begins to form. Treatment is aimed at reducing the pulmonary vascular pressures, usually with diuretics.

Following Airway Obstruction

Patients with obstructed airways sometimes develop pulmonary edema. The etiology is thought to be due to the tremendous negative pressure generated which literally sucks fluid out of the capillary. Once the obstruction is relieved, the force driving the edema is gone, and the edema should resolve quickly.

Adult Respiratory Distress Syndrome (ARDS)

ARDS is a complex response of the lung to a number of insults. ARDS is composed of pulmonary edema, decreased compliance, and refractory hypoxemia. There is increased lung permeability in patients with ARDS. This means that for a given capillary pressure, more edema is formed than if the permeability was normal. Thus, it is important to maintain pulmonary vascular pressures as low as hemodynamic concerns allow. This concept is somewhat supported by a recent article in which patients with a reduction in PCWP exhibited an improved survival (7).

Fluid Resuscitation

Much effort has gone into the question of which fluid to give for intravascular volume resuscitation. There are many problems with clini-cal studies of the issue such as what end-points to measure, no reliable way to measure lung water clinically, and the inability to measure many of the Starling forces in patients. However, the first goal of fluid resuscitation is not the avoidance of pulmonary edema but euvolemia. Most likely, the nature of the fluid is not as important as how high the pulmonary vascular pressures are raised during the resuscitation.

Neurogenic Pulmonary Edema

This type of pulmonary edema is temporally related to a neurologic insult. Neurologic injury is associated with a huge release of catecholamines, especially norepinephrine. The vasoactive hormones cause a transient but extreme increase in the pulmonary capillary pressure. If the pressure spike is long enough or high enough, enough fluid leaks out of the capillaries and edema accumulates. Generally, the capillary pressure spike resolves but the edema does not disappear as fast. In addition to this mechanism, there are probably other, as yet unspecified, mediators which may enhance to development of pulmonary edema and ARDS in these patients.

Increased Peak Inspiratory Pressure Edema

Laboratory studies have indicated that high levels of positive airway pressure induces pulmonary edema by both raising capillary pressure and increasing permeability. The edema formation appears to be related most closely to the peak airway pressure and whether the lung has suffered an insult (8). The significance of this phenomenon in humans is unclear.

PLEURAL EFFUSIONS

After a hiatus of about 30 years, attention has been refocussed on understanding pleural fluid physiology in normal and abnormal situations. It appears that pleural fluid arises from parietal and visceral pleural filtration, primarily from the former. The fluid is reabsorbed by a number of pathways but mainly through lymphatics which open as stoma in the parietal pleura and drain eventually into the superior vena cava as shown in Figure 8 (9).

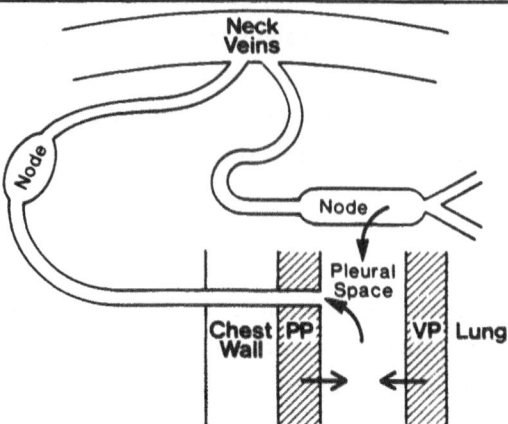

Figure 8. Diagram of pleural fluid formation and removal. Pleural fluid passes from the parietal (PP) or visceral pleura (VP), and is removed by lymphatics which originate on the PP and drain into neck veins. Pleural fluid formation can be increased by pulmonary edema fluid which passes into the pleural space and by leakage of lymph out of the thoracic duct which travels though the chest. Ref. #12.

Left atrial pressure (LAP). Increased LAP has long been associated with pleural effusions although experiment evidence has been conflicting. As pleural effusions tend to accompany congestive heart failure, the pleural space may serve as a pathway for pulmonary edema fluid removal. That is, the ability to form effusions may act to reduce the amount of pulmonary edema which might otherwise develop. Broaddus et al. found that visceral pleural fluid flow rates increased in sheep subjected to volume loading (10). Their data supports the concept that edema fluid leaks into the pleural space. We increased LAP (which increases capillary pressure) to various levels in unanesthetized sheep and measured the subsequent amount of pulmonary edema and volume of pleural effusions (11).

We found that the volume of pleural effusion correlated with capillary pressure. More compelling, we found that no effusions occurred unless a significant amount of pulmonary edema had occurred (Fig. 9). Thus, in the presence of increased LAP, pleural effusions occur secondary to the development of pulmonary edema. Further, as we did not see effusions with smaller amounts of pulmonary edema, the amount of edema fluid which was passing into the pleural space was removed by the parietal pleural lymphatics. With higher amounts of edema, the rate at which fluid entered the pleural space exceeded the rate of lymphatic removal and effusions formed.

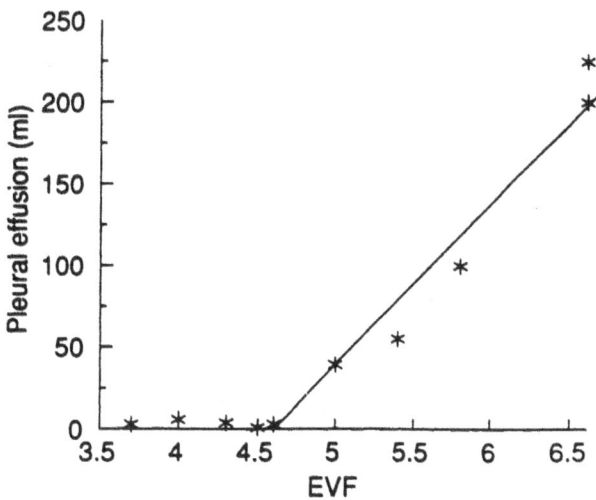

Figure 9. Relation of amount of edema (EVF) and pleural effusion volume. Note that pulmonary edema has to increase to >4.7 before effusions start to form. Ref. #11.

Central Venous Pressure

From the previous discussion, increases in lymphatic outflow pressure (caused by high central venous pressures) might impair drainage of pleural fluid and result in pleural effusions. To test this hypothesis, we increased only superior vena caval pressure (so as to avoid impairment of venous return to the heart) for 24 hours in unanesthetized sheep and then measured the volume of pleural effusions (10). We found that venous pressures below 15 mmHg were not associated with effusions in these otherwise healthy animals (Fig. 10) (12). On the other hand, venous pressures above 15 mmHg resulted in a progressive increase in the effusion. At the higher venous pressures, the effusion volumes were clearly larger than what would be expected from pulmonary sources alone. Most likely lymph fluid leaks out of the lymphatic trunks, such as the thoracic duct, which pass through the thorax.

Although we demonstrated that increased venous pressures produced effusions over 24 hours, clinical entities associated with long term venous pressure elevation are not usually associated with effusions. Superior vena caval syndrome is only occasionally complicated by

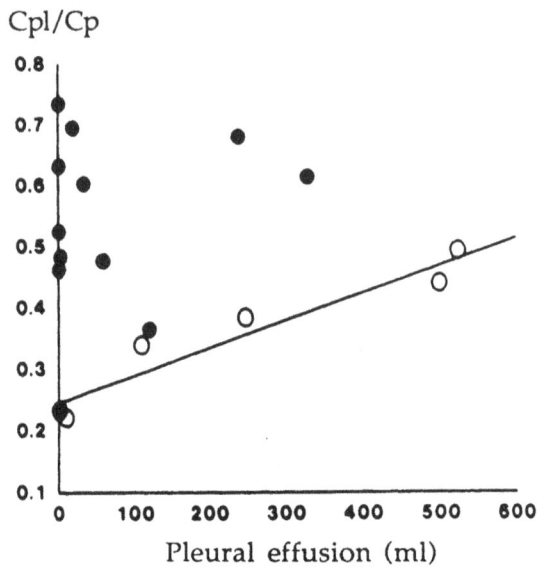

Figure 10. Effect of superior vena caval pressure (SVCP) on pleural effusion formation. There is no effusion present until SVCP is ≥ 15 mmHg. Ref. #12.

significant effusions. Further, investigators have studied patients with chronic elevations of central venous pressure and failed to find effusions (13). However the venous pressure increases found in these chronic patients were lower than either those produced in our sheep or those found in critically ill patients.

Thoracic duct drainage should also decrease the volume of pleural effusions by enhancing lymphatic drainage of both the pleural space and the lung parenchyma. Returning to a previously mentioned study, Figure 7 shows that pleural effusions were also decreased when pulmonary edema was produced by increased LAP.

FUTURE

Certainly, better techniques for measuring and decreasing pulmonary capillary pressure need to be developed. These techniques would provide the clinician better control of the rate of fluid leaking out of the capillary. Some laboratory investigators have pharmacologically *decreased* permeability. This may offer another method for managing pulmonary edema. Enhancing the removal of edema fluid is also a potentially viable option. This could be done with agents that augment lymph flow (lymphagogues) or by draining the thoracic duct (6).

Very little is understood about how the pulmonary interstitium adapts to the presence of extra fluid. In other tissues, such as skin, chronic edema is associated with structural organization. Whether an analogous process occurs in the lungs is not known. Initial studies into the chemical components of the pulmonary interstitium have begun. One such compound, hyaluronan (hyaluronic acid) possesses unique water binding properties. We have shown that hyaluronan may play a role in pulmonary water balance in newborn lungs (14), while Nettelbladt et al. have suggested the same in adult lungs (15). Manipulation of hyaluronan may play a role in the management of pulmonary edema.

REFERENCES

1. Allen SJ, Laine GA, Drake RE, et al: Lowered pulmonary arterial pressure prevents edema after endotoxin in sheep. J Appl Physiol 63:1008-11, 1987

2. Gattinoni L, Pesenti A, Bombino M, et al: Relationships between lung computed tomographic density, gas exchange, and PEEP in Acute Respiratory Failure. Anesth 69:824-32, 1988

3. Allen SJ, Drake RE, Williams WP, et al: Recent advances in pulmonary edema. Crit Care Med 15:963-70, 1987

4. Laine GA, Allen SJ, Katz J, et al: Effect of systemic venous pressure elevation on lymph flow and lung edema formation. J Appl Physiol 61:1634-38, 1986

5. Allen SJ, Drake RE, Katz J, et al: Elevation of superior vena caval pressure increases extravascular lung water following endotoxemia. J Appl Physiol 62:1006-9, 1987

6. Allen SJ, Drake RE, Gabel JC: Effect of thoracic duct drainage on hydrostatic pulmonary edema and pleural effusion in the sheep. J Appl Physiol, 1991, in press

7. Humphrey H, Hall J, Sznajder I, et al: Improved survival in ARDS patients associated with a reduction in pulmonary capillary wedge pressure. Chest 97:1176-80, 1990

8. Hernandez LA, Coker PJ, May S, et al: Mechanical ventilation increases microvascular permeability in oleic acid-injured lungs. J Appl Physiol 69:2057-61, 1990

9. Wiener-Kronish JP, Berthiaume Y, Albertine KH: Pleural effusions and pulmonary edema. Clinics in Chest Med 6:509-19, 1985

10. Broaddus VC, Wiener-Kronish JP, Staub NC: Clearance of lung edema into the pleural space of volume-loaded anesthetized sheep. J Appl Physiol 68:2623-30, 1990

11. Allen S, Gabel J, Drake R: Left atrial hypertension causes pleural effusion formation in unanesthetized sheep. Am J Physiol 257(Heart Circ Physiol 26):H690-2, 1989

12. Allen SJ, Laine GA, Drake RE, et al: Superior vena caval pressure elevation causes pleural effusion formation in sheep. Am J Physiol 255(Heart Circ Physiol 24):H492-5, 1988.

13. Wiener-Kronish JP, Goldstein R, Matthay RA: Lack of association of pleural effusion with chronic pulmonary arterial and right atrial hypertension. Chest 92:967-70, 1987

14. Allen SJ, Sedin EG, Jonzon A, et al: Lung hyaluronan during development: a quantitative and morphological study. Am J Physiol 260(Heart Circ Physiol 29):H1449-54, 1991

15. Nettelbladt O, Bergh J, Schenholm M, et al: Accumulation of hyaluronic acid in the alveolar interstitial tissue in bleomycin-induced alveolitis. Am Rev Respir Dis 139:759-62, 1989

OXYGEN CONSUMPTION MEASUREMENTS DURING ARTIFICIAL VENTILATION

J. F. Nunn

Oxygen consumption ($\dot{V}O_2$) is highly informative measurement, but one which has, in the past, been excluded from anesthesia and intensive care by technical difficulties. To be of any real value the measurement requires scrupulous attention to detail if the results are to be valid, and many factors combine to make it particularly difficult in sick patients undergoing artificial ventilation. To a large extent these technical difficulties have now been overcome, and there are now practical methods of validating the results which are obtained.

VALUE OF THE MEASUREMENT

$\dot{V}O_2$ is the most reliable measurement to indicate the very high metabolic rates in some patients undergoing intensive therapy (1), and, therefore, provides a rational basis for their supportive therapy. Observations of reduction in $\dot{V}O_2$ are of even greater importance, since reduced or inadequate $\dot{V}O_2$ is the common denominator of all circulatory shock syndromes and is the earliest pathophysiological event, preceding the initial hypotensive crisis (2,3).

Many centres have now reported studies relating $\dot{V}O_2$ to oxygen delivery ($\dot{D}O_2$). Below the critical $\dot{D}O_2$, $\dot{V}O_2$ decreases in proportion to $\dot{D}O_2$ (supply-dependent oxygenation) and therapy can then be directed towards maximizing these variables (2,4,5,6,7). Limitation of either $\dot{D}O_2$ or $\dot{V}O_2$ appears to be a powerful predictor of an unfavorable outcome (8).

The difference between methods of measurement including and excluding the lung will indicate the oxygen consumption of the lung itself (9). $\dot{V}O_2$ may be very large in the infected lung, and its measurement

83

T. H. Stanley and R. J. Sperry (eds.), Anesthesia and the Lung 1992. 83–90.
© 1992 Kluwer Academic Publishers.

seems likely to provide a valuable tool for relatively non-invasive investigation of pathological processes in the diseased lung.

MEASUREMENT OF $\dot{V}O_2$

It is possible to identify two approaches to the measurement of $\dot{V}O_2$ during artificial ventilation and intensive care.

The Reversed Fick Method

By far the commonest approach is the reversed Fick procedure, by which $\dot{V}O_2$ is calculated as the product of cardiac output and arterial/mixed venous oxygen content difference. This requires little additional effort or expense if a patient already has Swan-Ganz and arterial lines in place and cardiac output is being measured by dye or thermodilution. The reversed Fick method also has the advantage that the primary measurements also yield $\dot{D}O_2$ (cardiac output x arterial oxygen content), although these are two shared variables in the derivation of each measurement and the validity of comparison is therefore compromised.

Gasometric Methods

The second approach is to measure the deficit between the volumes of inspired and expired oxygen. While this is very easy in the subject breathing spontaneously, it requires considerable ingenuity when applied to a patient being ventilated artificially.

There are two sub-groups of the gasometric methods. The first measures either oxygen withdrawal from a closed circuit or, alternatively, the rate of replenishment required to maintain the total quantity of oxygen (10). Alternatively, an open circuit may be adapted using the principle of replenishment (11). The second sub-group of gasometric methods measures $\dot{V}O_2$ as the actual difference between the inspired and expired volumes of oxygen (i.e., the product of inspired minute volume and inspired oxygen concentration less the product of expired minute volume and mixed expired oxygen concentration).

The classical approach to the first group is the use of spirometer (Fig. 1) and, a workable system can be assembled at minimal cost (10). It has been shown to have no significant systemic error, and a standard deviation of random error of about 8 ml/min. It has been used in the intensive care unit (9), but it is undeniably inconvenient in such a situation, and it is demanding in the technical skills required for safe operation.

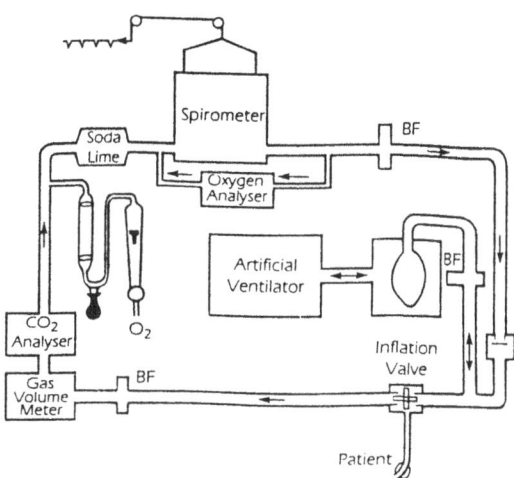

Figure 1. BF Bacterial Filter. An oxygen replenishment closed circuit spirometer system used during artificial ventilation. Reproduced from reference 9 with permission of the editor of Critical Care Medicine.

The second sub-group of gasometric methods is challenging because large minute volumes and high inspired oxygen concentrations increase the volume of both inspired and expired oxygen, and so magnify any errors in the measurement of the difference between them (12,13). Thus under typical ventilatory conditions which might be encountered in the intensive care unit, a 1% error in any of the four primary measurements may introduce a 30% error in the calculated $\dot{V}O_2$. Such considerations are daunting to the do-it-yourself investigator but, rather surprisingly, several commercial systems have now been shown to have an acceptable level of accuracy during mechanical ventilation with large minute volumes and high inspired oxygen concentrations (14-16).

The three best known commercial systems are the Datex Deltatrac, SensorMedics MMC Horizon and the Engstrom Metabolic Computer (EMC) (Fig. 2). The Deltatrac avoids measurement of minute volume by collecting and measuring expired CO_2 and then dividing by the respiratory quotient (RQ) to give $\dot{V}O_2$. The MMC an entirely conventional Haldane approach, with measurement of expired minute volume and the composition of both inspired and mixed-expired gas. Inspired minute volume is derived by multiplying the expired minute volume by the Haldane transformation factor (expired nitrogen concentration/inspired oxygen nitrogen concentration). The EMC can be used only with the Erica ventilator. It uses the conventional Haldane approach except that inspired minute volume is measured, and expired minute volume calculated by multiplication by the reversed Haldane transformation factor (inspired nitrogen concentration/expired nitrogen concentration).

VALIDATION OF TECHNIQUES OF MEASUREMENT OF $\dot{V}O_2$

It is crucially important to validate the accuracy of equipment which measures oxygen consumption, because very large errors can easily occur if some part of the system is not functioning correctly. Such errors may not be apparent in automated equipment. The technique of validation should simulate the clinical conditions in terms of intermittent positive pressure ventilation, high oxygen concentrations and other factors which complicate the measurement. There are two groups of methods available, metabolic simulators and the creation of a mock expired gas mixture.

Metabolic Simulators

Methanol and ethanol can be burned to give an RQ of 0.67. The quantity consumed can be determined by weighing or it would presumably be possible to deliver a known quantity of liquid by an automatic syringe. Both butane (10) and hydrogen (17) have been used, the former giving a RQ of 0.615. In the case of hydrogen, carbon dioxide can be added to the combustion chamber to give any required RQ.

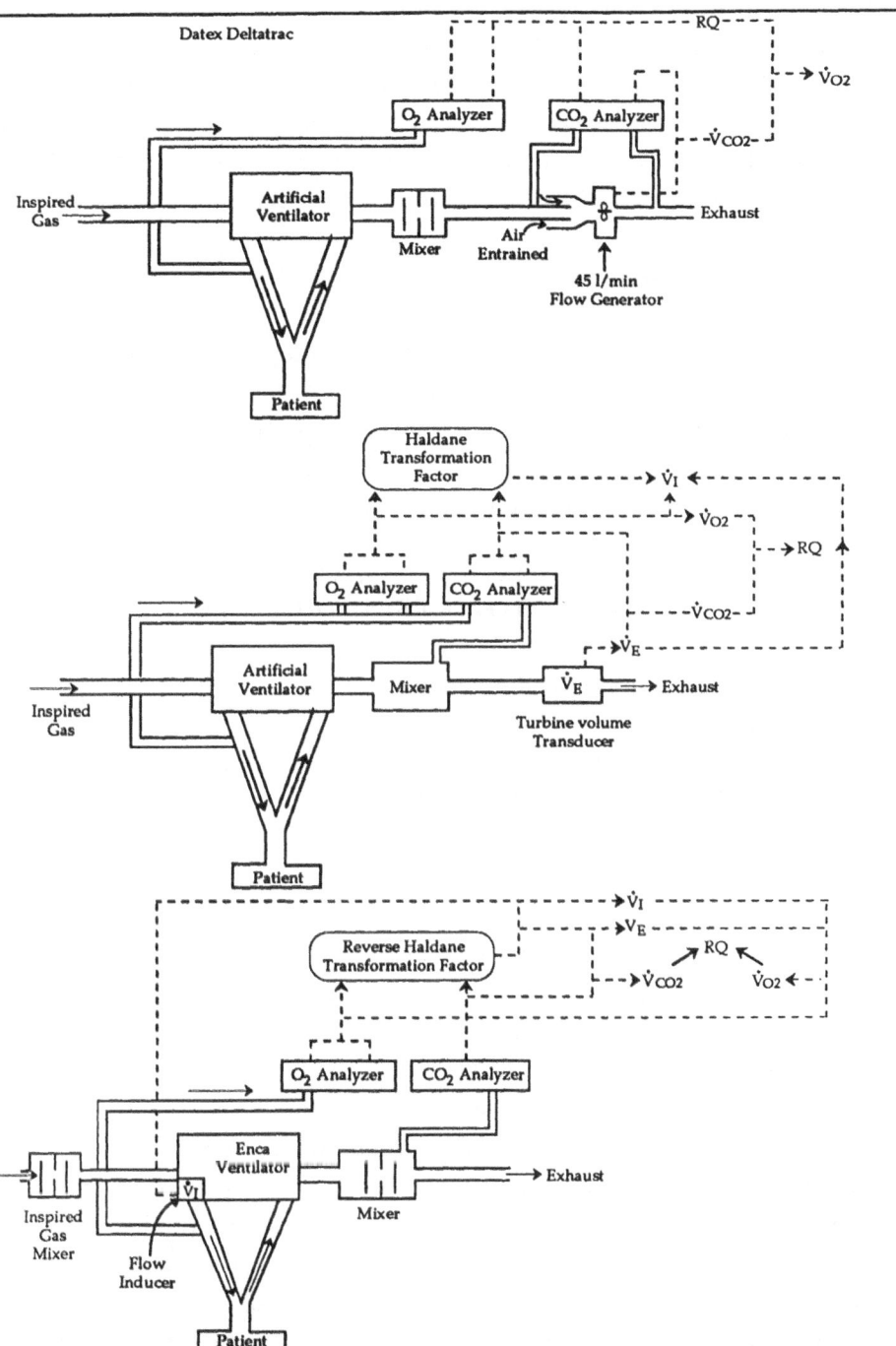

Figure 2. Schematic flow diagrams of three commercially available indirect calorimeters. Reproduced from reference 16 with permission of the editor of Critical Care Medicine.

Measurement of the flow rate of the combustible gas can easily be made with a level of accuracy well in excess of requirement. Combustion of inflammable gases in high concentrations of oxygen presents certain technical problems. However, these can be overcome and it is possible to predict $\dot{V}O_2$ and $\dot{V}CO_2$ of such model systems with an accuracy which is an order of magnitude better than that required for clinical measurement.

Mock Expired Gas Mixtures

Much care has been devoted to the development of systems that create a mock expired gas mixture which corresponds to highly predictable values for $\dot{V}O_2$ and $\dot{V}CO_2$ (15). Such systems are complex and expensive to develop. However, once assembled it is relatively easy to make large numbers of observations under a wide range of circumstances.

VALIDATION AND MEANING OF $\dot{V}O_2$ MEASURED BY THE REVERSED FICK PROCEDURE

Oxygen consumption is derived as:

$\dot{Q}$ (CaO$_2$ - C$\bar{v}$O$_2$)

The blood oxygen contents are usually calculated as saturation x hemoglobin concentration + dissolved oxygen.

There is no simple method of validation of any of the primary measurements, or of $\dot{V}O_2$ itself.

The reversed Fick method measures $\dot{V}O_2$ of the body *excluding the lung,* while the gasometric methods measure $\dot{V}O_2$ of the whole body *including the lung.* Under normal circumstances $\dot{V}O_2$ of the lung makes only an insignificant contribution to $\dot{V}O_2$ of the whole body and, therefore, the difference is insignificant (18,19). However, Light (18) clearly showed that, in contrast to healthy dogs, there was a very large oxygen consumption by the lungs of dogs with pneumonia. Several groups have now made simultaneous measurements of $\dot{V}O_2$ by gasometric and reversed Fick methods, and shown that, in patients undergoing intensive care, there may be large differences (Fig. 3), indicating very high values for pulmonary $\dot{V}O_2$ in the human infected lung (9,14,20). It seems unlikely that these values can be explained solely on account of increased metabolic activity and they may well indicate formation of oxygen-derived free

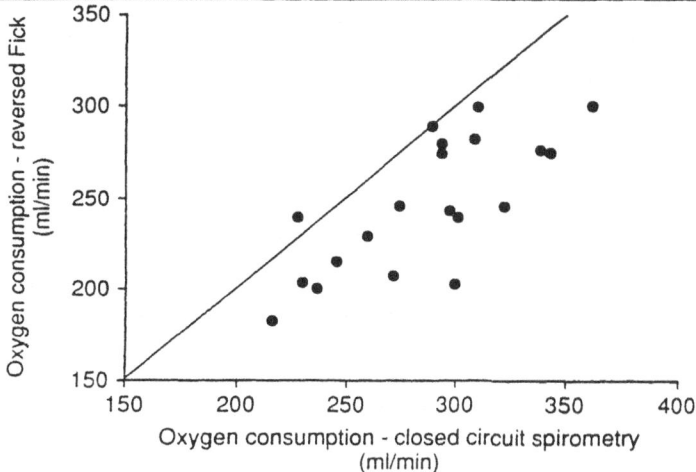

Figure 3. Simultaneous measurements of $\dot{V}O_2$ by a method which includes the lung (abscissa) and another which excludes the lung (ordinate). Reproduced from reference 9 with permission of the editor of Critical Care Medicine.

radicals and related species. This could be confirmed be measurement of pulmonary $\dot{V}O_2$ (also as the difference between gasometric and reversed Fick methods), since free radical formation should have an RQ of zero. This would then provide a valuable technique to measure free radical production in the lung.

REFERENCES

1. Skootsky SA, Abraham E: Continuous oxygen consumption measurement during initial emergency department resuscitation of critically ill patients. Crit Care Med 16:706, 1988
2. Shoemaker WC: Relation of oxygen transport patterns to the pathophysiology and therapy of shock states. Intensive Care Med 13:230, 1987
3. Shoemaker WC: What should be monitored? The past, present, and future of physiological monitoring. Clin Chem 36:1536, 1990
4. Wolf YG, Cotev S, Perel A, Manny J: Dependence of oxygen consumption on cardiac output in sepsis. Crit Care Med 15:198-203, 1987
5. Astiz ME, Rackow EC, Falk JL, Kaufman BS, Weil MH: Oxygen delivery and consumption in patients with hyperdynamic septic shock. Crit Care Med 15:26-8, 1987

6. Edwards JD, Brown GCS, Nightingale P, Slater RM, Faragher EB. Use of survivors' cardiorespiratory values as therapeutic goals in septic shock. Crit Care Med 17:1098-103, 1989

7. Shoemaker WC, Appel PL, Kram HB, Duarte D, Harrier HD, Ocampo HA: Comparison of hemodynamic and oxygen transport effects of dopamine and dobutamine in critically ill surgical patients. Chest 96:120, 1989

8. Shoemaker WC, Bland RD, Appel PL: Controversies in the pathophysiology and fluid management of postoperative adult respiratory distress syndrome. Surg Clin North Am 65:811, 1985

9. Smithies MN, Royston B, Makita K, Koniezko, K Nunn JF: Comparison of oxygen consumption measurements: Indirect calorimetry versus the reversed Fick method. Crit Care Med (in press)

10. Nunn JF, Makita K, Royston B: Validation of oxygen consumption measurements during artificial ventilation. J Appl Physiol 67:2129-34, 198

11. Westenskow DR, Roberts SE, Pace NL: Evaluation of replenishment type oxygen consumption monitor. Crit Care Med 17:798-802, 1989

12. Nunn JF, Pouliot JC: The measurement of gaseous exchange during nitrous oxide anesthesia. Br J Anaesth 34:752, 1962

13. Ultman JS, Bursztein S: Analysis of error in the determination of respiratory gas exchange at varying FIO2. J Appl Physiol 50:210, 1981

14. Takala J, Keinanen O, Vaisanen P, Kari A: Measurement of gas exchange in intensive care: Laboratory and clinical validation of a new device. Crit Care Med 17:1041-7, 1989

15. Bruan U, Zundel J, Freiboth K, Weyland W, Turner E, Heidelmeyer CF, Hellige G: Evaluation of methods for indirect calorimetry with a ventilated lung model. Int Care Med 15:196-202, 1989

16. Makita K, Nunn JF, Royston B: Evaluation of metabolic measuring instruments for use in critically ill patients. Crit Care Med 18:638-44, 1990

17. Swenson KL, Sonander HG, Stenqvist O: Validation of a system for measurement of metabolic gas exchange during anaesthesia with controlled ventilation in an oxygen consumption lung model. Br J Anaesth 64:311-9, 1990

18. Light RB: Intrapulmonary oxygen consumption in experimental pneumococcal pneumonia. J Appl Physiol 64:2490-5, 1988

19. Bihari DJ, Smithies M, Pozniak A, Gimson A: A compoarison of direct and indirect measurements of oxygen delivery and consumption: The effects of prostacyclin in two human volunteers. Scand J Clin Lab Invest 47(suppl)188:37-45, 1987

20. Behrendt W, Weiland C, Kalff J, Giani G: Continuous measurement of oxygen uptake. Acta Anaesth Scand 31:10-4, 1987

THE HYPOXIC BRAIN

T. F. Hornbein

INTRODUCTION

We cherish our brains as the essence of what we are, how we think and feel, and the determiner of what we do. The sleep of acute, severe hypoxia is not necessarily reversible, as exemplified by the consequences of high altitude balloon flights of intrepid explorers of the upper atmosphere over a century ago (1,2). J.B.S. Haldane was the one who said that hypoxia not only stops the machine but wrecks the machinery. My purpose will be to review the causes of hypoxia to the brain and to explore the limits of safe trespass and how one might try to recognize when one is approaching those limits. For general reviews of cerebral hypoxia, its metabolic correlates, clinical and pathological consequences and brain protection, see references 3 and 4.

THE ETIOLOGY OF BRAIN HYPOXIA

Metabolic Considerations

The brain's metabolic substrates are oxygen and glucose. As in other organs, hypoxia ensues when the organs' oxygen need exceeds supply. The overall oxygen utilization of the brain is about 3 ml^{-1}·100 gm·min^{-1}, a value that changes minimally with sleep or increased mental activity. Even so, measurements of focal metabolic activity indicate enhanced metabolism and oxygen requirement when local areas of the brain are activated. When oxygen supply falls short of need, such functional activity ceases prior to hypoxic encroachment on the maintenance of basic cellular integrity. Functional loss is reflected by loss

91

T. H. Stanley and R. J. Sperry (eds.), Anesthesia and the Lung 1992, 91–96.
© 1992 *Kluwer Academic Publishers.*

of consciousness and the absence of electrical activity as measured by the electroencephalogram or evoked electrical responses.

Biochemical Correlates of Progressive Brain Hypoxia

There is an increase in glucose utilization as the brain strives to sustain its energy (ATP) production through a less efficient, non-aerobic pathway. Lactic acid is produced instead of carbon dioxide and water. Depletion of energy stores follows, with conversion of ATP to ADP to AMP and depletion of phosphocreatine. As the energy required to sustain membrane function is lost, potassium leaks from cells into the extracellular fluid and cerebrospinal fluid, a sign we have come to correlate clinically with irreversible cell damage. Calcium is lost, and other evidence of extrusion of cellular contents occurs, such as brain creatinekinase into the extracellular fluid and cerebral spinal fluid.

CLINICAL CAUSES

Ventilatory Failure

I will forsake a review of the physiology of arterial hypoxemia for the moment to turn to the clinical occurrences with which we are most familiar. These are failure of air entry to the lungs due to airway obstruction or failure of ventilation; inadvertent administration of a hypoxic gas mixture; and shunt or severe ventilation/perfusion abnormality as a consequence of chronic lung disease and/or acute lung disorders such as atelectasis and pulmonary edema.

Circulatory Failure

Brain oxygenation depends upon delivery of sufficient oxygen from lungs to brain, which is in turn dependent upon an adequate blood flow to the brain and sufficient oxygen carriage by that blood. Blood flow may be compromised by inadequate cerebral perfusion pressure (the difference between mean arterial pressure and cerebral venous pressure) or by an increased resistance to flow. Autoregulation preserves near normality of cerebral blood flow in humans down to mean cerebral perfusion pressures below 50 mmHg. Loss of oxygen content in the perfusing blood, assuming arterial to be satisfactory, is a consequence of loss of functional hemoglobin, either through hemodilution or chemical complexing that renders the hemoglobin unable to carry oxygen, as for example with carbon monoxide poisoning.

THE CLINICAL APPEARANCE OF BRAIN HYPOXIA

Signs and Symptoms

Inspired hypoxia produces a pleasantly progressive loss of consciousness—that is, an anesthetic state. Loss of night vision is one of the earliest signs of minimal hypoxia, along with subtle impairment of thought processes including problem-solving abilities and judgment. Restriction of the visual fields and progressive motor weakness ensue. Even as vision and muscle power are lost, hearing and recall may remain remarkably unimpaired as a last touch with reality prior to loss of consciousness (1,2).

LIMITS OF HYPOXIA

Arterial Hypoxemia

PaO_2's below 40 mmHg may be tolerated acutely without harm. A PaO_2 of 30 mmHg, equivalent to about 8% inspired oxygen or an altitude in excess of 24,000 feet, will result in loss of consciousness, followed by brain injury, followed by death over the course of minutes. While more severe arterial hypoxemia may be tolerated momentarily, even less severe hypoxia may be harmful if sustained for a longer time.

Hypotension and Hemodilution

I will review the outcome of a study in non-human primates designed to address the question of safe limits for controlled hypotension, for hemodilution, and for the combination of the two (5). The primary purpose of this study was to identify the electrical correlates of brain hypoxia to a level sufficient to produce mild brain injury as assessed histopathologically. These animals were anesthetized with halothane, had normal acid base status, arterial blood oxygenation, and body temperature.

1. With hypotension alone to mean arterial pressures below 20 mmHg, none of the animals who survived the stress exhibited brain injury. The same was true of hemodilution alone to hematocrits in the range of 15%.

2. Combined hypotension and hemodilution was capable of producing brain damage in approximately half the animals in whom the product of mean arterial blood pressure and hematocrit was less than 600. Nevertheless neither arterial blood pressure nor hematocrit nor their product predicted which animals would sustain injury.

3. The degree of hypotension, hemodilution, and their combination was sufficient to eliminate all but delta (slow wave, 0 to 4 Hz) activity on the electroencephalogram in both injured and noninjured animals. The stress imposed did not produce either burst-suppression or a flat electroencephalogram in any of the animals in spite of subsequent injury in 7 of 16 experiencing combined hypotension/hemodilution. The electroencephalogram, like blood pressure and hematocrit, permitted no real time prediction of outcome, but the rate of recovery of the electroencephalogram after return to normal conditions was significantly slower in those animals who sustained injury.

4. The magnitude of the wave of the cortical somatosensory evoked response was depressed by hypoxia. So long as the amplitude of this wave remained above 60% of control, brain injury did not occur. If the evoked potential after 15 minutes of a 30 minute stress fell below 60% of control, a greater than 50% chance of injury existed. The cortical evoked potential may therefore have value as a monitor for safe levels of controlled hypotension and/or hemodilution in humans.

LIMITS WITH CHRONIC HYPOXIA

What limits performance at the extreme of earthbound hypoxia, namely the summit of Mt. Everest? While diffusion limitation in the lung may represent the rate-limiting step, the target organ limiting function appears to be the central nervous system. This proposal is based on anecdotal experience and also on studies of muscle function and metabolism during severe hypoxia performed during Operation Everest II. Extrapolating from the studies of non-human primates that I have just described to humans exposed to extreme environmental hypoxia, I will review briefly findings we obtained utilizing neurobehavioral assessments of function instead of brain histopathology in climbers to high altitude both before ascent and after return to sea level.

The major and still most significant observations were those reported previously in relation to the American Medical Research Expedition to Everest (6). Three primary lingering alterations were observed in these individuals on return to sea level: 1) impairment of both short and long-term memory storage and recall as assessed by the Wechsler Memory Scale; 2) aphasic impairments in response to simple commands; 3) impairment in single finger tapping speed, which was characterized by an inability to sustain the rate of tapping over a 15-second period. Of these three tests, the finger-tapping test continued to be abnormal in some of those evaluated a year later.

Subsequently, we have made similar observations on a total of 41 individuals upon return from high altitude (although we have not obtained additional long-term follow-up) including 6 subjects of Operation Everest II (7). Regard et al. report somewhat more consequential, longer lasting residuals in five of eight elite Himalayan mountaineers, all of whom climbed to above 8,500 meters without use of supplemental oxygen (8).

Of particular interest was a correlation of neurobehavioral impairment with measures of ventilatory drive, such as hypoxic ventilatory response (7). Those who had the most vigorous ventilatory response [and, therefore, might be presumed to be able to sustain a better performance at extreme altitude (9,10)] were also those who demonstrated the greatest degree of neurobehavioral impairment upon return to low altitude. Is it possible that a greater degree of hypocapnia in these individuals, while enhancing arterial oxygenation and physical performance at high altitude, might also cause greater cerebral vasoconstriction and hence a greater degree of brain hypoxia, sufficient to yield greater impairment of subsequent cerebral function?

REFERENCES

1. Glaisher J, Flammarion C , DeFonvielle W, Tissandier G: Travels in the Air, J Glaisher (ed.). Philadelphia, JB Lippincott, 1971
2. Bert P: Barometric Pressure: Researches in Experimental Physiology, trans. from French by MA Hitchcock and FA Hitchcock. Columbus: College Book Company, 1943
3. Fahn S, Davis JN, Rowland LP (eds.). Cerebral Hypoxia and Its Consequences, Vol. 26 of Advances in Neurology. New York, Raven Press, 1979, 350 pp
4. Hornbein P: Hypoxia and the brain. The Lung: Scientific Foundations, Crystal RG, West JB, et al (eds.). New York, Raven Press, 1991, pp 1535-40
5. Dong WK, Bledsoe SW, Chadwick HS, Shaw CM, Hornbein TF: Electrical correlates of brain injury resulting from severe hypotension and hemodilution in monkeys. Anesthesiology 65:617-25, 1986
6. Townes BD, Hornbein TF, Schoene RB, Sarnquist FH, Grant I: Human cerebral function at extreme altitude. In High Altitude and Man, JB West (ed.). Baltimore, Williams & Wilkins, 1984, chapt. 3, pp 31-36
7. Hornbein TF, Townes BD, Schoene RB, Sutton JR, Houston CS: The cost to the central nervous system of climbing to extremely high altitude. New Engl J Med 321:1714-19, 1989
8. Regard M, Oelz O, Brugger P, Landis T: Persistent cognitive impairment in climbers after repeated exposure to extreme altitude. Neurology 39:310-3, 1989
9. Masuyama S, Kimura H, Sugita T, Kuriyama T, Tatsumi K, Kunitomo F, Okita S, Tojima H, Yuguchi Y, Watanabe S, Honda Y: Control of ventilation in extreme-altitude climbers. J Appl Physiol 61:500-6, 1986
10. Schoene RB, Lahiri S, Hackett PH, Peters RM Jr, Milledge JS, Maret CJ, West JB: Relationship of hypoxic ventilatory response to exercise performance on Mount Everest. J Appl Physiol 56:1478-83, 1984

SEVERE HYPOXIA: INSIGHTS FROM EXTREME ALTITUDE

J. B. West

Severe tissue hypoxia is frequently a feature of patients in the intensive care setting, and two major experiments during the last ten years have greatly clarified the physiological effects of severe hypoxia in man. They are the 1981 American Medical Research Expedition to Everest (AMREE) (1) and Operation Everest II (OE II) in which eight subjects lived for 40 days in a low pressure chamber in a simulated climb of the mountain (2). In this brief presentation, I shall summarize some of the most interesting results from both experiments.

Climbers at very great altitudes develop enormous degrees of hyperventilation. On AMREE, the alveolar PCO_2 of a climber on the summit was less than 8 mmHg indicating the tremendous hyperventilation resulting from stimulation of the peripheral chemoreceptors by the very severe hypoxemia. Even so, the alveolar PO_2 was only approximately 35 mmHg, and the calculated arterial PO_2 was less than 30 mmHg. Direct measurements from arterial blood on OE II gave similar values. The reduction of arterial PO_2 below the alveolar value can be explained by diffusion limitation of oxygen transfer within the lung under these exceptional conditions. Calculations show that the arterial PO_2 rises very slowly along the pulmonary capillary because of the very steep slope of the oxygen dissociation curve. This comes about because the PO_2 values are very low on the curve, and in addition, there is considerable polycythemia.

As a result of the very low PCO_2, the calculated arterial pH on the summit during AMREE exceeded 7.7. The value in OE II was not so high because the PCO_2 values were not so low. These differences are consistent with the different periods of acclimatization in the two experiments. The

T. H. Stanley and R. J. Sperry (eds.), Anesthesia and the Lung 1992, 97–100.

measured base excess values for the two studies were almost identical. The extreme degree of respiratory alkalosis benefits oxygen transfer from the air to the mitochondria by accelerating the loading of oxygen by the pulmonary capillaries under conditions of diffusion limitation. Although the consequent left-shifted oxygen dissociation curve also interferes with the unloading of oxygen in peripheral capillaries, model studies show that the benefits of the enhanced central loading of oxygen in the lung outweigh the disadvantages of the slowed unloading of oxygen in peripheral capillaries.

Although the ventilation is enormously increased at these great altitudes, it is remarkable that the other great convection system, the blood circulation, changes little at high altitudes. In fact, the cardiac output for a given work level in acclimatized subjects is the same as it is at sea level. This contrasts greatly with a situation in acute hypoxia where cardiac output is greatly increased. The reason for the return of the cardiac output/oxygen uptake relationship to its sea level value is unclear. Perhaps it is related to the phenomenon of stress failure in pulmonary capillaries discussed in a companion presentation. Because of the hypoxic pulmonary vasoconstriction, some capillaries may be exposed to high pressures and an increase in cardiac output might cause the wall stresses to rise too high. Incidentally, although the cardiac output in relation to work level is returned to the sea level value in acclimatized subjects, hemoglobin flow is higher because of the polycythemia.

One of the most interesting results from OE II was that myocardial contractility was well maintained up to the most extreme altitudes where the arterial PO_2 was approximately 30 mmHg. These measurements were made by cardiac catheterization and also by two dimensional echocardiography. This surprising result emphasizes the tolerance of the normal myocardium to extreme hypoxemia. It also brings out the difference between hypoxemia and ischemia, the latter being well known to interfere with myocardial contractility.

Maximum oxygen consumption is greatly reduced as acclimatized subjects go to higher and higher altitudes, and on the summit of Mt. Everest was only approximately one l/min, some 20-25% of the sea level value. The results obtained in AMREE and OE II agreed very closely in spite of the different periods of acclimatization. One might expect that with such a great reduction in aerobic work capacity, and the accompanying extreme tissue hypoxia, the body would make great use of anaerobic glycolysis. However, paradoxically, the rise in blood lactate concentrations during maximal work at extreme altitude in acclimatized subjects is very small. Indeed extrapolation from results obtained at over 6300 m in well acclimatized subjects suggests that on the summit during maximal work, there will be no rise in blood lactate at all, surely an extraordinary prediction. The mechanism of the small increase in blood lactate is unclear, but may be related to inhibition of enzymes such as phosphofructokinase in the glycolytic chain. This hypothesis has yet to be tested.

The severe arterial hypoxemia of extreme high altitude has effects on many organs including the central nervous system (CNS). In view of the known vulnerability of the CNS to acute hypoxemia, it is not surprising that CNS function is impaired at great altitudes. However, perhaps a surprising finding is that climbers returning to sea level after long periods of residence at high altitude show residual impairment of CNS function compared with preexpedition measurements. The impairment was seen both in short term memory and a test of manipulative skill (finger-tapping) and the last remained abnormal in some expedition members for years after they returned to sea level.

An interesting feature of the impairment of CNS function was that is was most marked in the climbers who had the greatest hypoxic ventilatory responses. Presumably these people had the highest alveolar and arterial PO_2 values, and therefore, we have the paradoxical finding of more severe CNS changes in the presence of higher arterial PO_2 values. The explanation is probably the lower PCO_2 values in the climbers with the highest ventilations, and the fact that the reduced PCO_2 caused greater cerebral vasoconstriction with the result that brain hypoxia was more severe in the face of the higher arterial PO_2 values.

The severe hypoxia of extreme altitude is naturally an unusual situation. However, the remarkable physiological responses throw light on the way in which the body can adapt to prolonged very severe hypoxia, and help us to understand how some patients with chronic hypoxemia can maintain modest levels of physical activity.

ACKNOWLEDGEMENTS

This work was supported by NIH program project HL17331-16.

REFERENCES

1. West JB, Human physiology at extreme altitudes on Mount Everest. Science 223:748-88, 1984
2. Houston CS, Sutton JR, Cymerman A, Reeves JT: Operation Everest II: man at extreme altitude. J Appl Physiol 63:877-882, 1987

RESPIRATORY CONTROL RELATED TO ALTITUDE AND ANESTHESIA

J. W. Severinghaus

SYNOPSIS

This discussion includes a review of physiology and pharmacology of the normal and abnormal regulation of breathing as it relates to both anesthesia (1) and high altitude (2,3), and discusses several recent relevant advances in understanding. During days to weeks of hypoxia the ventilation is gradually stimulated not only by a fall of CSF HCO_3^- but also by a rise in hypoxic drive, probably due to a greater carotid body sensitivity. The central CO_2 chemoreceptor neurons have been histologically identified in rats by c-fos staining after hypercapnia. They apparently generate acid in hypoxia which may be detected on the local surface in ECF. This presumed intracellular lactic acidosis may underlie hypoxic ventilatory depression, which occurs after 5-20 minutes of hypoxia. This complicates understanding of altitude acclimatization while offering new insight into the mechanism of CO_2 and pH detection as a transmembrane pH gradient change. The effects of anesthesia on hypoxic response is in part due to the raising of PCO_2 threshold by both the anesthetic and hypoxia and the flattening of CO_2 response which hypoxia multiplies. After anesthesia, respiration may be compromised by interactions between the effects of residual depressant drugs, lack of lung-pump strength and airway patency, and hypoventilation at normal PCO_2 due to repaying a deficit of body CO_2 stores.

PART I. BACKGROUND PHYSIOLOGY

I. The CO_2 Response

About 2/3 of mammalian total ventilatory drive at rest awake arises in CO_2 chemoreceptors near the medullary ventral surface (MVS). The

101

T. H. Stanley and R. J. Sperry (eds.), Anesthesia and the Lung 1992, 101–115.
© 1992 Kluwer Academic Publishers.

other 1/3 arises in the carotid bodies and the cortex. MVS chemoreceptors are stimulated by increased PCO_2 and decreased HCO_3^-, the controllers of their pHecf (4-8). New observations (see below) suggest they are probably depressed or reset by intracellular (hypoxic lactic) acidosis. CSF HCO_3^- is influenced by the blood brain barrier, by regional metabolism and partially and slowly by renal or other blood acid-base balance changes (9). The normal HCO_3^- concentration is the same as blood, 24 mM/L. Chemoreceptor tissue PCO_2 is 4 to 8 mmHg above P_aCO_2 and its blood flow is about 0.5 to 1.0 $ml \cdot gm^{-1} \cdot min^{-1}$, which results in a delay of 1 to 2 minutes of the response (to 63% of completion, the time constant) after a step change of PCO_2 (10). The chemoreceptor's effective ECF HCO_3^- concentration is little affected by acid or alkaline changes in blood, at least for many hours.

HCVR, the Hypercapnic Ventilatory Response, is the slope of the CO_2 response, which in normal adults averages 3 ± 2 $l \cdot min^{-1} \cdot mmHg^{-1}$ PCO_2. In the normal range 1 mmHg rise of PCO_2 approximates a fall of CSF and ECF pH of 0.01 units. Furthermore, CO_2 rise acidifies ICF about 2/3 as much as ECF. If the stimulus proves to be transmembrane H^+ gradient, the CO_2 response calculates to be about 3 $liters \cdot min^{-1}$ for a gradient change of 0.0033 pH!

II. Hypoxic Ventilatory Response, HVR

Carotid body chemoreceptors respond to pH and PO_2 rather than O_2 saturation or content. Anemia and carbon monoxide fail to stimulate them. Before 1975, most studies of hypoxic sensitivity reported the hyperbolic (or exponential) relationship of ventilation to end-tidal or arterial PO_2, as parameter 'A' (11) or as $\Delta \dot{V}_{40}$ (12). However, the demonstration by Rebuck and Campbell (13) that in isocapnic hypoxia, ventilation is a linear function of arterial oxygen desaturation facilitated and simplified quantification of hypoxic sensitivity as HVR = $\Delta \dot{V}_I / \Delta \dot{V}S_aO_2$. While this linearity may be accidental, it supports the concept that the carotid body oxygen transducer is a hemoglobin-like pigment (cytochrome) described in carotid body extracts by Mills and Jöbsis (14).

Using an oximeter, a capnometer and a pneumotachygraph, the sensitivity to hypoxia can be described by measurement of response at 75% saturation at constant normal PCO_2. Normal HVR is 1.0 $liter \cdot min^{-1} \cdot$% desaturation in a 70 kg adult (13). Arterial oxygen saturation by pulse oximetry provides a continuous, non-invasive measure of the stimulus without the errors inherent in estimating P_aO_2 from $P_{ET}O_2$ (especially at high altitude where subclinical pulmonary edema often results in large (A-a) O_2 differences). Oximetry may introduce its own errors (15).

III. Interaction of Hypoxic and CO_2 Responses

When normal subjects at rest close their eyes and breathe oxygen, PCO_2 rises 1 to 3 mmHg, stimulating central chemoreceptors sufficiently to take over essentially 100% of the drive to breathe. HVR depends on the level of PCO_2. Hypoxia has little ability to stimulate ventilation when PCO_2 is below normal, a matter of greatest concern to anesthesiologists during recovery from anesthesia with hyperventilation. This has killed underwater swimmers who hyperventilated before beginning. As PCO_2 rises, hypoxia multiplies or steepens the CO_2 response. This interaction is thought to be partly within the peripheral chemoreceptors, partly central.

IV. Hypoxic Ventilatory Depression

During isocapnic hypoxia, the ventilatory response begins to fade after about 5 minutes (16,17). After 30 minutes at about 75% S_aO_2, half or more of the hypoxic ventilatory response disappears. This has been called hypoxic ventilatory depression. The degree of fade varies between individuals. HVR remains depressed for 10 to 20 minutes of subsequent normoxia (18). This depression has introduced a variability between laboratories in normal responses because some sea level control studies of HVR have been done before HVD occurs, others during its development as when slowly progressive hypoxia is the test method (19), or after 12 minutes of hypoxia (2). HVR studies at altitude may begin with 5 to 15 minutes of hyperoxia which may partially reverse HVD if present. The CO_2 response has been thought to be reduced during the post hypoxic period (20). Van Beek et al. (21) showed that hypoxic perfusion of the brain with systemic normoxia did not attenuate the slopes of ventilatory responses to either CO_2 or peripheral chemoreceptor hypoxia. As described below, we found subjects to have undepressed incremental response to further hypoxia even when hypoxic depression had developed.

This depression is not due to endorphin release (17). Anthonisen and colleagues (18) identified adenosine and GABA as possible mediators. The effect is not in the carotid bodies. Neubauer, Simohe and Edelman suggest that HVD is related to brain lactic acid generation since it could be prevented by high doses of dichloroacetate, a stimulant of oxidative metabolism which reduces lactate production (22). We now suspect that HVD may be an upward shift of the set point of the central CO_2 chemoreceptors due to intracellular acidosis in those specific medullary ventral special cells, to be described below.

Hypoxic depression is clinically significant. A hypoxic patient will breathe more during the first 5 to 10 minutes of hypoxia than he will if hypoxia continues.

V. Chronic Hypoxic Blunting of the Hypoxic Drive

HVR falls irreversibly over years of exposure to hypoxia, such as high altitude, congenital cyanotic heart disease or and some COPD patients (called blue bloaters) (12,23-28). The carotid body at altitude has been reported to be enlarged. The responses to hypoxia of patients vary widely, which may place some at greater risk.

VI. Denervation of Peripheral Chemoreceptors

Denervation of the carotid bodies raises resting PCO_2 by about 6 mmHg for at least 6 months (29), probably permanently. In anesthetized animals, after bilateral chemoreceptor denervation, hypoxia may induce apnea (30). The carotid body drive during hypoxia is responsible for dyspnea (31), which may be regarded as the respiratory center's equivalent of pain. Some patients with bad lung disease have claimed to feel much better after carotid body resection or denervation. After denervation, they breathe less and thus are less well oxygenated. They have proceeded to "sell" the operation to others with COPD. Most have lived for months or years thereafter. A few died in the days or weeks after denervation. The distress of severe dyspnea merits more consideration by physicians.

VII. Acclimatization

Early changes during residence at altitude are called acclimatization, late changes adaptation. Acclimatization changes include a gradual increase of ventilation, fall of PCO_2, rise of PO_2, decrease in symptoms of headache, nausea, nose bleeding, and somewhat later, a rise in hematocrit.

Hypoxic peripheral drive increases ventilation, which promptly lowers P_aCO_2 and decreases central ventilatory drive. Over hours to days, CSF HCO_3^- and P_aCO_2 fall proportionally, and ventilation increases (32), while CSF pH (and presumably medullary ECF pH) remain alkaline (27,33).

The measure of acclimatization is the reduction of $P_{ET}CO_2$ or P_aCO_2 compared to sea level control, determined after breathing oxygen for 5 to 15 minutes. This fall of PCO_2 is proportional to the reduction of CSF HCO_3^- (33). The role of CSF HCO_3^- is contested (27).

In the operating room or intensive care unit patients may "acclimatize" slowly during prolonged hyperventilation. Eger et al. (34) found that 8 hours of hypoxic hyperventilation in normal awake subjects caused a downward shift of their subsequent resting PCO_2 of 36% of the imposed PCO_2 fall, while without hypoxia the same hypocapnia caused only half as much "acclimatization". This suggests that little acclimatization will occur during long hyperventilation of anesthetized subjects if they are well oxygenated.

If the fall of hyperoxic PCO_2 during acclimatization were due only to the CSF HCO_3^- reduction, CSF pH would be expected to fall as acclimatization increases arterial PO_2 and decreases peripheral chemoreceptor drive. Observations of a gradual increase in CSF pH with time at altitude suggest increased peripheral chemoreceptor drive at constant PO_2 and PCO_2. Sørensen and Cruz (23) found almost 3 times greater peripheral chemoreceptor responses to single breaths of CO_2 at altitude than at sea level, in both sea level and high altitude natives. Forster et al. (26) found a doubling of $\Delta\dot{V}_{40}$ at 3100m altitude in normal men. However, a serious problem with that study was that $\Delta\dot{V}_{40}$ remained at the altitude level 45 days after return to sea level, leaving it unclear whether a) a long-term potentiation had occurred, or b) the final values more accurately represented sea level controls. Forster et al. (35) also showed a 2- to 3-fold increase in response to Doxapram, a peripheral chemoreceptor stimulant, after 2 to 3 weeks at 3100m altitude. Vizek, Pickett and Weil (19) found increased HVR in cats after 48 hours at 15,000 ft (P_b=440 mmHg), both measured as whole animal responses and as carotid sinus nerve traffic. They reported no increase in the central integrator "gain." Barnard et al. (36) reported increased carotid sinus nerve traffic after 28 days at P_IO_2=70 mmHg in cats. On the other hand, Tatsumi, Pickett and Weil (28) more recently reported in cats decreased responses of both carotid body impulse traffic and ventilation to acute hypoxia after 3 to 4 weeks exposure to 5500m altitude (28). Bisgard et al. (37) and his associates Nielsen and Vidruk (38) and Engwall (39) have shown in goats an increased sensitivity of carotid chemoreceptors after chronic hypoxia, increased ventilatory responses to hypoxia, and a role of dopamine in this response.

Forster and Dempsey (27) concluded that "ISF (H^+) in the environment of the medullary chemoreceptor does not mediate either acclimatization to or deacclimatization from altitude sojourn." Because the only human study of this possible hypersensitization was flawed, we repeated and confirmed this effect in men in 1990 and again in 1991 (below). The acclimatization process is interactive (33,40), a major component resulting from the gradual reduction of CSF HCO_3^-, with a gradual increase in peripheral chemoreceptor drive.

THREE NEW OBSERVATIONS BY UCSF INVESTIGATORS

I. Medullary CO_2 Chemoreceptor Neuron Histologic Identification

To identify and count CO_2 chemoreceptor neurons in the brain stem, in Sprague-Dawley rats after 1 hour exposure to 13 to 15% PCO_2, Sato et al. (41) used an immunocytochemical staining method to identify the expression of c-fos in those cells where high CO_2 increased neuronal activity. Fos-immunoreactive cells were found in the area of the nucleus tractus solitarius (NTS) and in a thin layer near the ventral medullary surface but not elsewhere in the medulla. In the MVS, he found 321 ± 146 neurons/rat, of which 67% were within 50 μm of the surface, more than 90% lay between 1.0 and 3.0 mm from the midline, and about 60% were in the rostral half of the medulla. Morphine (10 mg/kg s.c.) did not suppress CO_2-evoked FLI in either the VMS or the NTS, although it eliminated excitement and hyperventilation. The distribution was similar to that first identified as chemoreceptive in cats by Mitchell and Loeschcke (4).

II. Acidification of Ventral Medullary Surface by Hypoxia

It has generally been assumed that hypoxic hyperventilation, mediated by peripheral chemoreceptors, would alkalinize the interstitial fluid of the MVS, as it does elsewhere (7,8). However, in 1982 Nolan et al. (42) reported acid shifts of the surface ECF on the medullary ventral surface during hypoxia. This has been confirmed by several other groups (30,43-

46). It had not been determined whether this acid was confined to the region of chemosensitivity or was more general.

Xu et al. (47) have repeated these studies in castrated male goats, in which 1 mm diameter glass bulb pH and reference electrodes on flexible catheters were chronically implanted through a posterior fossa craniotomy to lie in cerebrospinal fluid (csf) over the "rostral" medullary ventral surface (MVS) ventilatory "CO_2" chemoreceptors and pons. The fall of pH_{MVS} during isocapnic hypoxia was linearly proportional to desaturation. With 30-minute periods of steady hypoxia, pH_{MVS} fell rapidly at first, then slowly, becoming constant after 15 to 25 minutes. The time constants (to 63%) were 3.7 minutes for hypoxia and 2.0 minutes for recovery. The mean acid shift was 0.09 pH units at S_aO_2=70%, N=9. CO inhalation had the same effect. When $P_{ET}CO_2$ was permitted to fall with hypoxic hyperventilation, pH_{MVS} only began to fall when S_aO_2 fell below 80%. No acidosis was seen on the adjacent pons surface or the dorsal spinal cord at C1-C2. The levels and duration of hypoxia tested induced no systemic lactic acidosis. Xu has extended these studies to cats and determined that the acid secretion is localized to the chemosensitive areas of Mitchell and Loeschcke.

Implications of these studies on the nature of central chemoreception. This localized acid generation implies the presence of some metabolically active oxidative process in this region, topographically related to chemoreception. Since this acid fails to stimulate ventilation, pH_{ecf} appears not to be the unique signal of these chemoreceptors. Nor can it be intracellular pH alone, since both hypoxia and Diamox acidify initially the inside of cells. It now seems most likely that these cells are stimulated by a change in their transmembrane (H^+) gradient, as when pH_{ecf} falls more than pH_{icf} with either rising PCO_2 or falling HCO_3^-. This resembles a glass pH electrode, the membrane of which is permeable only to H^+. Inward diffusion of the positively charged protons reduces membrane potential toward the threshold of depolarization. With hypoxia, ICF pH must fall more than ECF, and depress activity or reset the cell threshold to higher PCO_2.

III. Effect of Acclimatization on HVR in Man (48)

Isocapnic hypoxic ventilatory response, HVR, was tested in six normal males at sea level (SL), after 1 to 5 days at 3810m altitude (AL1-3), and again at sea level. HVR tests at both altitudes were done with a special test P_{CO_2} (end-tidal) which set $\dot{V}_I = 140$ ml·kg^{-1}·min^{-1} during initial hyperoxia, assuring equal central ventilatory drive in the hyperoxic control state. HVR rose from 0.91 ± 0.38 at sea level to 1.27 ± 0.57 after 3.2 ± 0.8 days, and to 1.46 ± 0.59 after 4.8 ± 0.4 days at altitude. It slowly fell to within the normal range after the 4 to 7 days back at sea level. This confirmed the idea that carotid body drive is somehow increased by chronic hypoxia.

Hypoxic ventilatory depression (HVD) on ambient air. At altitude on day 3-4 while breathing ambient air ($S_pO_2 \simeq 88\%$) when HVR was tested without preoxygenation it was found to be "depressed" by ambient hypoxia to about half the preoxygenated HVR. At both sea level and high altitude, 25 minutes of isocapnic hypoxia ($S_aO_2 \simeq 77\%$) reduced HVR 45 to 63% from its early peak (2.5-5 min). However, at 25 minutes, a further S_aO_2 decrease from 77 to 65% raised ventilation along a normal slope giving a "differential" HVR of 111 to 127% of control. This normal response during evident hypoxic depression cannot be explained in terms of a GABA mediated global depression in response of brain respiratory centers to incoming peripheral chemoreceptor stimuli (49). The observations suggest that HVD represents a resetting of the central CO_2 (CSF pH) chemoreceptor to a higher P_{CO_2} comparable to the effect of raising ECF HCO_3^-. Such resetting should not reduce the slopes of response to further increase of either peripheral or central drive, in agreement with the studies of separate brain stem hypoxia reported by Van Beek et al. (21). This resetting of the $\dot{V}_I$·pH^{-1} relationship of central chemoreceptors may be related to the acid these medullary ventral cells generate in hypoxia.

The cause of the increased HVR occurring over days to weeks at altitude cannot be attributed to known factors related to central chemosensitivity. In natives of high altitude, decreased hypoxic peripheral chemosensitivity, called blunting, is associated with a transfer of drive to central chemoreceptors marked by a less alkaline CSF pH (12,25,33,40).

PART II. ANESTHETICS AND POST-ANESTHESIA PROBLEMS

Depression of Ventilation by Anesthetics

Ventilatory drive falls, P_{CO_2} rises and the slope of the CO_2 response is reduced in response to the inhalational anesthetics and to most of the injectable barbiturates, tranquilizers and narcotics. Exceptions are ketamine and N_2O. While PCO_2 rises approximately in proportion to depth of anesthesia, there are significant differences between drugs. This subject is fully covered in anesthesia and pharmacology textbooks, and in Hickey's review (1).

In normal sleep, PCO_2 rises 2 to 4 mmHg, and ventilatory responses to CO_2 may be significantly depressed especially in younger subjects (50). While we often notice that re-awakening after anesthesia restores respiratory drive, this so-called wakeful stimulus is probably more dependent on the sudden appreciation of pain.

Effects of Anesthetics on HVR

HVR is more sensitive than HCVR to halothane (51). Hypoxia acts to multiply the CO_2 drive, so when CO_2 drive is depressed, the hypoxic response is equally depressed even when no specific effect of the drug on hypoxic drive can be shown. For studies of anesthetic effects, the isocapnic hypoxic response should be computed as the fractional increase in ventilation produced by hypoxia. Hypoxia appears to independently depress the slope of the CO_2 response with 1.1% halothane, to nearly zero (52).

Post-hyperventilation Hypoxia

Post-hyperventilation hypoxia is a common but misunderstood phenomenon. In the recovery room, O_2 saturation may be found to be below 80% while breathing air, without any pulmonary atelectasis or shunt and with normal P_aCO_2 (53,54). It is caused by loss of body CO_2 stores during preceding hyperventilation. In 2 hours of hyperventilation to 20 mmHg PCO_2, expired gas may carry away 5 liters of CO_2 from stores, about equal to 25 minutes of metabolic CO_2 production, which must be paid back later by hypoventilation. The estimated half time for restoration of stores is 20 minutes, and full recovery requires hours. While the stores are being refilled from metabolically produced CO_2, pulmonary CO_2 excretion will be reduced, i.e., R, the ratio of $\dot{V}CO_2/\dot{V}O_2$, will be low. Ventilation, being primarily driven by CO_2 excretion, will therefore be inadequate for oxygen supply while breathing air, even though P_aCO_2 may be normal. It is thus especially important to administer nasal or mask O_2 after anesthesia when PCO_2 has been reduced, and this applies particularly during transport from the OR to recovery, the time when the ventilation will be minimum.

Narcotic Rebound Respiratory Depression

Narcotic respiratory depression may re-occur after the drug has been thought to be eliminated. Studying 29 patients given fentanyl, Becker et al. (55) showed that, after the CO_2 response slope had normalized in the recovery room, it fell again to 55% of normal during the following 30 to 90 minute period, without an accompanying rise of PCO_2. In two patients the slope of the CO_2 response fell as low as 10% of control during this recovery period. This might be responsible for occasional unexplained post-operative deaths. This is another reason to use O_2 for a few hours after general anesthesia.

Interaction of Narcotics and Vapors

Ventilatory depression from narcotics persists after analgesia disappears. In four anesthetized animal species, Steffey et al. (56) administered a bolus dose of 1 to 2 mg/kg of morphine, and then kept the animal at 1 MAC by reducing the alveolar halothane or isoflurane concentration. Morphine raised PCO_2 by about 20 mmHg, even though MAC was constant. As morphine wore off, the vapor concentration had to be increased to keep the animal at 1 MAC. When vapor concentration had returned to control, suggesting that all the analgetic effect of the narcotic was gone, PCO_2 was still elevated to 55 to 60 mmHg. At this point, naloxone administration immediately restored PCO_2 to about 40 mmHg. Naloxone had no effect on MAC. The clinical significance is obvious: post-operative patients will have significant respiratory depression from narcotics after the analgesic effects have gone.

Other Dangerous Interactions

In anesthesia we ordinarily use many drugs together, whereas most studies of the respiratory effects are done separately. Drugs may synergise in their depressant effects, either with each other or with mechanical factors such as a partially obstructed airway. The PCO_2 at 1.0 MAC halothane rose to 72 to 82 in patients with COPD whose FEV_{-1} was less than 0.5 $l \cdot min^{-1}$ (57). Depression of ventilation produced by a narcotic may occasionally be greater after addition of a tranquilizer which, by itself, does not depress CO_2 response, whereas studies in volunteers have not shown this interaction. During recovery from neuromuscular block, when twitch and tetanus responses of the adductor pollicis have returned to normal, up to 75% of the neuromuscular junctions may still be blocked. Johansen and Osgood (58) studied in dogs the effects of combining several minor respiratory impairments, each of which by itself had almost no effect of ventilation, PO_2 or PCO_2. These stresses were a small airway resistance, a reduced compliance, added dead space or partial curarization. When dead space and airway resistance were combined with partial curarization, PCO_2 rose to about 140 mmHg when O_2 was breathed. When air was breathed for 2 to 3 minutes, apnea occurred from hypoxic depression at a PCO_2 of 85 and PO_2 of 26 mmHg. Small doses of curare in awake normal humans have been shown to increase the breathholding time, increasing tolerance to hypoxia and hypercapnia.

Chronically hypoxic patients may be more liable to become apneic with narcotics, sedatives and anesthetics. This may be a cause of post-anaesthetic apnea, sleep apnea and sudden infant death.

Mechanism of Hypoxic Damage

The cause of cellular damage by hypoxia has been thought to be acid. However, Cohen et al. (59) showed by magnetic resonance spectroscopy that brain high energy compounds were fully maintained in rats exposed for 30 minutes to $PCO_2 = 400$ mmHg in O_2, which reduced intracellular pH to 6.3. The rats recovered and behaved normally for a week. The experiments have recently been extended by Litt to over 700 mmHg PCO_2 in a pressure chamber, again with no evidence for damage by carbonic acidosis. My suspicion is that hypoxia causes the tissue osmotic pressure to rise due to breakdown of sugar, leading to water entry and mechanical distention and explosion of mitochondria in particular. In certain highly vulnerable cell layers it is thought that hypoxia leads to increased activity causing damage where intracellular calcium binding is deficient.

CONCLUSION

The mechanisms of hypoxic accidents are often a mix of drug effects, pathophysiologic pulmonary impairment, airway obstruction, and the depressant interactions of hypoxia and CO_2 with these other factors. Study of the physiology of hypoxia continues to provide new insights.

REFERENCES

1. Hickey RF, Severinghaus JW: Regulation of breathing: drug effects. In Regulation of Breathing, Hornbein T (ed.). Part II. New York, M Dekker, 1981, pp 1251-1312

2. Cunningham DJC: Integrative aspects of the regulation of breathing: A personal view. In Respiratory Physiology, Guyton and Widdicombe (eds.). Physiology Series 1, Vol 2, MTP International Review of Science. London, Butterworths, 1974, pp 303-370

3. Berger A, Mitchell R, Severinghaus JW: Regulation of respiration. N Eng J Med 297:92-97, 138-43, 194-201, 1977

4. Mitchell RA, Loeschcke HH, Massion WH, Severinghaus JW: Respiratory responses mediated through superficial chemosensitive areas on the medulla. J Appl Physiol 18:523-33, 1963

5. Schlafke ME, See WR, Loeschcke HH: Ventilatory response to alterations of H^+ ion concentration in small areas of the ventral medullary surface. Resp Physiol 10:198-212, 1977

6. Shams, H: Differential effects of CO_2 and H^+ as central stimuli of respiration in the cat. J Appl Physiol 58:257-364, 1985

7. Teppema, LJ, Barts PWJA, Folgering HT, Evers JAM: Effect of respiratory and (isocapnic) metabolic arterial acid-base disturbances on medullary fluid pH and ventilation in cats. Resp Physiol 53:379-95, 1983

8. Ahmad HR, Loeschcke HH: Transient and steady state responses of pulmonary ventilation to the medullary extracellular pH after approximately rectangular changes in alveolar PCO_2. Pflügers Archiv 395:285-92, 1982

9. Irsigler GB, Severinghaus JW: Respiratory regulation of cerebrospinal fluid and peripheral acid-base balance. In The Kidney: Physiology and Pathology of Electrolyte Metabolism, Seldin DW, Giebisch G (eds.). Boston, Raven Press, 1985, pp 1459-70

10. Feustel PJ, Stafford MJ, Allen JS, Severinghaus JW: Ventrolateral medullary surface blood flow determined by hydrogen clearance. J Appl Physiol 56:150-54, 1984

11. Weil JV, Byrne-Quinn E, Sodal ID, et al: Hypoxic ventilatory drive in normal man. J Clin Invest 49:1061-72, 1970

12. Severinghaus JW, Bainton CR, Carcelen A: Respiratory insensitivity to hypoxia in chronically hypoxic man. Resp Physiol 1:308-34, 1966

13. Rebuck AS, Campbell EJM: A clinical method for assessing the ventilatory response to hypoxia. Amer Rev Resp Dis 109:345-50, 1974

14. Mills E, Jöbsis, FF: Mitochondrial respiratory chain of carotid body and chemoreceptor response to changes in oxygen tension. J Neurophysiol 35:405-28, 1972

15. Severinghaus JW, Naifeh KH, Koh SO: Errors during profound hypoxia in 14 pulse oximeters. J Clin Monit 5:72-81, 1989

16. Weil JV, Zwillich CW: Assessment of ventilatory response to hypoxia. Chest 70 (Suppl):124-28, 1976
17. Kagawa S, Stafford MJ, Waggener TB, Severinghaus JW: No effect of naloxone on hypoxia induced ventilatory depression in adults. J Appl Physiol 52:1030-34, 1982
18. Easton PA, Anthonisen NR: Ventilatory response to sustained hypoxia after pretreatment with aminophylline. J Appl Physiol 64:1445-50, 1988
19. Vizek M, Pickett CK, Weil, JV: Increased carotid body hypoxic sensitivity during acclimatization to hypobaric hypoxia. J Appl Physiol 63:2403-10, 1987
20. Sato M: Hypoxic ventilatory response during recovery period from sustained hypoxia. Jikeikai Medical Journal 37:481-88, 1990
21. Van Beek JHGM, Berkenbosch A, DeGoede J, Olievier CN: Effects of brain stem hypoxaemia on the regulation of breathing. Respiration Physiol 57:171-88, 1984
22. Neubauer JA, Simohe A, Edelman NH: Role of brain lactic acidosis in hypoxic depression of respiration. J Appl Physiol 65:1324-31, 1988
23. Sørensen SC, Cruz J: Ventilatory response to a single breath of CO_2 in O_2 in normal man at sea level and high altitude. J Appl Physiol 27:186-90, 1969
24. Lahiri S: Dynamic aspects of regulation of ventilation in man during acclimatization to high altitude. Resp Physiol 16:245-58, 1972
25. Severinghaus JW: Hypoxic respiratory drive and its loss during chronic hypoxia. Clin Physiol (Japan) 2:57-79, 1972
26. Forster HV, Dempsey JA, Birnbaum ML, Reddan WG, Thoden J, Grover RF, Rankin R: Effect of chronic exposure to hypoxia on ventilatory response to CO_2 and hypoxia. J Appl Physiol 31:586-92, 1971
27. Forster HV, Dempsey JA: Ventilatory adaptations. In Regulation of Breathing, Hornbein T (ed.). Part II. New York, M Dekker, pp 845-904
28. Tatsumi K, Pickett CK, Weil JV: Attenuated carotid body hypoxic sensitivity after prolonged hypoxic exposure. J Appl Physiol 70:748-55, 1991
29. Wade JG, Larson CP, Hickey RF, Ehrenfeld WK, Severinghaus JW: Effect of carotid endarterectomy on carotid chemoreceptor and baroreceptor function in man. N Eng J Med 282:823-29, 1970
30. Millhorn, DE, Eldridge FL, Kiley JP, Waldrop TJ: Prolonged inhibition of respiration following acute hypoxia in glomectomized cats. Resp Physiol 57: 331-40, 1984
31. Stulbarg MS, Winn WR, Kellett LE: Bilateral carotid body resection for the relief of dyspnea in severe chronic obstructive pulmonary disease. Physiologic and clinical observations in three patients. Chest 95:1123-8, 1989 (with editorial: Severinghaus JW: Carotid body resection for COPD? Chest 95:1128-9, 1989)
32. Severinghaus JW, Mitchell RA, Richardson BW, Singer MM: Respiratory control at high altitude suggesting active transport regulation of CSF pH. J Appl Physiol 18:1155-66, 1963

33. Crawford RD, Severinghaus JW: CSF pH and ventilatory acclimatization to altitude. J Appl Physiol 45:275-83, 1978
34. Eger EI, Kellogg RH, Mines AH, Lima-Ostos M, Morrill CG, Kent DW: Influence of CO_2 on ventilatory acclimatization to altitude. J Appl Physiol 24:607, 1968
35. Forster HV, Dempsey, JA, Vidruk E, DoPico G: Evidence of altered regulation of ventilation during exposure to hypoxia. Resp Physiol 20:379-92, 1974
36. Barnard P, Andronikou S, Pokorski M, Smatresk N, Mokashi A, Lahiri S: Time-dependent effect of hypoxia on carotid body chemosensory function. J Appl Physiol 63: 685-91, 1987
37. Bisgard GE, Kressin NA, Nielsen AM, Daristotle L, Smith CA, Forster HV: Dopamine blockade alters ventilatory acclimatization to hypoxia in goats. Resp Physiol 69:245-55, 1987
38. Nielsen AM, Bisgard GE, Vidruk EH: Carotid chemoreceptor activity during acute and sustained hypoxia in goats. J Appl Physiol 65:1796-1802, 1988
39. Engwall MJA, Bisgard GE: Ventilatory responses to chemoreceptor stimulation after hypoxic acclimatization in awake goats. J Appl Physiol 69:1236-43, 1990
40. Severinghaus JW, Crawford RD: Carotid chemoreceptor role in CSF alkalosis at altitude. Chest 73:249-51, 1978
41. Sato M, Severinghaus JW, Basbaum AI: Medullary CO_2 chemoreceptor neurone identification by c-fos immunocytochemistry. FASEB Journal 5:4348, 1991
42. Nolan, WF, Houck PC, Thomas JL, Davies DG: Ventral medullary extracellular fluid pH and blood flow during hypoxia. Am J Physiol 242 (Regulatory Integrative Comp Physiol 11): R159-R198, 1982
43. Kiwull-Schone H, Kiwull P: Hypoxic modulation of central chemosensitivity. In Central Neurone Environment. (Schlafke ME, Koepchen HP, See WR, eds.): Springer-Verlag, Berlin and Heidelberg 1983, pp 88-95
44. Brown DL, Lawson EE: Brain stem extracellular fluid pH and respiratory drive during hypoxia in newborn pigs. J Appl Physiol 64: 1055-59, 1988
45. Neubauer JA, Melton JE, Edelman NH: Modulation of respiration during brain hypoxia. J Appl Physiol 68:441-51, 1990
46. Javaheri S, Teppema LJ: Ventral medullary extracellular fluid pH and PCO_2 during hypoxemia. J Appl Physiol 63(4):1567-71, 1987
47. Xu F, Severinghaus JW, Spellman M, Sato M: Hypoxia uniquely acidifies medullary ventral surface ECF. FASEB Journal 5:4342, 1991
48. Severinghaus JW, Sato M, Powell F, Jensen JB, Sperling B, Lassen NA: Altitude acclimatization slowly augments hypoxic responses of ventilation and cerebral circulation. Clin Res 39:387A, 1991
49. Easton PA, Anthonisen NR: Ventilatory response to sustained hypoxia after pretreatment with aminophylline. J Appl Physiol 64:1445-50, 1988

50. Naifeh KH, Severinghaus JW, Kamiya J, Krafft M: Effect of aging on estimates of hypercapnic ventilatory response during sleep. J Appl Physiol 66:1956-64, 1989

51. Knill RL, Gelb AW: Ventilatory response to hypoxia and hypercapnia during halothane sedation and anesthesia in man. Anesthesiology 49:244-51, 1978

52. Weiskopf RB, Raymond LW, Severinghaus JW: Effects of halothane on canine respiratory response to hypoxia with and without hypercarbia. Anesthesiology 41:350-60, 1974

53. Salvatore AJ, Sullivan SF, Papper EM: Postoperative hypoventilation and hypoxemia in man after hyperventilation. N Engl J Med 280:467-70, 1969

54. Canel J, Ricos M, Vidal F: Early postoperative arterial desaturation. Anesth Analg 69:207-12, 1989

55. Becker LD, Paulson BA, Miller RD, Severinghaus JW, Eger EI: Biphasic respiratory depression after fentanyl-droperidol or fentanyl alone used to supplement nitrous oxide anesthesia. Anesthesiology 44:291-95, 1976

56. Steffey EP, Jarvis KA, Elliott AR, Willits N, Wolliner MJ: Morphine induced hypercapnia in anesthetized swine, monkeys and dogs. Physiologist 32:24.16 (A) 1989

57. Pietak S, Weenig CS, Hickey RF, Fairley HB: Anesthetic effects on ventilation in patients with chronic obstructive pulmonary disease. Anesthesiology 42:160-66, 1975

58. Johansen SH, Osgood P: Ventilatory reserve in the dog during partial curarization. Anesthesiology 33:222, 1970

59. Cohen Y, Chang FM, Litt L, Severinghaus JW, Weinstein PR, Davis RL, James TL: Stability of brain intracellular lactate, and ^{31}P metabolite levels at reduced intracellular pH during prolonged hypercapnia in rats. J Cereb Blood Flow Metab 10:277-84, 1990

LACTIC ACIDOSIS, TYPE A

T. F. Hornbein

INTRODUCTION

Lactic acidosis is a metabolic acidosis caused by accumulation of lactate and hydrogen ion, accompanied by elevated blood lactate concentration. That lactic acidosis which is due to inadequate tissue oxygenation, termed Type A lactic acidosis, is one of the more common causes of metabolic acidosis encountered in our anesthetic practice. Lactic acidosis falls into that category of metabolic acidosis associated with an increased acid content (reflected by an increased anion gap: $Na-(Cl + CO_2)$) rather than a decrease in base (normal anion gap). Lactic acidosis may also result from interference disruption of carbohydrate metabolism, termed Type B lactic acidosis. Lactic acidosis may or may not be associated with acidemia depending upon both the physiological and physiochemical buffering capabilities of the organism. We will focus our attention on Type A Lactic Acidosis as we proceed to review the metabolism (biochemistry and physiology), clinical manifestations, pathophysiology, and therapy [1,2], including recent concerns about the use of sodium bicarbonate.

METABOLISM

The lactate concentration in blood is normally less than 1 mM/L. The lactate existing in cells is in an equilibrium relationship with the pyruvate produced either by glycolysis of glucose or by alanine transamination:

$$\sim 1 \text{ mM} \xrightleftharpoons[]{\text{LDH}} \sim 0.1 \text{ mM}$$
$$\text{Lactate} + \text{NAD} \rightleftharpoons \text{Pyruvate} + \text{NADH} + \text{H}^+$$

T. H. Stanley and R. J. Sperry (eds.), Anesthesia and the Lung 1992, 117–124.
© 1992 *Kluwer Academic Publishers.*

Lactate is a moderately strong acid, possessing a pK of about 3.8. Thus at a pH of 7.1 only about 1/2,000 of the lactate will be lactic acid, a major portion being in the basic form.

By the mass action relationship, therefore

$$[\text{Lactate}] = [\text{Pyruvate}] \cdot K \cdot [\text{NADH}]/[\text{NAD}] \cdot H^+$$

where NAD and NADH are the oxidized and reduced forms of nicotinamide-adenine dinucleotide. Biochemically therefore, lactate concentration may be increased either: (1) secondary to an increase in pyruvate without change in the redox state, e.g., with alkalosis activating the glycolytic enzyme, phosphofructokinase; (2) due to anaerobic metabolism with increased NADH/NAD; or (3) as a consequence of increased H^+ without change in the redox state. In clinical situations any mix of the these three factors may be contributing to the increase in lactate concentration. The change in redox state as a consequence of hypoxia and decrease in energy substrate (ATP) and the increase in hydrogen ion concentration result in lactate concentration increasing disproportionately to the increase in pyruvate concentration.

Lactate may be produced or consumed by all cells, but skeletal muscle, skin, gut, brain and blood normally represent the major producers of about 10 to 20 mM/kg/day in adults. The liver is the major organ clearing lactate from the blood, converting it to bicarbonate as glycogen stores are repleted or as pyruvate is oxidized to CO_2 during aerobic metabolism. Lactic may also be excreted by the kidney. The capacity of this system to handle lactate production in the adult is about 17 mols/day. Lactic acidosis occurs when the rate of lactate acid production exceeds the capacity for its utilization. Increased blood lactate level most commonly reflects diminished utilization as well as increased production.

Table 1 illustrates examples of blood lactate levels observed in a variety of states. Maximum exercise above the anaerobic threshold can yield lactate levels of 10 to 20 mM/L under conditions that might be considered as physiologic but clearly cannot be sustained. In pathologic clinical situations, increasing blood lactate levels have been associated with an increasing mortality. For example, in patients with shock, while a blood lactate concentration between 1.4 and 4.4 mM/L resulted in a mortality of only 2%, between 4.4 and 8.9 mM/L it was 78%, from 8.9 to 13.3 mM/L mortality was 93% and above 13.3 mM/L it was 100%. This mortality is

Table 1. Lactate levels—some examples.

Type		mM/Liter
	Normal Resting	<1.2
A	Exercise	10-22
A	Anemia (severe)	2 (to 5.2)
A	Arterial hypoxemia (P_aO_2 < 35)	4
A	Hyperventilation	2 (8-10?)
A	Shock	35
A	Epinephrine	4
B1	Leukemia	24
B3	Glycogen Storage Disease	14
B1	Diabetes Mellitus	<5 (to 31)
B2	Phenformin	31
B2	Ethanol	8
B2	Fructose	7

not primarily a consequence of the increase in lactate ion *per se* but lactate concentration becomes a monitor of the state of tissue oxygenation and metabolic acid production.

Lactic acidosis can be suspected in the presence of an increased anion gap that is not accounted for by some other cause such as uremia or the presence of ketones. Lactate concentrations can now be measured rapidly using ion-specific electrodes. Respiratory or circulatory failure are the most common causes of Type A lactic acidosis, that due to inadequate tissue oxygenation. Less common are the type B causes, not clearly associated with tissue hypoxia but possibly related to abnormalities of pyruvate metabolism. This category includes the lactatemia of diabetes, liver failure, infection, renal failure, perhaps leukemia, certain hereditary (or idiopathic) forms, and that caused by certain drugs, including salicylates, methanol, ethanol, rapid fructose or sorbitol infusion, biguanides, and most notably (until recently) the oral hypoglycemic agent, phenformin. Although high blood lactate concentrations are associated with a high mortality, with acute lactic acidosis secondary to hypoxia, it is likely that therapy that successfully addresses the underlying cause can result in a successful outcome.

Increased production and decreased utilization can both contribute to the development of lactic acidosis. The balance of the role of these two factors likely varies depending on the nature and the acuity of the derangement causing the lactic acidosis. While the capacity of those organs that utilize lactate to do so seems to far exceed the maximum rate of production under normal circumstances, when the organs primarily responsible for lactate clearance—liver, kidney, muscle, etc.—are themselves not functioning optimally because of lack of oxygen delivery, then all bets are off and the relative roles of production versus utilization in the development of lactic acidosis may change.

CLINICAL MANIFESTATION

So far as is known the consequences of lactic acidosis are similar to those of other forms of metabolic acidosis, suggesting that the perturbation in pH is the primary cause of derangement of oxygen function. In general, a surfeit of H+ causes depression of function (3). The direct effects of H^+ on cardiac muscle, vascular smooth muscle or bronchial smooth muscle exemplify this phenomenon. Myocardial contractility is depressed and cardiac output may be decreased. In the presence of acidosis, blood vessels dilate and become less responsive to vasoconstrictor drugs such as catecholamines. The low voltage pattern of ventricular fibrillations seen on the electrocardiogram and the inability to defibrillate successfully by electrical counter shock until acidosis has been corrected is another, albeit poorly documented, example of the cost of acidosis. Similarly, the bronchodilating actions of drugs such as isoproterenol and aminophylline may be attenuated when H^+ is elevated. Dysrhythmias are more common. These effects are generally not severe at an arterial pH greater than 7.2 but become progressively so as pH falls below that level. Pharmacologic block of sympathetic nervous system responses may enhance the effect of acidosis.

PATHOPHYSIOLOGY OF TYPE A LACTIC ACIDOSIS

Type A lactic acidosis is a consequence of inadequate tissue oxygenation resulting in a state of anaerobiosis that results in increased lactic acid production and a consequent rise in serum lactate concentration, ultimately associated with metabolic acidemia. An inadequate supply of oxygen to feed the mitochondrial electron transport chain is a consequence of a deficit in oxygen supply relative to oxygen demand. Increased oxygen demands are associated, for example, with exercise, seizures, and, in theory at least, uncoupling of oxidative phosphorylation as is thought to occur with malignant hyperthermia. The supply of oxygen is by way of the lungs and cardiovascular system. Limitations in the ability of these two organ systems' function may result in lactic acidosis.

Respiratory failure, either acute or chronic, may mimic inspired hypoxia in causing a decrease in arterial oxygen content; this hypoxemia may or may not be associated with elevation of CO_2 depending on the underlying pulmonary pathology. Cardiovascular failure may range from total ischemia, e.g. cardiac arrest, to partial ischemia, as with the hypotension of hemorrhagic shock or cardiac failure, or excessive vasoconstriction, often pharmacologically induced. In these instances, arterial oxygen content may be normal but its delivery to tissues is insufficient to meet the need. These events may appear globally but often some organs are more affected than others. In contrast to arterial hypoxemia, diminished perfusion will result in inadequate removal of CO_2 as well as delivery of oxygen; tissue respiratory acidosis results, reflected usually by a rise in mixed venous PCO_2. The presence of tissue hypercapnic acidosis, whether of respiratory or circulatory origin (or both) is of theoretical concern in relation to the use of sodium bicarbonate for treatment, as shall be discussed below.

TREATMENT OF LACTIC ACIDOSIS

The primary treatment for Type A lactic acidosis is to improve tissue oxygenation, mainly by improving oxygen delivery. Thus the goal is to treat the primary disorder leading to lactic acidosis, most commonly respiratory or circulatory failure. Depending upon the etiology of the problem, therapeutic approaches may include increasing the F_IO_2, alterations in ventilation, enhancement of oxygen carrying capacity of the blood by transfusion, or increasing blood flow through volume expansion or use of cardiovascular active drugs. Oxygen demand may, under certain circumstances, also be manipulated, such as by temperature control.

Because a surfeit of acidosis can itself impair cardiovascular function and therefore oxygen delivery, when acidemia becomes sufficiently great that this possibility is a concern, then alkali therapy may be indicated (1). Sodium bicarbonate is still the drug of choice. The efficacy of sodium lactate is dependent upon its metabolism to bicarbonate by a functioning liver. THAM (trishydroxmethylaminomethane) has the theoretical advantage of not adding a sodium load and of lowering rather than raising the PCO_2 as compared to sodium bicarbonate, but has not been shown to have greater efficacy in the treatment of acidosis. Recently proposed is a mixture of 0.3 M sodium bicarbonate and 0.3 M sodium carbonate; this mixture has been shown not to raise the PCO_2 when used to treat metabolic acidosis. It's theoretical advantage over sodium bicarbonate alone has yet to be clearly documented.

Recently the value of bicarbonate therapy for treatment of lactic acidosis, including resuscitation from cardiac arrest, has been questioned based on the observation that its administration can result in hypernatremia, hyperosmolarity, and hypercapnia (4,5,6). The osmolarity and sodium concentration of the usual clinical preparation of sodium bicarbonate (50 mEq/50 mL) are both approximately six times the normal values in plasma. When sodium bicarbonate reacts with acid, carbon dioxide is produced, which, if not excreted, may result in elevation of carbon dioxide tension, mitigating the alkalinizing effect of the sodium bicarbonate. Because the bicarbonate ion crosses the blood brain barrier and cell membranes slowly, brain and intracellular pH may fall even while blood pH is increased, resulting in a further decrement of function. Bicarbonate administration may be particularly a problem in situations where CO_2 excretion is compromised, as for example in the presence of cardiac arrest or severe airway obstruction. As a result of these several concerns, the advocacy of bicarbonate for treatment of cardiac arrest and the advanced cardiac life support guidelines for its use have been modified to encourage greater restraint in bicarbonate administration (7). Among the factors leading to this recommendation for a more conservative use of sodium bicarbonate in the treatment of cardiac arrest is the finding that in-hospital arrests are frequently associated with minimal metabolic acidosis because resuscitation efforts are begun quickly. Also the efficacy of sodium bicarbonate treatment has been questioned based upon several studies in animals suggesting that sodium bicarbonate treatment might at times make the situation worse. Indeed, some of the studies demonstrating efficacy for sodium bicarbonate in the treatment of metabolic acidosis have suggested that the major benefit may accrue from the volume expanding effect of hyperosmolar sodium bicarbonate rather than from correction of the acid base derangement itself.

In reviewing this literature, I have come to several conclusions regarding sodium bicarbonate therapy, all of which may require modification as more information becomes available:

1. Metabolic acidosis can have detrimental effects on cardiovascular and other organ function. Titrated alkali therapy may be beneficial.

2. Sodium bicarbonate should be administered slowly and carefully, especially in the absence of confirmed documentation of metabolic acidosis and physiologic responses that might be attributable to the acidosis itself. Sodium bicarbonate administration can result in a rise in PCO_2, especially if the drug is administered rapidly or if CO_2 elimination is compromised. The possibly greater efficacy and non-CO_2 generating buffers such as THAM and the carbonate-bicarbonate mixture, have not yet been documented.

3. Continued sodium bicarbonate therapy should be titrated based upon repeated measurements of blood acid-base status and plasma sodium concentration and osmolarity.

4. Cardiac arrest of brief duration may not be associated with significant metabolic acidosis and may therefore not require sodium bicarbonate administration.

GENERAL REFERENCES

1. Hornbein TF: Acid-base balance. In Anesthesia, Miller R (ed.). Vol. 2, 2nd edition. Churchill Livingstone, 1986, pp. 1289-1312.
2. Kreisberg RA: Pathogenesis and management of lactic acidosis. Annu Rev Med 35:181-93, 1984
3. Pavlin EG, Hornbein TF: Organ and tissue disturbances produced by acid-base abnormalities. In Extrapulmonary Manifestations of

Respiratory Disease, Robin E (ed). Marcel Dekker, New York, 1978, pp 363

4. Hindman BJ: Sodium bicarbonate in the treatment of subtypes of acute lactic acidosis: Physiologic considerations. Anesthesiology 72:1064-76, 1990

5. Narins RG, Cohen JJ: Bicarbonate therapy for organic acidosis: The case for its continued use (editorial). Ann Intern Med 106:615-8, 1987

6. Stacpoole PW: Lactic acidosis: The case against bicarbonate therapy (editorial). Ann Intern Med 105:276-78, 1986

7. Standards and guidelines for cardiopulmonary resuscitation (CPR) and emergency cardiac care (ECC). JAMA 255:2942, 1986.

RIB CAGE CONTRIBUTION TO VENTILATION DURING ANESTHESIA

A. B. Lumb and J. F. Nunn

The effects of general anesthesia on the respiratory muscles have interested anesthetists for 130 years, and are still not clearly understood. John Snow was the first to report changes in ribcage (RC) and abdominal (AB) motion during anesthesia. In his comprehensive description of chloroform anesthesia published in 1858 (1) he described reduced movement of the RC in most patients, and regarded this as a sign that "a little more chloroform had been inhaled than was necessary." In a more recent study (1925) (2), Miller described five types of respiration during ether anesthesia, varying from predominantly RC motion to predominantly AB motion. He described RC motion as decreasing progressively with deepening anesthesia, and reported that at division 2 of Guedel's stage 2 anesthesia, respiration was mainly by the diaphragm in most patients. Interestingly, he found no such changes with nitrous oxide-air anesthesia.

MEASUREMENT OF RIBCAGE CONTRIBUTION

Techniques

There are several methods available, many of which have been used during anesthesia:

1. *Observation* of thoracic and abdominal motion was used with excellent results by the anesthetists in the preceding paragraph. However, this does not enable quantification of the contributions of different compartments, and is difficult at the small tidal volumes and rapid respiratory rates seen during anesthesia with newer agents.

2. *Electromyography* (EMG) is an attractive technique as this measures actual muscular activity, whilst most other methods record movement of

T. H. Stanley and R. J. Sperry (eds.), Anesthesia and the Lung 1992, 125–133.
© 1992 Kluwer Academic Publishers.

the body surface. RC and AB motion do not necessarily reflect intercostal/diaphragmatic muscle activity respectively, as movement of the body surface will be the result of activity in several, possibly opposing muscle groups. For instance, in the upright position, the lower part of the thoracic cage is expanded not only by intercostal activity, but also by the diaphragm contracting and using the abdominal contents as a fulcrum on which to elevate the lower ribs. However, electromyography of respiratory muscles is technically difficult. With the exception of sternomastoid, the respiratory muscles are inaccessible, and lie very close to other, often antagonistic muscles, e.g., the external and internal intercostals, or the crural diaphragm and erector spinae muscles. Nevertheless, EMGs of the parasternal intercostal muscles have been recorded during anesthesia, and were reported to be completely abolished by halothane (3). Diaphragmatic EMG has been recorded in two ways. Firstly, intra-esophageal electrodes have been positioned behind the crura of the diaphragm, and secondly, surface electrodes have been placed over the costal margin with posterior intercostal nerve blocks to abolish the overlying intercostal muscle signal. The latter technique has been used to demonstrate tonic activity in the diaphragm when awake, and in one subject this was seen to be reduced by halothane anesthesia (4).

3. *Magnetometers* have been used to measure anteroposterior, transverse, and cephalo-caudad dimensions of the chest and abdomen. If all three dimensions are recorded simultaneously, an accurate assessment of ventilation can be obtained (5), but this is a cumbersome set-up which has not been used during anesthesia. Single pairs of magnetometers, sited anteroposteriorly have been used many times during anesthesia (see below), but changes in the shape of body compartments on induction of anesthesia may invalidate this technique.

4. *Circumferential Strain Gauges* have been used during anesthesia, and by measuring circumferences partly overcome the error caused by changes in body cavity shape (6).

5. *Respiratory Inductive Plethysmography* (RIP) measures the cross-sectional area of the body, and has been shown to give accurate readings regardless of changes of shape in the physiological range (7). An example of RIP recordings is shown in Figure 1. This technique has been used for many studies during anesthesia, and is discussed further below.

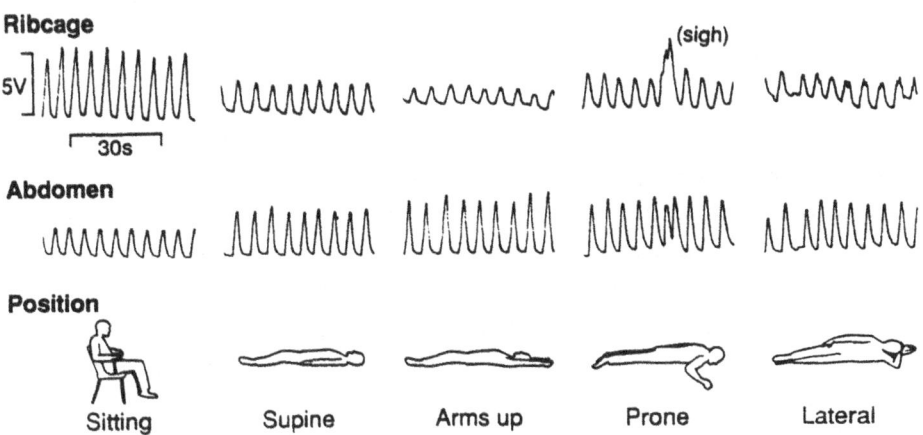

Figure 1. RIP recordings from a normal awake subject in five different postures. Note that the spontaneous sigh is entirely RC in origin. Reproduced from reference 10 with permission of the editor of Anesthesia and Analgesia.

6. *Computerized Tomographic Scans* (CT) may be used to obtain cross sectional views of the chest and abdomen. In its simplest form, several "slices" are recorded at fixed points, cross sectional areas calculated, and these related to respiratory volumes (8) to calculate the RC contribution. The Dynamic Spatial Reconstructor is a more complex CT system which can perform multiple scans simultaneously to produce a 3-dimensional computer reconstruction of the chest, from which volume changes resulting from chest wall or diaphragm movements can be calculated (9).

Both these techniques require the subjects to hold their breath for at least 4 seconds, which may therefore alter normal respiratory muscle activity, and prevents their use in spontaneously breathing anesthetized subjects. Also, CT scanning requires the subjects' arms to be above their heads, a maneuver which we have found to increase functional residual capacity by 250 ml, but not to alter RC contribution to ventilation (10).

7. *Optical Method.* The most recent application of this involves a low energy laser beam scanning the body surface, with a video camera recording the shape of the resulting lines (11). Computer analysis of the shape of the line can reconstruct a 3-dimensional image of the body compartments, and hence with appropriate calibration derive volume changes. This technique will, therefore, take some complex changes in body shape into

account, but cannot view the sides or posterior aspects of the body. It has not yet been applied to subjects during anesthesia.

Calibration During Anesthesia

For partitioning of ventilation into RC and AB compartments from body surface measurements, the isovolume maneuver remains the simplest calibration method. However, this does involve the subject performing a voluntary respiratory maneuver, and assumes that Konno and Mead's (12) description of the respiratory system behaving with only two degrees of freedom is true. The latter may not be true during anesthesia, when for instance spinal movement may occur causing flexion or extension of the chest or abdomen, and a voluntary maneuver clearly cannot be performed by the patient. Various ways round this problem have been used. Firstly, an isovolume maneuver has been imitated by obstructing the endotracheal tube during anesthesia (3,13), but this results in distortion of the body compartments, and compression/expansion of the gas within the lung, invalidating Konno and Mead's assumptions (12). Secondly, the system may be calibrated with the subject awake, and care then taken not to change the position of the subject during induction and maintenance of anesthesia (14, 15), but minor changes in body compartment shape may still occur. Finally, computerized techniques of calibration are now available which can calibrate the RIP during normal breathing, by using the normal variation in RC contribution which occurs between different breaths of the same tidal volume (16). This has not yet been used during anesthesia.

EFFECT OF POSTURE

RC contribution to ventilation is most easily expressed as the percentage RC, i.e., the contribution of the RC as a proportion of the total breath size. There is a large variation in the %RC between subjects both when awake and anesthetized (Fig. 2), with mean values awake of 70% sitting, and 30% when supine. Interestingly, when awake, the %RC in other horizontal postures used during anesthesia (e.g., lateral/prone) do not differ significantly from supine (Fig. 1) (10).

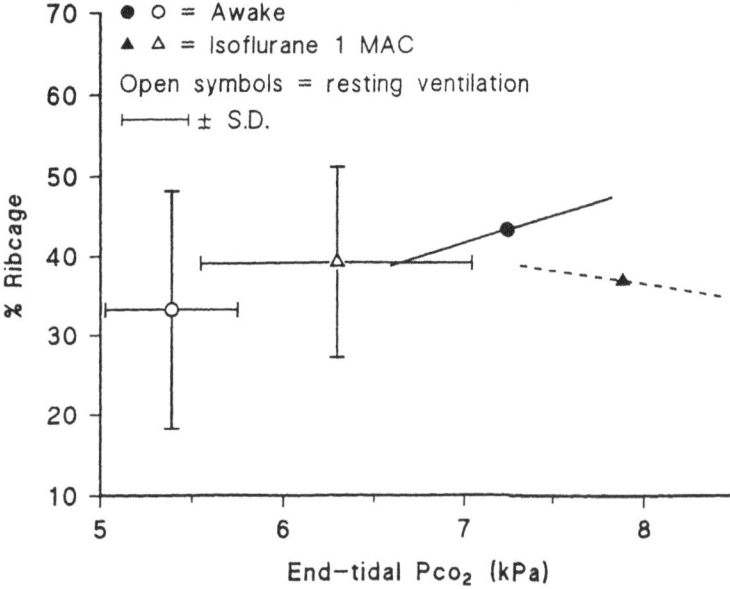

Figure 2. Mean RC contribution to resting and CO_2 stimulated ventilation in 15 subjects, both awake and during anesthesia. Reproduced form reference 14 with permission of the editor of the British Journal of Anaesthesia.

EFFECT OF ANESTHESIA ON RIBCAGE CONTRIBUTION

Effects on Respiratory Pattern

The magnitude of tidal volume (V_T) has been shown to affect the RC contribution to ventilation, voluntary increases in V_T in normal awake subjects causing an increased contribution of the RC to each breath (17). However, voluntary reductions in V_T have not been studied, and reduced V_T *per se* may be a factor in changes caused by anesthetic agents (see below). A further complication in studies of RC contribution during anesthesia is the onset of abnormal phase relationships between the RC and AB. A difference in phase between AB and RC contribution during early inspiration commonly occurs during the high minute ventilations seen with CO_2 rebreathing (18). Similar respiratory patterns during anesthesia with unstimulated breathing were originally described by Miller in

1925 (2), and have been reported since in some patients (14). Phase differences during anesthesia occur in all patients if the airway is obstructed (19), so these observations may simply reflect undetected mild degrees of airway obstruction.

Effects of Different Anesthetic Agents

1. *Paralysis and IPPV* increase the RC motion during ventilation regardless of the type of agent used (depolarizing or non-depolarizing), or the anesthetic drugs given (6,13,20).

2. *Opiates.* Morphine reduces the RC contribution to ventilation during both quiet breathing and CO_2 rebreathing, despite little change in V_T (21). However, meperidine, given in conjunction with benzodiazepines, caused an increase in the %RC, this observation being completely reversed with naloxone (22). There is, therefore, no clear picture of the effects of opiates on compartmental ventilation, but from the study with meperidine it would appear that opiate receptors can affect the %RC.

3. *Benzodiazepines.* Midazolam (0.1 mg/kg) given intravenously to volunteers resulted in %RC increasing from 33% to 46%, with a mean reduction in V_T of 39% (23). Moderate doses of intravenous midazolam (0.05 mg/kg) or diazepam (0.15 mg/kg) caused a large increase in %RC from 30% to 45%, with a substantial reduction in mean V_T from 500 to 360 ml. There was little further change with a repeated dose of either drug, and the change was unaffected by naloxone (22). The findings of these two studies are in close agreement, indicating a rapid and non-dose dependent *increase* in %RC in spite of a substantial reduction in V_T. This is in contrast to the physiological studies above in which increasing V_T also increased %RC.

4. *Intravenous Anesthetics.* Ketamine anesthesia, using a bolus followed by infusion, resulted in an *increase* in %RC from 34% to 59%, with an increase in V_T from 300 to 400 ml (24). A similar regimen using methohexitone found no change in %RC, presumably with reduced V_T though these data are not provided (15). In 12 subjects, we found a large change in mean %RC immediately following a bolus of 2.5 mg/kg of propofol, the %RC increasing from 32% awake to 46% when spontaneous ventilation returned after induction (unpublished observations).

5. *Inhalational Anesthesia.* Early studies described selective reduction of RC motion with deeper planes of anesthesia, whilst no such effect was seen with nitrous oxide, presumably because of its inability to produce deep anesthesia (1,2). Halothane has been studied twice, using different techniques for assessment of RC motion. The first study used 1.4 MAC of halothane in oxygen and reported a reduction in %RC from 43% awake to 19% asleep (3). The second study used between 1.3 and 3.3 MAC (Halothane plus N_2O) resulting in %RC decreasing from 15% awake to between 5-8% anesthetized, with some evidence of progressive decreases in %RC with deepening anesthesia (6). Isoflurane given at between 0.5 and 1.5 MAC caused non-significant but progressive reductions in %RC in a small study of 7 patients (19). However, one MAC of isoflurane in air/oxygen in a larger study of unpremedicated patients resulted in no change of RC contribution to non-stimulated ventilation (14).

CO_2 STIMULATION

The RC contribution increases with end-tidal CO_2 at an average rate of 1% per mmHg CO_2, regardless of the method of CO_2 stimulation used (rebreathing or steady state), and this increase is greatest in subjects with a large increase in VT with CO_2 (25). During anesthesia, halothane (1.4 MAC) and isoflurane (1 MAC) both cause total abolition of this *proportional* increase in RC contribution during CO_2 rebreathing, but both compartments continue to contribute to the *absolute* increase in ventilation (14,3) (Fig. 2).

CONCLUSIONS

Partitioning of ventilation into RC and AB compartments during anesthesia is difficult, mainly because of problems with calibrating the equipment currently available, though more elegant systems are now being investigated. The relationship between different respiratory muscle groups is complex, and body surface measurements of the RC and AB do not necessarily reflect activity of the intercostal muscles and diaphragm, but EMG studies of these muscles are also technically difficult. It appears that regardless of their effects on the magnitude of V_T, benzodiazepines and intravenous anesthetic agents increase the RC contribution to breathing. Inhalational agents tend to depress RC motion, particularly at large tidal volumes such as during CO_2 stimulated hyperpnea. During non-stimulated breathing, RC motion is depressed in a dose-dependent manner such that at levels of anesthesia of 1 MAC or less the effect is undetectable and so of little relevance clinically. It is both interesting and inexplicable that intravenous and inhalational anesthetic agents, which have similar effects on most body systems, should have such opposing actions on the different respiratory muscle groups. Perhaps John Snow was correct in 1858 when he regarded loss of RC motion as indicative of unnecessarily deep anesthesia.

REFERENCES

1. Snow J: On chloroform and other anaesthetics. Churchill, London, 1858
2. Miller AH: Ascending respiratory paralysis under general anesthesia. J Amer Med Assoc 84(3):201, 1925
3. Tusiewicz K, Bryan AC, Froese AB: Contributions of changing rib cage diaphragm interactions to the ventilatory depression of halothane anesthesia. Anesthesiology 47:327, 1977
4. Muller N, Volgyesi G, Becker L, Bryan MH, Bryan AC: J Appl Physiol 47(2):279, 1979
5. McCool FD, Kelly KB, Loring SH, Greaves IA, Mead J: Estimates of ventilation from body surface measurements in unrestrained subjects. J Appl Physiol 61(3):1114-9, 1986
6. Jones JG, Faithfull D, Jordan C, Minty B: Rib cage movement during halothane anaesthesia in man. Br J Anaesth 51:399, 1979
7. Watson HL, Poole DA, Sackner MA: Accuracy of respiratory inductive plethysmographic cross-sectional areas. J Appl Physiol 65(1):306-8, 1988
8. Hedenstierna G, Strandberg A, Brismar B, Lundquist H, Svensson L, Tokics L: Functional residual capacity, thoracoabdominal dimensions, and central blood volume during general anesthesia with muscle paralysis and mechanical ventilation. Anesthesiology 62:247-54, 1985
9. Krayer S, Rehder K, Beck KC, Cameron PD, Didier EP, Hoffman EA: Quantification of thoracic volumes by three-dimensional imaging. J Appl Physiol 62(2):591, 1987
10. Lumb AB, Nunn JF: Respiratory function and ribcage contribution to ventilation in body positions commonly used during anesthesia. Anesth Analg (in press)

11. Drummond GB, McGowan S, Duffy ND: A rapid method to assess chest wall shape and volume change. Br J Anaesth 67:204P, 1991

12. Konno K, Mead J: Measurement of the separate volume change of rib cage and abdomen during breathing. J Appl Physiol 22(3):407, 1967

13. Vellody VPS, Nassery M, Balasaraswathi K, Goldberg NB, Sharp JT: Compliances of human rib cage and diaphragms abdomen pathways in relaxed versus paralyzed state. Am Rev Resp Dis 118:479, 1978

14. Lumb AB, Petros AJ, Nunn JF: Ribcage contribution to resting and carbon dioxide stimulated ventilation during 1 MAC isoflurane anaesthesia. Br J Anaesth (in press)

15. Bickler PE, Dueck R, Prutow RJ: Effects of barbiturate anesthesia on functional residual capacity and ribcage/diaphragm contributions to ventilation. Anesthesiology 66:147, 1987

16. Sackner MA, Watson H, Belsito AS, Feinerman D, Suarez M, Gonzalez G, Bizousky F, Krieger B: Calibration of respiratory inductive plethysmograph during natural breathing. J Appl Physiol 66(1):410, 1989

17. Sharp JT, Goldberg NB, Druz WS, Danon J: Relative contributions of rib cage and abdomen to breathing in normal subjects. J Appl Physiol 39(4):608, 1975

18. Pengelly LD, Tarshis AM, Rebuck AS: Contribution of rib cage and abdomen diaphragm to tidal volume during C_2 rebreathing. J Appl Physiol 46(4):709, 1979

19. Cantineau JP, Mankikian B, Poete P, Sartene R, Clergue F, Viars P: Ventilatory patterns and chest wall mechanics during isoflurane anesthesia. Anesthesiology 63: A551, 1985

20. Hedenstierna G, Lofstrom B, Lundh R: Thoracic gas volume and chest-abdomen dimensions during anesthesia and muscle paralysis. Anesthesiology 55:499, 1981

21. Rigg JRA, Rondi P: Change in rib cage and diaphragm contribution to ventilation after morphine. Anesthesiology 55:507, 1981

22. Berggren L, Eriksson I, Mollenholt P: Changes in breathing pattern and chest wall mechanics after benzodiazepines in combination with meperidine. Acta Anaesth Scand 31:381-6, 1987

23. Morel DR, Forster A, Bachmann M, Suter PM: Effect of intravenous midazolam on breathing pattern and chest wall mechanics in humans. J Appl Physiol 57(4):1104, 1984

24. Mankikian B, Cantineau JP, Sartene R, Clergue F, Viars P: Ventilatory pattern and chest wall mechanics during ketamine anesthesia in humans. Anesthesiology 65:492, 1986

25. Lumb AB, Nunn JF: Ribcage contribution to CO_2 response during rebreathing and steady state methods. Resp Physiol 85:97-110, 1991

OXYGEN — THE BREATH OF LIFE

J. F. Nunn

Surely the most important responsibility of an anesthetist is to ensure that oxygen continues to reach the vital organs of his patients. Without oxygen these organs can neither function nor survive. So deeply is this engrained that we tend to make two assumptions. Firstly, it is all too easy to accept oxygen as a natural if not inevitable constituent of our atmosphere. Secondly, oxygen is often considered to be universally beneficial to living creatures under all circumstances. Neither assumption could be farther from the truth.

In fact, the earth is the only body in solar system—planet or satellite —to have oxygen in its atmosphere. It is there by a complex chain of circumstances in which physical, chemical and biological influences have all played a part. It is likely that further changes will occur in the future and human intervention may well be a major factor. Although oxygen is essential for the function and survival of all but the simplest animals, it is in fact a highly toxic gas. Coexistence of an organism with oxygen depends on elaborate defence mechanisms which have evolved over some thousands of millions of years.

THE ORIGIN OF THE ATMOSPHERE

It is believed that the earth was formed by the gravitational accretion of cold material 4600 million years ago, when the solar system was formed. However, the earth was rapidly heated by three mechanisms —the kinetic energy of the accreting masses, radioactive decay and solar radiation. This resulted in vaporization of immense quantities of water and there was also thermal and radioactive decomposition of various

135

T. H. Stanley and R. J. Sperry (eds.), Anesthesia and the Lung 1992, 135–139.
© 1992 Kluwer Academic Publishers.

constitutes of the earth, with outgassing to the surface by volcanoes and fumaroles. This phenomenon is widespread in the solar system, and active volcanoes have been observed on Mars and Io, a satellite of Jupiter. In the case of the earth, evidence from Hawaiian volcanoes suggests that the outgassing consisted mainly of water vapor with carbon dioxide, nitrogen, oxides of sulfur, argon and hydrogen, but no oxygen.

Important physico-chemical changes then occurred in the primitive atmosphere. Helium and hydrogen tended to be lost from the earth's gravitational field, while heavier gases were retained. Some carbon dioxide was reduced by hydrogen to methane, but very large quantities reacted with surface silicates and became trapped as carbonates while forming silica. Carbon dioxide has probably remained in the atmosphere throughout the life of the earth, and it now forms more than 90 per cent of the atmospheres of Venus and Mars. The atmosphere probably remained without oxygen for at least the first thousand million years of the life of the earth.

The surface of the earth cooled rapidly by radiation. Solidification of the crust of the earth probably occurred only 600 million years after the formation of the earth. Not long afterwards, most of the water vapor condensed to form the oceans. Clouds resulted in recirculation of water, producing rivers, freshwater lakes and lagoons. This produced an environment compatible with the evolution of life, an event of immense complexity about which only speculation is possible.

It is established that a wide range of organic compounds can be formed without the intervention of life. Certain meteorites (carbonaceous chondrites) contain organic compounds, including amino acids, which can no longer be considered the exclusive product of living organisms. These compounds could have been formed under the conditions which prevailed on the earth some 3500-4000 million years ago. Encapsulation of organic compounds within lipid membranes can easily be achieved in the laboratory, and it is now possible to envisage the formation of lifeless "protocells" as probable, if not inevitable.

The next stage in the evolution of life is less easy to understand and has not been tested in the laboratory. However, time, space, and variety of environment were all available in abundance, and it has been postulated that random sequencing of ribonucleic acid (RNA) eventually produced by chance a template for the formation of a "useful" protein which conferred some biochemical advantage on a particular "protocell." This enabled it to compete effectively with its neighbors, as well as to replicate the RNA. It is conceivable that this process progressed, with a steadily increasing repertoire of useful proteins being encoded by self replicating RNA, until transmission of the genetic code was eventually taken over by deoxyribonucleic acid (DNA) in organisms with the greatest potential. The problem has always been to understand how useful proteins could be formed without the appropriate sequences in RNA or DNA, and how RNA and DNA could be polymerized without the appropriate enzymes. Nevertheless, life undoubtedly did evolve, and the earliest geological evidence of life is the appearance of stromatolites (microbial deposits), dated to 3400-3500 million years ago.

There was only limited potential for the anaerobic life which is presumed to have evolved in the soup of abiogenically preformed organic compounds. The original input of energy into the ecosystem was the conversion of inorganic into organic compounds under the influence of solar ultra-violet radiation and electrical discharge (e.g. from lightening). It is likely that the explosion of living organisms eventually outstripped their energetic basis, and a new energy source was needed. It appears that a radical change occurred approximately 3000-3500 million years ago, when there was the first evidence of the utilization of visible light as an energy source for photosynthesis, with production of oxygen as a byproduct.

The evidence for this early production of oxygen is strong and can be approximately dated. There are numerous reports of stromatolites dated 2700-3500 million years ago, and some are likely to be deposited from algae or cyanobacteria capable of photosynthesis. The earliest true fossils of algae are in the gun flint cherts on the north shore of Lake Superior, and are dated to 1900 million years ago. In the earliest rock, iron was deposited in reduced form, such as the banded iron deposits dated 3800 million years ago. During the last 2600 million years, iron has been deposited in ferric form, as in the "red beds," and this is taken to indicate an oxidizing environment.

It seems likely that appreciable quantities of oxygen began to accumulate in the atmosphere about 2200 million years ago. It is impossible to say how quickly its concentration increased, but it is generally assumed to have risen steeply just before the beginning of the overt fossil record in the Cambrian period (570 million years ago). There may well have been a further rise in the Devonian period when ultra-violet screening by oxygen and ozone first permitted the land to be colonized. Carbon deposits from forest fires suggest that the atmospheric oxygen concentration cannot have changed very much since the beginning of the Carboniferous period (345 million years ago).

THE IMPACT OF AN OXIDIZING ATMOSPHERE

The appearance of molecular oxygen in the environment would not have been welcomed by the anaerobic organisms. Oxygen is an extremely toxic gas capable of partial reduction to a wide range of highly reactive free radicals and related species. Primitive anaerobes were unlikely to have had defenses and three lines of response can be identified. Firstly, some anaerobes sought an anaerobic micro-environment, in which to remain and survive. Secondly, the vast majority of organisms developed biochemical defences in depth against oxygen and its derived free radicals, and such defences are now currently found in all living organisms except obligatory anaerobes. The third response was the adoption of aerobic metabolism, which gave them enormous energetic advantages over organisms relying on a aerobic metabolism. The increased availability of biological energy was essential for the evolution and survival of all forms of life more complex than primitive micro-organisms. Photosynthesis and aerobic metabolism established a cycle of energy exchange between plants and animals, with an ultimate energy input in the form of solar visible light which can be interrupted only under exceptional circumstances.

A sufficiently high concentration of oxygen will kill any living organism, mainly by attacking DNA, lipids and sulph-hydryl containing proteins. It also enhances damage caused by ionizing radiation and poisons such as paraquat. However, the toxicity of oxygen and its derived free radicals is not an unmitigated evil. Certain free radicals and related compounds such as hypochlorous acid (household bleach) are utilized within the body for bacterial killing by polymorphs and macrophages.

Congenital lack of the enzymes required for their production results in greatly weakened resistance to bacterial attack.

Oxygen has had a profound effect on evolution by ultra-violet screening. Oxygen itself absorbs ultra-violet radiation to a certain extent, but ozone (O_3) is far more effective. It is formed from oxygen in the stratosphere where it undergoes photodissociation. Life first evolved in water which provided adequate screening from ultra-violet radiation. Colonization of dry land by plants and animals, in the Devonian period (345-395 million years ago), must have depended on ozone having reached a level at which the degree of ultra-violet shielding permitted organisms to leave the shelter of an aqueous environment.

Oxygen is thus seen as both friend and foe. On the credit side oxygen confers the energetic advantages necessary for evolution beyond the stage of the simplest organisms. It also provides the body with powerful defence mechanisms against bacterial attack. Thirdly, it provides the ultra-violet screening necessary for terrestrial existence. On the debit side it has powerful toxic potential which will kill any organism without the defence mechanisms which have evolved in depth for the protection of all aerobic organisms.

MANAGEMENT OF THE PATIENT WITH REACTIVE AIRWAY DISEASE

S. J. Allen

Asthma is a condition that affects 10% of the population and thus, patients at risk for perioperative bronchospasm present frequently for anesthesia care. Although most events are mild, the occasional life-threatening episode presents a major challenge for the anesthesiologist. The impact of asthma on perianesthetic morbidity is unclear. Converse and Smotrilla noted that intraoperative deaths were more likely to occur in asthmatics as non asthmatics. Gold and Helrich found no deaths but a higher incidence of respiratory complications. Contemporary optimal management of asthma requires knowledge of 1) the pathophysiology, 2) the effect of various anesthetic agents and maneuvers, as well as 3) the various bronchodilator drugs.

PATHOPHYSIOLOGY OF ASTHMA

Perhaps the biggest change in our understanding of asthma is the realization that it is an inflammatory response quite similar to other inflammatory processes. In other words, asthma is more than just bronchospasm.

Triggers

Studies in recent years have markedly expanded our understanding of what factors may trigger bronchospasm. These factors not only include antigens (extrinsic asthma) but a number of "nonspecific" agents that do not trigger through immunologic mechanisms. This latter class of bronchospasm triggers (intrinsic asthma) includes aerosols of distilled or

141

T. H. Stanley and R. J. Sperry (eds.), Anesthesia and the Lung 1992, 141–155.
© 1992 Kluwer Academic Publishers.

hypertonic water, sulfur dioxide, ammonia, aspirin (and other non-steroidal anti inflammatory agents), sulfites, beta blockers, exercise, emotional disturbance, as well as others. The ability of triggers to stimulate bronchospasm depends on the state of reactivity of the airways. By definition, asthmatics have abnormal bronchial reactivity which may increase over time due to illness or other factors.

Cells and Mediators

The cells involved in producing triggers are eosinophils and mast cells. At some point in the past, the patient became sensitized to some antigen and now produces IgE. The IgE attaches to the surface of a mast cell. At the start of an asthma attack, the antigen attaches to the IgE and the mast cell releases its preformed mediators (degranulation) and starts making additional mediators. The effects of mast cell derived mediators are immediate and myriad. They include increased vascular permeability, smooth muscle contraction, mucus secretion, and leukocyte chemoattraction. Over time, further changes occur including mucosal edema and cellular infiltration, desquamation of epithelial cells, thickening of basement membrane, and hyperplasia of goblet cells. These latter events may be due to mast cell contents or cells attracted to the site. Mast cells may also degranulate in response to other stimuli besides immunologic agents. Hypoxia, opiates, certain drugs and neuropeptides and changes in local osmolarity can cause mast cell degranulation in vitro. The presence of bronchospasm also appears to increase the bronchial reactivity further, thus making another attack more likely. Eosinophils also play a role in stimulating mast cell degranulation and producing asthma mediators.

Asthmatic patients who are bronchoscoped following antigenic challenge show extensive *mucosal edema*. Airway mucosal edema is due to the increased vascular permeability. Histamine, prostaglandin, leukotriene C4, LTD4, platelet activating factor, and bradykinin can induce mucosal edema. However, the contribution of mucosal edema to bronchospasm is not clear. The airway mucosa often contains infiltrates of eosinophils, neutrophils, macrophages, lymphocytes, and plasma cells. In the lumen itself, the secretions may contain eosinophils, neutrophils, and desquamated epithelial cells. Numerous mediators of allergy and inflammation could play a role in these infiltrates. Again, the clinical significance of these infiltrates is not clear.

Increase in *mucus secretion* plays a major role in the clinical picture of asthma. Allergic mediators increase mucus and stimulate active fluid secretion by the surface epithelium. However, airway mucus transport rates are lower in asthmatics. In severe asthma attacks, the airway epithelial surface may become denuded with replacement by goblet cells. The mechanism for the sloughing of epithelial cells is not known.

CLINICAL PRESENTATION

Airway narrowing causes most of the clinical manifestations in asthmatic attacks. Airway narrowing in asthmatics probably involves all of the tracheobronchial tree. In the early response to antigen, airway narrowing is due to bronchial smooth muscle constriction and is generally promptly reversible with beta adrenergic drugs. However, in the late antigen response, mucus and mucosal edema contribute to airway narrowing and bronchodilators have less of an effect. In fact, the mucus retention leads to the characteristic obstruction of smaller airways seen in severe asthma.

Pulmonary Mechanics

The airway narrowing results in relative obstruction of airflow through the tracheobronchial tree. Patients may have marked bronchospasm and still be asymptomatic. However, any worsening of the airway narrowing may result in critical deterioration. The obstruction to airflow imposed by airway narrowing results in air trapping. Thus, during an acute attack, both residual volume (RV) and functional residual capacity (FRC) are increased. In most instances these abnormalities return to normal after the attack subsides, but may persist long after the airway narrowing has resolved in some patients. Total lung capacity (TLC) probably does not change significantly during attacks. Similarly, elastic recoil is relatively unaffected in asthma.

Alterations in Pulmonary Circulation

The degree of bronchospasm varies throughout an affected patient's airway. This results in uneven distribution of ventilation. Hypoxic pulmonary vasoconstriction (HPV) develops in lung units where ventilation is inadequate and results in redistribution of pulmonary blood flow to lung units where ventilation is better. Due to HPV, pulmonary hypertension may develop during severe asthma and may be evident on EKG by a reversible "p pulmonale" pattern.

Alterations in Gas Exchange

The uneven ventilation distribution may lead to mild hypoxemia which is a common finding in severe asthmatic attacks. A recent study of $\dot{V}/\dot{Q}$ distribution in severe asthma found a broad spectrum of $\dot{V}/\dot{Q}$ ratios <1.0 but almost no shunt and surprisingly little dead space. When the patients were allowed to breathe F_IO_2 1.0 for 30 minutes, significant increases in shunt were found. Bronchodilators such as isoproterenol may worsen hypoxemia by affecting pulmonary blood flow distribution. Indeed, investigators have documented worsening P_aO_2 following beta adrenergic treatment even as bronchospasm improved. The tachypnea associated with asthma often results in hypocapnia and respiratory alkalosis. The development of normocapnia or hypercapnia is an ominous sign of respiratory collapse and requires intervention.

Cardiovascular Effects

The cardiovascular effects of asthma are not trivial. The more negative pleural pressure required for ventilation results in enhancement of the central blood volume. Pulmonary vascular resistance may be increased by 1) HPV (see above), 2) hyperinflation of the lung, and 3) acidosis. Thus, right ventricular function may be compromised by volume and pressure sufficiently to decrease cardiac output. Similarly, the more negative pleural pressure results in a relatively greater afterload for the left ventricle. These may be possible mechanisms for the exaggerated decrease in blood pressure during inspiration (pulsus paradoxus) that is often seen in severe asthma.

PHARMACOLOGY OF BRONCHODILATORS

Beta agonists are currently the drugs of choice in the treatment of asthma. Bronchial smooth muscle possess beta-2 receptors which, when stimulated, produce bronchodilatation. Newer agents are more selective of beta-2 sites and have a longer duration of action than the older drugs used for asthma. The agents may be given by inhalation, IV, orally, or IM. Inhalation appears to be the best route of administration for producing rapid onset and few systemic side effects. Inhalation may be accomplished by a metered-dose inhaler or by aerosolization with compressed gas. *Epinephrine* and *isoetharine* are available for inhalation and subcutaneous (epinephrine only) administration. They are much shorter acting than the newer beta-2 selective agents and are associated with more adverse side effects. *Isoproterenol (Isuprel)* is also a nonspecific beta agonist and is available for inhalation. It may be used intravenously in children. However, the associated tachycardia and ventricular ectopy limit IV isoproterenol in adults. Albuterol (Proventil, Ventolin) is beta-2 selective and may be administered orally or inhalationally. *Terbutaline (Brethine)* is a selective beta-2 and is available for inhalation, oral, and subcutaneous administration. *Bitolterol (Tornalate)* is the latest selective beta-2 agent and is available for inhalation. *Metaproterenol (Alupent)* is not as selective a beta-2 drug as terbutaline, resulting in more cardiac stimulation.

Corticosteroids have been used increasingly in asthmatic attacks that do not respond to adrenergic agents. Steroids probably induce their antiasthmatic effect by reducing the inflammatory reaction that is inherent in the pathophysiology of airway narrowing. The drugs may be given in high doses for short terms (<2 weeks) and toxicity is rare. Inhaled steroids include *beclomethasone (Vanceril), Flunisolide (Aerobid), and triamcinolone (Azmacort).* Of importance to note is that enough inhaled drug is absorbed that adrenal suppression may be induced.

Ipratropium (Atrovent) is an anticholinergic drug that enhances the bronchodilating action of adrenergic agents. It is administered by inhalation. Similarly, *atropine* has been reported to improve asthmatic patients when given by inhalation. Although anticholinergics may increase the tenacity of secretions, this is more than offset by their bronchodilating action. Anticholinergics improve certain subgroups of asthmatics.

Theophylline, once used extensively to treat bronchospasm, has dropped in popularity in recent years due to associated toxicity and its questionable effectiveness when compared to the newer adrenergic agents. In one study, asthmatic patients were treated with an inhalation beta agonist every 3 hours. The addition of therapeutic levels of theophylline did not improve the bronchospasm and increased the frequency of side effects. Toxicity of theophylline is related to serum concentrations. Blood levels below 10 µg/ml are not generally associated with toxicity while between 10 and 20 µg/ml is often associated with jitteriness as well as behavioral changes. Above 20 µg/ml, nausea, vomiting, diarrhea, insomnia, cardiac rhythm irregularities, seizures, and death may occur.

Cromolyn (Intal) acts to stabilize mast cells and inhibit release of asthma mediators. It is of no use in an acute episode once the mast cells have degranulated. Cromolyn is administered by an inhaler and must be taken regularly for effective prophylaxis.

New Drugs

New beta-2 agonists, such as procaterol, are undergoing clinical trials. The advantages sought in these newer agents is longer duration and more beta-2 selectivity. Ketotifen is an antihistamine and possesses very mild antiasthma activity. To minimize the use of steroids in severe asthmatics, clinicians have use a variety of anti-inflammatory agents such as methotrexate and gold.

PERIOPERATIVE MANAGEMENT OF PATIENT WITH HISTORY OF BRONCHOSPASM

Preoperative evaluation of the patient with asthma requires an understanding of severity of disease and effectiveness of current management, as well as whether further therapy should be instituted prior to surgery. The goal of preoperative evaluation is to formulate a plan that will prevent or ameliorate airway narrowing. Preoperative evaluation begins with a careful history to elicit the severity of disease. Particular aspects of the history relative to patients with asthma are listed in Table 1.

Table 1. Important historical points to be elicited in preoperative evaluation of asthmatic patients.

Age of onset

Associated triggers

Details of an attack-initiating events

Ever hospitalized? (Number of times?)

Known allergies

Cough, sputum, change in sputum color

Previous anesthetic history

Medications

Pulmonary Function Tests

There are three parameters that are generally used to quantitate the degree of airway narrowing:

Forced vital capacity (FVC) is the maximal volume that can be forcibly exhaled after inspiration to total lung capacity. When FVC is plotted over time, the volume expired over the first second (FEV1) and the *Forced expiratory flow 25 to 75%* (FEF 25-75%) may be calculated. An asthma attack is associated with an obstructive pattern demonstrating delayed expiration with a consequent decrease in FVC, FEV1, FEV1/FVC, and FEF 25 to 75%. The FEF 25 to 75% is felt to be a more sensitive indicator of airway narrowing in the smaller bronchioles.

Peak (maximum) expiratory flow rate (PEFR) can be calculated from a spirogram or by using a peak expiratory flow meter. PEFR is markedly decreased in asthma attacks. For example, normal PEFR is >600 l/min which may be reduced to 100 l/min in a severe asthma attack.

Patients with a history of asthma may be divided into three groups. Individuals in the first group have had no attacks in recent years, take no bronchodilator medications, and physical examination reveals no wheezing. The second group have recurrent attacks and take prophylactic bronchodilator medications but are not actively wheezing. The third group consists of patients who are actively wheezing at the time of examination or who report deterioration in their pulmonary status.

The first group requires no other workup. The third group needs preoperative PFTs to document their baseline and should not undergo elective surgery until their bronchodilator therapy has been optimized. Controversy exists concerning the preoperative management of the second group. Some authors recommend obtaining PFT's in these patients. These clinicians recommend delay of elective surgery and further bronchodilator therapy if the FEV1, PEFR, and FEF 25 to 75% are less than 80% of predicted or there has been a deterioration from previous measurements. This does not appear to be universal practice.

As any patient with a history of asthma may develop perioperative bronchospasm, all such patients should be administered a technique that has the least risk of triggering an attack.

Anesthetic Management

Although regional anesthesia remains the anesthetic technique of choice for patients with a history of asthma, it is not completely free of risk. One study found that 1.9% of asthmatic patients receiving regional anesthesia still developed bronchospasm during surgery. There are many instances where a regional anesthetic is not appropriate and a general anesthetic must be administered. The anesthesiologist must understand which anesthetic techniques and drugs possess the potential for inducing bronchospasm.

Premedication. Few studies have been performed to ascertain the relative benefit of one premedicant regimen over another. However, practical considerations dictate careful administration of any respiratory depressant, such as narcotics, in patients with significant bronchospastic disease. Diazepam does not increase airway resistance in patients with asthma. Hydroxyzine and droperidol are probably safe as well. If the patient has been receiving corticosteroid therapy, a plan for continuation should be developed.

Induction. Controversy has existed concerning the triggering potential of *thiopental*. The evidence suggests that too little thiopental (light anesthesia) is the more likely culprit rather than thiopental itself. However, reflex triggered bronchospasm may still occur even with appropriate dosing of thiopental and administration of potent volatile anesthetics may necessary. After intubation, it may be difficult to differentiate light anesthesia from bronchospasm as the cause of a "tight chest." Succinylcholine will relieve the difficulty in ventilation due to light anesthesia but will have no effect on bronchospasm. *Ketamine* has the advantage of possessing sympathomimetic action and enhance bronchodilation in asthmatics. *Lidocaine*, 1 mg/kg IV, has been found to be beneficial in the induction of asthmatic patients. Intravenous local anesthetics ameliorate reflex induced bronchospasm, probably by a central mechanism. Aerosol administration is felt by some to increase the risk of bronchospasm while others believe it is the most effective route. Some authors recommend IV atropine prior to stimulating the airway to block cholinergic mediated bronchoconstriction.

Maintenance.

Inhalation agents. Halothane, enflurane, and isoflurane are equally effective bronchodilators. However, halothane has been shown to sensitize the myocardium to catecholamines and toxic levels of aminophylline may interact with halothane to produce cardiac arrhythmias and cardiac arrest.

Nitrous oxide/narcotic. There is a paucity of studies evaluating narcotics in asthmatic patients. In contrast to the volatile agents, narcotics do not possess bronchodilating properties.

Muscle relaxants and antagonists. D-tubocurarine is associated with histamine release and, theoretically, would be less desirable than a sympathomimetic muscle relaxant such as pancuronium. However, the data is conflicting and both asthmatic and nonasthmatic patients have developed bronchospasm with pancuronium. Atracurium is also associated with histamine release. The risk of bronchospasm with this drug is still unclear. Succinylcholine appears as safe as any other muscle relaxant in asthmatics. Neostigmine increases cholinergic activity and may induce bronchospasm. This can be prevented by atropine.

An optimal anesthetic plan designed to prevent the development of bronchospasm must be tailored to each patient. However, for the elective patient at significant risk for bronchospasm who has no other medical problems, the following suggestions may be useful.

After monitors have been placed, administer

atropine 1 mg or iprotropium 4 puffs by inhalation
metaproterenol 4 puffs or albuterol 4 puffs by inhalation

While breathing 100% O_2

    thiopental 3-5 mg/kg or ketamine 1-2 mg/kg IV

    mask induction with enflurane or isoflurane

    lidocaine 1.5 mg/kg IV bolus and 2 mg/min infusion

Intubation when patient deeply anesthetized

Management of intraoperative bronchospasm. Wheezing and increased inflation pressures are the signs of the onset of bronchospasm. Adequacy of oxygenation and ventilation are the first priorities. The work of breathing may increase several fold and spontaneous ventilation may not be adequate. Ventilation by mechanical means may be difficult to maintain due to 1) the high inflation pressures required to move air past the narrow airways and 2) the long expiratory phase needed to prevent air trapping. Many ventilators available on anesthetic machines will not be suitable and manual ventilation may be necessary. Positive end expiratory pressure may worsen air trapping and is generally avoided in acute asthma. Pulse oximetry and ABG's should be used to guide adjustments of F_IO_2 and minute ventilation.

Suppression of bronchospasm may be accomplished by 1) by giving IV lidocaine or ketamine, 2) increasing the concentration of the volatile anesthetic or 3) administering a nonanesthetic bronchodilator. IV lidocaine has been reported to reverse intraoperative bronchospasm with a single bolus of 100 mg. Similarly, ketamine has been effective even in the presence of halothane anesthesia. Increasing the volatile anesthetic concentration may improve the bronchospasm but the cardiovascular depression may be unacceptable.

Administration of *beta-2 selective adrenergic agents* are often effective in treating intraoperative bronchospasm. An adapter for the metered dose inhaler can be placed in the anesthesia circuit. However, due to precipitation in the endotracheal tube, several puffs may be required. Terbutaline, 0.25 mg SQ, may also be effective. Despite its popularity *theophylline* is short on benefit and long on adverse side effects. Interestingly, most of the studies in the anesthetic literature concerning theophylline are about the side effects encountered. Theophylline has been reported to antagonize the action of morphine, benzodiazepines, and barbiturates.

Corticosteroids have been used intraoperatively for treatment of acute bronchospasm. Although a minimum of 3 to 4 hours would be expected after injection before any benefit might be seen, there are reports of almost immediate response. As a single dose of steroids poses little risk to the patient, there is little reason not to give them in a critical situation.

Emergence. The endotracheal tube in a lightly anesthetized patient with asthma poses the greatest stimulus for inducing or exacerbating bronchospasm. Thus, many clinicians extubate while the patient is deeply anesthetized. In a patient who is actively wheezing, one has to decide whether the endotracheal tube is better left in or taken out. In severely affected patients, continued intubation and mechanical ventilation may be necessary to maintain adequate gas exchange until the airway narrowing improves. Even if extubation occurs uneventfully, the severe asthmatic can develop life threatening bronchospasm at anytime during the immediate postoperative period, and therefore, requires close observation until fully recovered.

Emergency Surgery

The combination of emergency surgery and asthma poses a particularly difficult to the anesthesiologist as many of the maneuvers used for airway protection may exacerbate asthma. Further, there is often insufficient time to attempt optimization of bronchodilator therapy prior to surgery. Regional anesthesia remains the technique of choice in asthma patients undergoing emergency surgery. However, the risk of this technique in these patients is not the block but the sedation with potential respiratory depression.

Intubation. Many, if not all, patients presenting for emergency surgery are at risk for aspiration of gastric contents. The lungs must be protected if airway reflexes are to be impaired by anesthetics. There are two ways to protect the airway during intubation, awake and rapid sequence. Both have disadvantages, particularly for patients with asthma. Awake intubation in a patient with a full stomach will stimulate laryngeal and tracheal reflexes which may induce bronchospasm. Rapid sequence induction and intubation may result in a lightly anesthetized patient at the time of intubation and induce bronchospasm. A slow induction may allow a more completely anesthetized patient but may also increase the risk of aspiration, which, in a severe asthmatic, may be life-threatening.

Induction. Thiopental is not associated with an increase in bronchospasm. However, *ketamine* is an alternative as it possesses sympathomimetic properties and is associated with improvement of bronchospasm. However, seizures have been reported in patients receiving aminophylline who were given ketamine. Regardless of the induction agent chosen, intravenous lidocaine 1 mg/kg should be given prior to laryngoscopy for reasons described above. If tachycardia is not a problem, atropine should also be given intravenously at this time.

Emergence. As deep extubation is not appropriate for the patient with a full stomach, patients should be awake prior to extubation. Pretreatment prior to extubation with intravenous lidocaine or ephedrine may help prevent problems.

Asthma and Pregnancy

The effect of pregnancy on preexisting asthma is variable. In fact, one third of asthmatic women will worsen, one third improve and the rest remain unchanged. A particular problem that arises in women at term is that beta-2 agents not only are bronchodilators, but tocolytics as well. Thus, albuterol and terbutaline could potentially inhibit the progress of labor. Anticholinergic drugs such as ipratropium may be of benefit. There is a report of improvement of asthma following the institution of epidural anesthesia. The authors felt that some degree of bronchospasm was due to the mother's anxiety of the pain of labor, which, once relieved, no longer contributed to airway narrowing.

Emergency caesarian sections generally require a general anesthetic. In order to prevent fetal depression, the anesthetic is usually kept light. However, a light anesthetic may induce bronchospasm in the mother. A suitable anesthetic plan has not been agreed upon for this situation. Fetal toxicity has been reported with the use of IV theophylline in the mother. Halothane or isoflurane appears to be a reasonable alternative. Uterine relaxation induced by a volatile inhalation agent may be treated with pitocin infusion.

Asthma and Coexisting Heart Disease

Patients with both asthma and coronary artery disease pose a difficult management problem. Therapies that are effective for treating one condition may exacerbate the other. Beta adrenergic drugs and the theophylline derivatives may enhance dysrhythmias or alter metabolism of cardiac drugs. On the other hand, beta blockers are popular agents in the treatment of cardiac disease and hypertension. This class of drugs may induce bronchospasm. If bronchospasm does develop intraoperatively, IV lidocaine as a bolus followed by an infusion can be effective. Preliminary work suggests that calcium entry blockers may be the best alternative for treatment of bronchospasm in these patients.

Management of Status Asthmaticus

Status asthmaticus is defined as unresolving bronchospasm that is severe enough to be considered life-threatening. Thus, patients in status should be monitored in an intensive care setting. Because of their expertise in airway and ventilator management, anesthesiologists may be called upon to assist with the care of a patient in status asthmaticus. A brief review of therapeutic points is presented below.

Oxygen. Hypoxemia is a major contributing factor to patients who die of asthma. Supplemental oxygen should always be administered and the adequacy of patient oxygenation monitored by pulse oximetry and ABG's. Humidification of delivered gas is highly desirable and heated saline is preferable.

Fluids. A decrease in the extracellular fluid volume is common in patients with severe asthma and may be reflected by increased hematocrit and BUN. This relative volume deficit may contribute to the tenacity of sputum and enhance airway obstruction. Hydration with intravenous fluids is usually indicated.

Baseline data. The following are appropriate aids to the management of status:

Peak flow measurement in order to quantify effects of therapy
Chest X-ray to check for pneumonia, atelectasis, pneumothorax
ABG's
H&H and electrolytes

ECG to follow right ventricular strain

Sputum Gram stain and culture

Intubation and mechanical ventilation is instituted usually for progressive alveolar hypoventilation and/or exhaustion. As these patients may suddenly develop apnea, intubation should be performed before respiratory arrest occurs. The minute ventilation is adjusted to correct respiratory acidosis. Profoundly elevated inspiratory pressure are often required in order to deliver an appropriate tidal volume. Further, the airway narrowing requires a prolonged expiratory phase to avoid aggravation of air trapping. Pulmonary toilet is helpful in treating and preventing the obstruction of airways with secretions.

Drugs. By definition, status asthmaticus is diagnosed when the patient has not responded to bronchodilators. Thus, beta adrenergics and theophylline have already been administered to maximal doses in these patients. The next step is *corticosteroids*. One gram hydrocortisone is administered IV followed by 4 mg/kg Q4H. Benefit is usually not evident for several hours. The use of *theophylline* is apparently undergoing transition. However, it is still administered in status asthmaticus. The loading dose is 5 to 6 mg/kg IV over 15 to 20 minutes, followed by 0.5 to 2 mg·kg·$^{-1}$hr^{-1} infusion. The metabolism of theophylline varies greatly among patients and monitoring of theophylline blood levels is wise.

There appear to be cholinergic receptors that result in the production of mediators. *Atropine and ipratrobium* given inhalationally may improve the occasional patient.

Antibiotics are given to treat documented infection.

General anesthesia. When conventional therapy fails, general anesthesia has been advocated in selected patients. Halothane, enflurane, and isoflurane have been used successfully to treat refractory status. As many of these patients are receiving maximal doses of potentially cardiac stimulating drugs, enflurane and isoflurane may be preferable. There is one case of 50 hours of general anesthesia for the treatment of status asthmaticus without adverse sequelae.

Fiberoptic bronchoscopic bronchial lavage with large amounts of saline is advocated by some clinicians for the removal of tenacious secretions in refractory status. There does not appear to wide spread acceptance of this potentially dangerous technique.

SUGGESTED READING

1. Drazen JM, Boushey HA, Holgate ST, et al: The pathogenesis of severe asthma: A consensus report from the Workshop of Pathogenesis. J Allergy Clin Immunol 80:428-37, 1987
2. Kingston HGC, Hirshman CA: Perioperative management of the patient with asthma. Anesth Analg 63:844-55, 1984
3. Fung DL: Emergency anesthesia for asthma patients. Clin Rev Allergy 3:127-41, 1985
4. Hopewell PC, Miller RT: Pathophysiology and Management of Severe Asthma. Clin Chest Med 5:623-34, 1984
5. Richards W, Thompson J, George L, et al: Cardiac arrest associated with halothane anesthesia in a patient receiving theophylline. Ann Allergy 61:83-4, 1988
6. Rodriguez-Roisin R, Ballester E, Rocca J, et al: Mechanisms of hypoxemia in patients with status asthmaticus requiring mechanical ventilation. Am Rev Respir Dis 139:732-9, 1989
7. Barnes PJ: A new approach to the treatment of asthma. N Engl J Med 321:1517-27, 1989

MANAGEMENT OF THE DIFFICULT AIRWAY PART I: EPIDEMIOLOGY, THE ASA ALGORITHM AND RECOGNITION

J. L. Benumof

I. EPIDEMIOLOGY: INCIDENCE OF DIFFERENT DEGREES OF A DIFFICULT AIRWAY

The most fundamental routine responsibility of an anesthesiologist to an anesthetized patient is to maintain adequate gas exchange. In order to do this, the airway must be managed in such a way so that it is almost continuously patent. The result of failure to maintain adequate airway patency and gas exchange for a critical amount of time is brain damage and whole body death. Thus, it is not surprising that over 85% of all respiratory-related closed malpractice claims involve a brain damaged or dead patient (1) and it has been estimated that inability to successfully manage very difficult airways has been responsible for up to 30% of deaths totally attributable to anesthesia (2-4).

The incidence of a difficult airway in the general surgical population varies greatly depending on the degree of difficulty in question (Table 1). Mildly to moderately difficult ETT intubation, as indicated by such events as requiring multiple attempts or laryngoscope blades, is relatively common and occurs in 100-1800/10,000 patients or 1-18% (5-11). If the degree of difficulty is increased to a Grade IV laryngoscopic view (Fig. 1), then the incidence is generally slightly less and ranges 100-400/10,000 patients or 1-4% (4,9). When the degree of difficulty is specified as definite failure of ETT intubation (i.e., very severe or impossible) the incidence is still less and ranges 5-35/10,000 patients or 0.05-0.35% (4,5,12-15). There are no data available regarding the incidence of difficulty with mask ventilation alone. However, the incidence of completely failed mask ventilation *and* ETT intubation is known, because such an airway failure combination heretofore frequently resulted in brain damage or death, and ranges 0.01-2.0/10,000 patients (2,3,16).

T. H. Stanley and R. J. Sperry (eds.), Anesthesia and the Lung 1992, 157–165.
© 1992 *Kluwer Academic Publishers.*

Table 1. Incidence of difficult conventional ETT intubation according to degree of difficulty.

Degree of Difficulty with ETT Intubation	Clinical Correlate	Range of Incidence		Reference
		Per 10,000	%	
Beginning of airway difficultly	ETT intubation successful but multiple attempts and/or laryngoscopic blades required; general difficulty	100-1800	1-18	5-11
On the increasing degree of difficulty continuum	ETT intubation successful but the laryngoscopic view was grade IV	100-400	1-4	4,9
The impossible extreme for ETT intubation	ETT intubation not successful	5-35	0.05-0.35	4,5,12-15
The impossible extreme—for ETT intubation and mask ventilation	Cannot ventilate by mask, plus Cannot ETT intubation; brain damage or death	0.01-2.0	0.0001-0.02	2,3,16

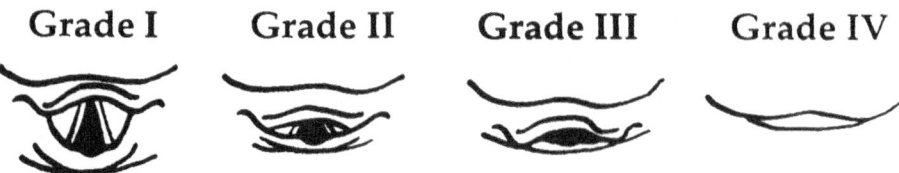

Figure 1. The four grades of laryngoscopic view, as defined by reference #5 are as follows: Grade I is visualization of the entire laryngeal aperture; Grade II is visualization of just the posterior portion of the laryngeal aperture; Grade III is visualization of only the epiglottis; Grade IV is visualization of just the soft palate. Reproduced with permission from reference #5.

II. ASA ALGORITHM

The specific management of the difficult airway should follow the ASA Task Force approved algorithm shown in Figure 2.

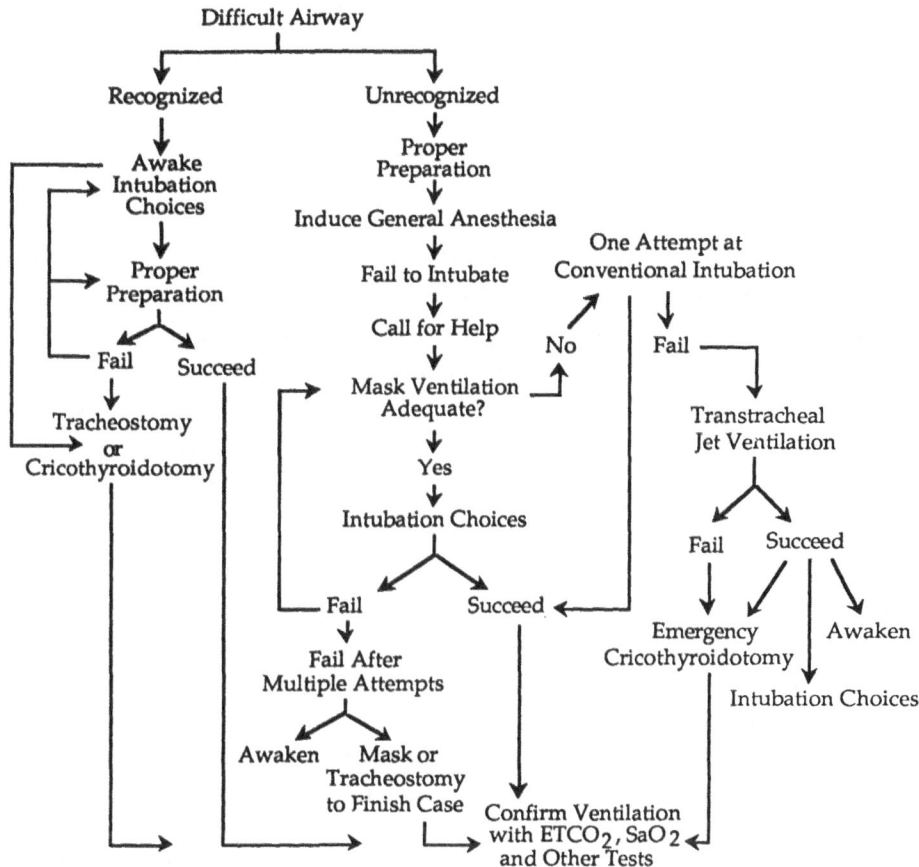

Figure 2. ASA Task Force Difficult Airway Management Algorithm. If an airway is recognized to be difficult, endotracheal tube (ETT) intubation should be performed awake, which demands proper preparation of the patient. When the patient is properly prepared any one of a number of ETT techniques can be successful. If unsuccessful, the patient may need to be better prepared, another ETT technique chosen, a combination of ETT techniques used or a surgical solution utilized. Once in a great while a tracheostomy or cricothyroidotomy may be the best first choice. If the patient refuses to be intubated awake, or a difficult airway is not recognized, and anesthesia is induced, then the airway will ordinarily be first controlled by mask ventilation prior to conventional laryngoscopy. If conventional laryngoscopy should fail, a call for help should be initiated and the airway should then be controlled by mask ventilation. If ETT by conventional laryngoscopy is still unsuccessful after a few attempts (perhaps using a different blade or head position) and special alternative techniques fail, the the patient should either be awakened, the case done by mask, or a semi-elective tracheostomy or cricothyroidotomy performed. If at any point mask ventilation becomes impossible and the patient still cannot be intubated, then transtracheal jet ventilation (TTJV) through a percutaneous IV catheter should be instituted. Once life sustaining gas exchange is again effected by TTJV, then the patient should either be awakened, a semi-elective tracheostomy or cricothyroidotomy performed or the patient intubated with a special ETT technique. At all times ETT, with any technique should be further confirmed by capnography, pulse oximetry and other tests.

III. RECOGNITION OF THE DIFFICULT AIRWAY

The algorithm begins with the most basic question of whether or not the presence of a difficult airway is recognized.

A. Gross Obvious Factors

An airway may be recognized as difficult on a very gross obvious, level, or the potential difficulty may be very subtle and require careful examination of the patient. The causes of obvious difficulties with the airway are very numerous and have been extensively detailed elsewhere (17-21). When an obvious condition is present, potential difficulty with a conventional approach to the airway is typically recognized. These conditions have not been responsible for many anesthesia related airway catastrophes (brain damage, death) (*,4,9,18,22,23).

Most airway catastrophes have occurred when recognition of the difficult airway has been a subtle issue; in other words, in the context of what was considered an adequate preoperative examination (looking for only gross abnormalities), the subsequent airway difficulty was fully unexpected (*,9,18,22-24).

It is clear that unexpected cases of difficulty occur commonly and some cases of anticipated difficulty turn out to be simple to manage; thus, better routine predictors of easy versus difficult airway are needed.

B. Relative Tongue/Pharyngeal Size

Fortunately, three recent, extremely easy to perform, zero cost, preoperative examinations appear to be much more accurate predictors of subtle ETT intubation difficulty than any criteria used in the past. First, the size of the tongue in relation to the size of the oral cavity can be very simply and visually graded by how much the pharynx is obscured by the tongue. The patient sits upright with the head in a neutral position and is asked to open the mouth as widely as possible [normal maximum mandibular opening is 50-60 mm (18) (maximum depth of the flange of a

---

*American Society of Anesthesiologists Committee on Professional Liability, Personal Communications, March, 1990.

Macintosh #3 laryngoscope is 20 mm)] and to protrude the tongue to a maximum. The observer then classifies the airway according to the pharyngeal structures seen (see Fig. 3).

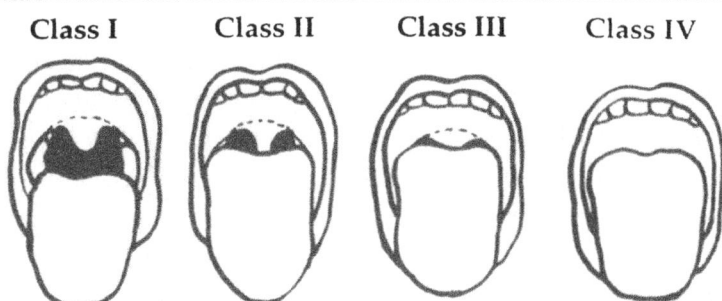

Class I   **Class II**   **Class III**   **Class IV**

Figure 3. Classification of the upper airway in terms of the size of the tongue relative to the size of the pharynx upon mouth opening. In Class I patients the soft palate, fauces, uvula and anterior and posterior tonsillar pillars can be seen; in Class II patients all of the above can be seen except the tonsillar pillars are hidden by the tongue; in Class III patients just the base of the uvula can be seen; in Class IV patients not even the uvula can be visualized. Reproduced with permission from reference #7.

A significant correlation has been noted between the ability to visualize the faucial pillars, soft palate and uvula and the ease of laryngoscopy (4,7). In patients with a Class I airway, the laryngoscopic view is Grade I 99-100% of the time (4,7,25) and in those with a Class IV airway, the laryngoscopic view is Grade III or IV 100% of the time (7,26). However, patients with intermediate tongue/pharynx size classifications of II and III were found to have a relatively uniform distribution of all grades of laryngoscopic view (I-IV) (7,25). Reasons for the lack of correlation between tongue/pharyngeal size classification and laryngoscopic grade include failure of the tongue/pharyngeal size classification to consider neck mobility, the size of the mandibular space and significant interobserver variability in classification (27). Sources of interobserver variability include use of the test in patients in the supine position and whether or not the patient phonates (says "Ah") during the test (which falsely improves the view) or arches their tongue (which obscures the uvula). Thus, despite widespread general agreement with the usefulness of the original findings (4,7,17,25,26), the test has a significant false-negative (27,28) and false-positive rate (27) and cannot be considered to be entirely predictive of severe ETT intubation difficulty.

C. Atlanto-Occipital Joint Extension

Second, it has long been well appreciated that when the neck is slightly to moderately flexed on the chest and the atlanto-occipital joint is well extended (head extended on the neck), the oral, pharyngeal and laryngeal axes are brought more nearly into a straight line (otherwise known as the "sniff" or McGill position) (29,30). To the extent that this is achieved, there will be less of the tongue obscuring the view of the larynx and consequently there will be much less of a need for strenuous effort to displace the tongue anteriorly. Thirty-five degrees of extension are possible at the normal atlanto-occipital joint (31). Bedside evaluation of the atlanto-occipital extension may be performed by having the patient sit straight with head held erect and facing directly to the front. In this position, the occlusal surface of the upper teeth is horizontal and parallel to the ground. The patient then extends the atlanto-occipital joint as much as possible and the examiner estimates the angle traversed by the occlusal surface of the upper teeth. Any reduction in extension can be expressed as a fraction of the normal and graded accordingly (3). When the atlanto-occipital joint cannot be extended (as might be caused by a very small occipital-C1 gap), vigorous attempts to do so will cause the convexity of the cervical spine to bulge further anteriorly, which will push the larynx anteriorly and compromise a conventional laryngoscopic view (32-34).

D. Mandibular Space

Third, the space anterior to the larynx (the mandibular space) has been easy to measure by ruler or by number of finger breadths and has been expressed as the inside of the mandible to the hyoid bone distance (Fig. 4), the thyromental distance and/or the horizontal length of the mandible. The mandibular space is important for two reasons. First, the space anterior to the larynx determines how readily the laryngeal axis will fall in line with the pharyngeal axis when the atlanto-occipital joint is extended. If the thyromental distance is very short, the laryngeal axis will make a more acute angle with the pharyngeal axis and it will be more difficult for atlanto-occipital extension to bring these two axes into line, and vice versa. The thyromental distance and horizontal length of the mandible have been found to inversely correlate extremely well with the class of pharynx described above (26,35). A thyromental distance greater than 6 cm and a horizontal length of the mandible greater than 9 cm are tightly associated with low tongue/pharyngeal size classification and strongly suggest that direct laryngoscopy will be relatively easy (18,26,35). Second, when there is a large mandibular space (larynx is relatively posterior), the tongue is easily compressed into a large compartment and does not have to be pulled maximally forward in order to reveal the larynx. When there is a very small mandibular space (larynx is relatively anterior) the tongue has to be compressed into a much smaller compartment and must be pulled maximally forward in order to view the larynx.

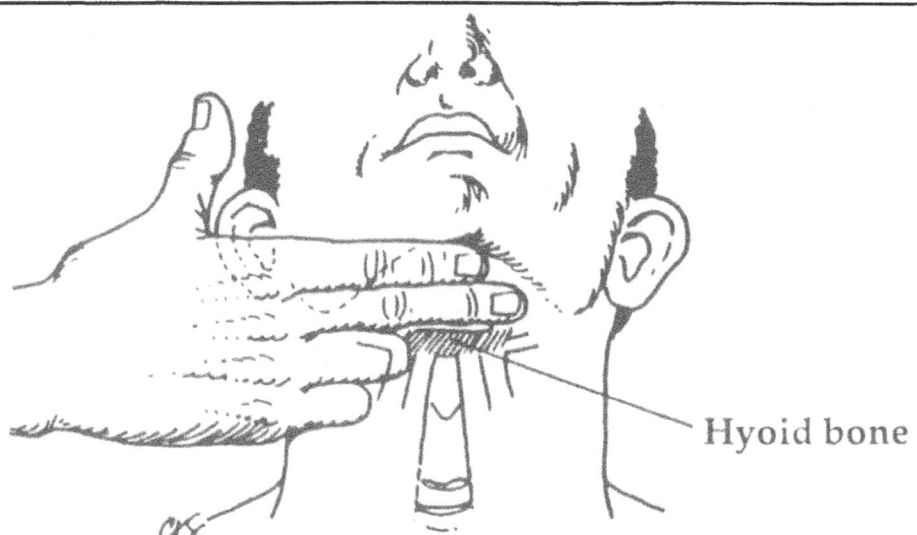

Hyoid bone

Figure 4. Schematic diagram showing the inside of the mandible-hyoid bone distance to be two finger breadths in an average patient.

These three tests (tongue versus pharyngeal size, anterior mandibular space, and atlanto-occipital extension) have great appeal as routine preoperative airway evaluation tests because they are so simple and quick to perform and hold promise for identifying patients who are at risk for getting into potentially life-threatening situations. Although there have been no studies using all three of these predictors of difficult ETT intubation, it seems logical that use of multiple predictors together would have much more power and accuracy than use of any one predictor alone (3,11).

Indeed, a 100% accuracy has been found by one investigator (3). Future careful studies are needed to document this highly promising, three-variable, difficult ETT intubation prediction scheme.

REFERENCES

1. Caplan RA, Posner KL, Ward RJ, et al: Adverse respiratory events in anesthesia: A closed claims analysis. Anesthesiology 723:828-33, 1990
2. Benumof JL, Scheller MS: The importance of transtracheal jet ventilation in the management of the difficult airway. Anesthesiology 71:769-778, 1989
3. Bellhouse CP, Dore' C: Criteria for estimating likelihood of difficulty of endotracheal intubation with Macintosh laryngoscope. Anaes Intens Care 16: 329-37, 1988
4. Samsoon GLT, Young JRB: Difficult tracheal intubation: A retrospective study. Anaesthesia 42:487-90, 1987
5. Cormack RS, Lehane J: Difficult tracheal intubation in obstetrics. Anaesthesia 39:1105-11, 1984
6. Aro L, Takki S, Aromaa U: Technique for difficult intubation. Br J Anesth 43:1081-83, 1971
7. Mallampati SR, Gatt SP, Gugino LD, et al: A clinical sign to predict difficult tracheal intubation: A prospective study. Can Anaes Soc J 32:429-34, 1985
8. Phillips OC, Duerksen RL: Endotracheal intubation. A new blade for direct laryngoscopy. Anesth Analg 52:691-98, 1973
9. Hirsch IA, Reagan JO, Sullivan N: Complications of direct laryngoscopy: A prospective analysis. Anesth Rev 17:34-40, 1990
10. Finucane BT, Santora AH: Principles of Airway Management. Philadelphia, FA Davis, 1988, p. 147
11. Deller A, Schreiber MN, Gromer J, et al: Difficult intubation: incidence and predictability. A prospective study of 8,284 adult patients. Anesthesiology 73:A1054, 1990
12. Bellhouse CP: An angulated laryngoscope for routine and difficult tracheal intubation. Anesthesiology 69:126-9, 1988
13. Lyons G: Failed intubation. Anaesthesia 40:759-62, 1985
14. Lyons G, MacDonald R: Difficult intubation in obstetrics. Anaesthesia 40:1016, 1985
15. Glassenburg R, Vaisrub N, Albright G: The incidence of failed intubation in obstetrics—Is there an irreducible minimum? Anesthesiology 73:A1061, 1990
16. Tunstall ME: Failed intubation in the parturient (editorial). Can J Anaesth 36:612-13, 1989
17. McIntyre JRW: The difficult intubation. Can J Anaesth 34:204-13, 1987

18. Finucane BT, Santora AH: Evaluation of the airway prior to intubation. Chapter 4 in Principles of Airway Management. Philadelphia, FA Davis, 1988, pp 69-83

19. Latto IP, Rosen M: Intubation Procedures and causes of difficult intubation. Chapter 5 in Difficulties in Tracheal Intubation. London, Bailliere Tindall, 1985, pp 76-89

20. Steward DJ: Manual of Pediatric Anesthesia, 2nd ed. New York, Churchill-Livingstone, 1985, pp 289-343

21. Jones AEP, Pelton DA: An index of syndromes and their anesthetic implications. Can Anaesth Soc J 23:207-26, 1976

22. Sica RL, Eden ET: How to avoid problems when using the fiberoptic bronchoscope for difficult intubations. Anaesthesia 36:74, 1988

23. Norton ML, Wilton H, Brown A: The difficult airway clinic. Anesth Rev 25:25-8, 1988

24. Latto IP, Rosen M: Management of difficult intubation. Chapter 7 in Difficulties in Tracheal Intubation. London, Bailliere Tindall, 1985, pp 99-141

25. Cohen SM, Zaurito CE, Segil LJ: Oral exam to predict difficult intubations: A large prospective study. Anesthesiology 71:A937, 1989

26. Mathew M, Hanna LS, Aldrete JA: Preoperative indices to anticipate a difficult tracheal intubation. Anesth Analg 68:S187, 1989

27. Wilson ME, John R: Problems with the Mallampati sign. Anaesthesia 45:486-487, 1990

28. Charters P, Perera S, Horton WA: Visibility of pharyngeal structures as a predictor of difficult intubation. Anaesthesia 42:1115, 1987

29. Magill IW: Technique in endotracheal anaesthesia. Br Med J 2:817-20, 1930

30. Salem MR, Mathrubhutham M, Bennett EJ: Difficult intubation. N Engl J Med 295:879-81, 1976

31. Brechner VL: Unusual problems in the management of airways 1. Flexion-extension mobility of the cervical spine. Anesth Analg 47:362-73, 1968

32. White A, Kander PL: Anatomical factors in difficult direct laryngoscopy. Br J Anaesth 47:488, 1975

33. Nichol HL, Zuck B: Difficult laryngoscopy—The 'anterior' larynx and the atlanto-occipital gap. Br J Anaesth 55:141, 1983

34. Roberts JT, Ali HH, Shorten GD, et al: Why cervical flexion facilitates laryngoscopy with a Macintosh laryngoscope but hinders it with a flexible fiberscope. Anesthesiology 73:A1012, 1990

35. Patil VU, Stehling LC, Zauder HL: Fiberoptic Endoscopy in Anesthesia. Chicago, Year Book Medical Publ, 1983

MANAGEMENT OF THE DIFFICULT AIRWAY PART II: PROPER PREPARATION FOR THE AWAKE INTUBATION, FIBEROPTIC AND RETROGRADE TECHNIQUES

J. L. Benumof

I. PROPER PREPARATION FOR THE AWAKE PATIENT

If it is recognized that the ETT intubation or mask ventilation is going to be difficult due to the presence of an obvious factor(s) or a combination of subtle factors (large tongue size, small mandibular space, restricted atlanto-occipital extension), then airway patency should be secured and guaranteed (usually by ETT intubation) while the patient is awake. Although this is generally much more time consuming for the anesthesiologist and a more unpleasant experience for the patient compared to a routine intravenous anesthetic induction, there are several compelling reasons why ETT intubation should be done while a patient with a recognized difficult airway is still awake. First, and most importantly, gas exchange is better maintained in most patients ("no bridges are burned"); this is simply good common sense. Second, and one of the basic reasons why gas exchange is maintained in the awake patient, is that muscle tone is maintained which keeps the relevant upper airway structures separated from one another and much easier to identify. In an awake patient, muscle tone clearly separates out the tongue, vallecula, epiglottis, larynx, esophagus and posterior pharyngeal wall from one another in a vertical plane (in that order, from top to bottom or anterior to posterior), whereas in the anesthetized and paralyzed patient loss of muscle tone tends to cause these structures to collapse in toward one another into a horizontal plane (e.g., the tongue moves posteriorly) which distorts the anatomy (the structures look more like a stack of pancakes) (1,2). Third, the larynx moves to a more anterior position with the induction of anesthesia and paralysis which makes conventional ETT intubation more difficult (3). Thus, if a difficult ETT intubation is clearly

167

T. H. Stanley and R. J. Sperry (eds.), Anesthesia and the Lung 1992, 167–178.
© 1992 *Kluwer Academic Publishers.*

recognized it strongly behooves the anesthesiologist to perform the ETT intubation while the patient is awake.

The most important determinant of the success of an awake ETT intubation is the proper preparation of the patient for an awake ETT intubation. It is very difficult to do an awake ETT intubation (with any method) in an objecting, fighting patient, who has an extremely reactive larynx, whereas almost any awake ETT intubation technique will work easily and smoothly in a quiet cooperative patient who has a nonreactive larynx. The components of properly preparing a patient for an awake intubation are shown in Table 1.

Table 1.   Components of properly preparing a patient for awake intubation.
          FOB = Fiberoptic bronchoscope

Component	Purpose/Special Comment
Psychological	Better cooperation
Maintain Oxygenation	Safety. With FOB, insufflate O_2 down suction port (see text)
Maintain Ventilation	Safety. On rare occasion may need TTJV
Drying Agent	Better visualization, better mucosal application of topical anesthesia spray, prevent laryngovagal reflexes
Topical Anesthesia	Main component to proper preparation; must allow sufficient time
Bilateral Lingual and Superior Laryngeal Nerve Blocks	Nerve blocks anesthetize sub-mucosal pressure receptors. The lingual nerve block allows laryngoscopy with MacIntosh blade and Superior Laryngeal Nerve Block allows laryngoscopy with a Miller blade
Sedation	Relieve anxiety, increase pain threshold.

As with any procedure, proper preparation begins with psychological preparation; awake ETT intubation will proceed easier in the patient who knows and agrees with what is going to happen. Whenever hypoxemia and/or hypercapnia is suspected to be pre-existing and/or develop during awake ETT intubation (e.g., patients with large upper airway masses and/or constrictions, concurrent pulmonary parenchymal diseases, etc), then steps to augment F_IO_2 and minute ventilation must be taken before beginning topical and nerve block anesthesia and sedation. Although there are many ways to augment F_IO_2 , perhaps the best way to augment F_IO_2 when using a FOB (Fiberoptic Bronchoscope) is to insufflate oxygen down the suction port while actually using the FOB; depending on O_2 flow rate, it increases the F_IO_2 , prevents fogging of the FOB tip and it blows the secretions away from the tip of the FOB. On rare occasions it may be most prudent and safe for the the patient to have minute ventilation (and oxygenation) assured before beginning an awake ETT intubation by passing an IV catheter through the cricothyroid membrane and instituting transtracheal jet ventilation (4-6). A drying agent, allows better application of local anesthetic spray to the mucosa, improves visualization and prevents laryngovagal reflexes.

Topical anesthesia is the main component to preparation of the patient for an awake ETT; if it is correctly done (proper spray system) it may be all that is needed in many patients (Fig. 1). However, no matter how and what local anesthetic is applied to the mucosa, sufficient time must be allowed to anesthetize *all* of the relevant anatomy. A good endpoint for topicalization is the ability to touch the epiglottis with the spray end of the atomizer without patient objection. If nasotracheal

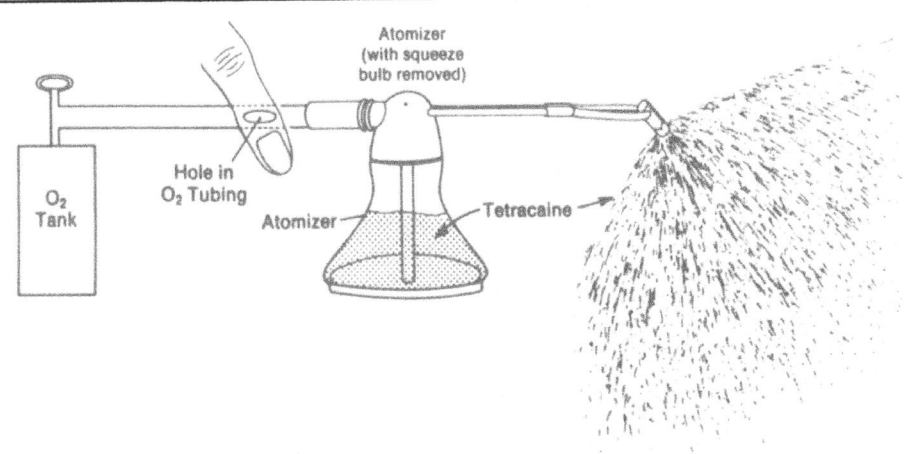

Figure 1. This schematic diagram shows the system for creating a fine mist of local anesthetic. Oxygen green tubing is connected to an oxygen tank. A hole is cut in the oxygen green tubing near the nebulization chamber. When oxygen is flowing in the green tubing and a finger is placed over the hole a fine dense mist from the nebulization chamber results. The size and velocity of spread of the mist is proportional to the oxygen flow rate. Reproduced with permission from reference 7.

intubation is planned, then the nose should be vasoconstricted and anesthetized. However, even careful prolonged spraying may be inadequate preparation for awake laryngoscopy because the pressure receptors that cause the gag reflex are submucosal and are not blocked by spraying; in this circumstance a bilateral lingual nerve block is required (see below).

There are two nerve blocks that are easy to perform, have virtually no risk of complications and have a high degree of potential benefit. The first is bilateral blockage of the lingual branch of the glossopharyngeal nerves (IX) (8). Firm pressure on the root of the tongue elicits a gag reflex which is mediated by pressure receptors which are submucosal and hence, not susceptible to topical anesthesia (9). The following technique is effective in eliminating the gag reflex and hemodynamic response to laryngoscopy, is easy to perform, has a high degree of patient acceptance and carries virtually no risk. The patient's tongue is gently retracted laterally (by pulling the tip of the tongue with gauze and by pushing it with a tongue blade), exposing the palatoglossal arch (which is also called the anterior tonsillar pillar) (Fig. 2). The base of the palatoglossal arch forms a U-shaped flap of tissue or bridge starting from the soft palate, running out from along the lateral pharyngeal wall to the lateral margin of the base of the tongue. The palatoglossal arch is pierced approximately 0.5 cm from the lateral margin of the root of the tongue at the point at which it joins the floor of the mouth (at the trough of the U-shaped band of tissue) using a 25-gauge spinal needle (the length of the spinal needle allows the local anesthetic syringe to be outside of the mouth and therefore not in the line of vision). The needle is inserted 0.5 cm and an aspiration test is performed. Air will enter the syringe if needle placement is too deep, as the tip of the needle may exit from the posterior aspect of the palatoglossal arch and enter the oropharynx. An aspiration test is also helpful in reducing the possibility of an intravascular injection which, while harmless, will result in a failed block. Two ml of 2% lidocaine are slowly injected and the procedure is repeated on the opposite side. Since the injection is made into loose sublingual tissue, there should be minimal resistance to injection. Within a few minutes the posterior third of the tongue and the pharyngeal side of the epiglottis should be adequately anesthetized to allow direct laryngoscopy with a Macintosh

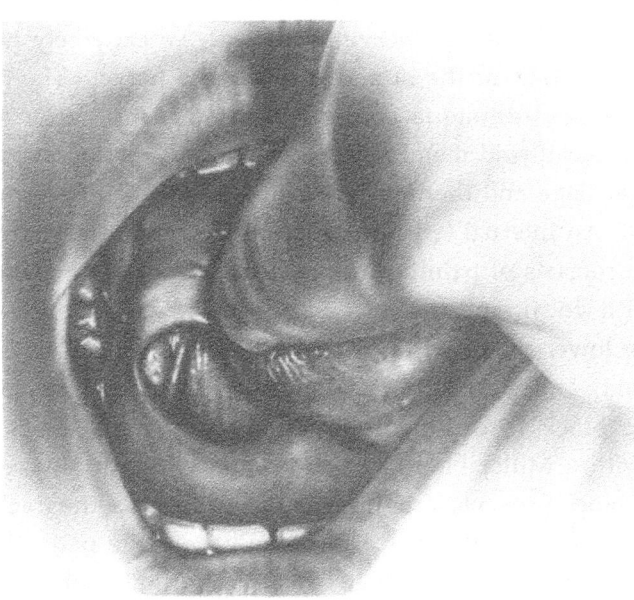

Figure 2. This photograph of pharyngeal anatomy shows the tongue being retracted to the patient's right side of the mouth by the index finger of the observer's left hand. A few of the upper and lower incisors are visualized as is the uvula and the posterior wall of the pharynx behind it. In front of the posterior wall of the pharynx is the posterior pillar and in front of the posterior pillar is the tonsil and in front of the tonsil is the anterior pillar The tip of the index finger is pointing to the trough of the curve formed by the band of tissue called the glossopalatine arch (which is also referred to as the anterior pillar). The block of the lingual branch of the glossopharyngeal nerve is made by injecting 2 ml of local anesthetic at the trough of the glossopalatine arch and in this picture the point of injection would be just lateral to the tip of the index finger.

blade with minimal discomfort or gagging. Although this block is directed primarily at the terminal portion of the glossopharyngeal nerve (lingual branch), studies using lidocaine and methylene blue dye have shown retrograde submucosal tracking of the agent and contact with proximal branches (pharyngeal and tonsillar). The larynx or laryngeal aspect of the epiglottis should not be touched since these areas are innervated by the superior laryngeal nerve (see next nerve block) which remains fully intact as do all other protective airway reflexes, if only a lingual nerve block is performed. The ease and safety of this block greatly increases the utilization and success rate of awake laryngoscopy. Coupled with topical anesthesia of the larynx and upper trachea, laryngoscopy and intubation can be performed with minimal hemodynamic consequences and without profound levels of central nervous system depression.

The second upper airway nerve block with an extremely favorable risk/benefit ratio is that of the superior laryngeal nerve. The superior laryngeal nerve block technique consists of needle application of local anesthetic to the thyrohyoid membrane between the superior lateral cornu of the thyroid cartilage and the inferior lateral margin of the cornu of the hyoid bone (10). An internal (within the mouth) superior laryngeal nerve block technique consists of painting the pyriform fossa with sponges that are soaked with local anesthetic. Superior laryngeal nerve block anesthetizes the lower pharynx, laryngeal epiglottis, vallecula, vestibule, aryepiglottic fold, and posterior rima glottis. Consequently, superior laryngeal nerve block in conjunction with lingual nerve block allows laryngoscopy with a Miller blade to be tolerated. In addition, superior laryngeal nerve block prevents coughing as the ETT enters the trachea.

Acute intravenous sedation can certainly help the patient tolerate all of the above. However, it is extremely important that meaningful contact be maintained between the anesthetist and the patient; meaningful contact is defined as the patient remains rational, oriented and obeying commands appropriately. Maintaining meaningful contact is important for two reasons. First, harmful respiratory depression will not occur during the various local anesthetic procedures. Second, an awake, rational, oriented and responsive patient will have a low likelihood of aspirating stomach contents. Thus, sedation should relieve anxiety and increase the pain threshold but not excessively diminish respiratory drive or eliminate protective reflexes.

II. FIBEROPTIC ENDOSCOPY-AIDED AWAKE INTUBATION (RELATIVELY NON-BLOODY NON-EMERGENT PROBLEM (12))

When the anesthesiologist is not able or does not expect to be able to see the vocal cords with conventional laryngoscopy, then the two primary special intubation techniques are fiberoptic bronchoscopy and retrograde techniques. For most anesthesiologists, fiberoptic bronchoscopy is most useful for a nonbloody, nonemergent problem and the more invasive retrograde technique is useful for either bloody or non-bloody problems.

A. Oral Fiberoptic Intubation

After adequate anesthesia of the airway is achieved, the airway intubator (#9 or #10) (11) is carefully inserted into the midline of the mouth (Fig. 3) (12). An approximately 4.9 mm OD fiberoptic bronchoscope is lubricated with clear lubricating fluid (American Cystoscope Co.) and inserted through an adaptorless endotracheal tube (8 mm ID or less if the #9 airway intubator is used, and 9 mm ID or less if the #10 airway intubator is used) so that the endotracheal tube jackets the proximal end of the bronchoscope (the endotracheal tube may be held in place on the proximal bronchoscope by tape).

The anesthesiologist should hold the fiberoptic bronchoscope so that the maneuverable tip lever and suction port are, with reference to the

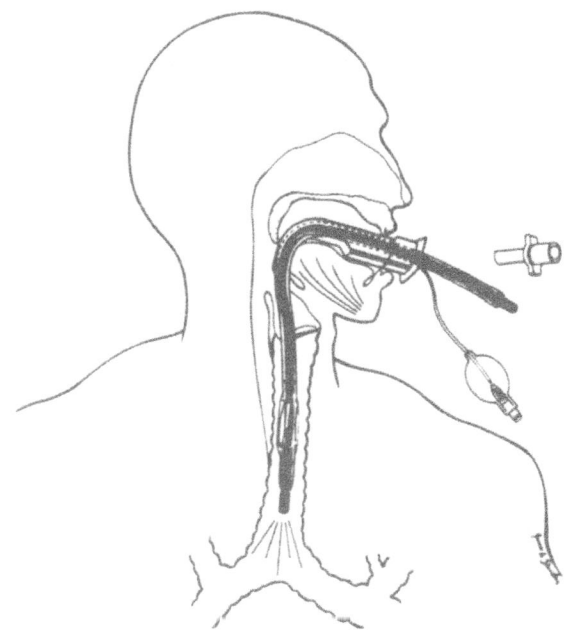

Figure 3. Schematic diagram showing the use of the oral airway intubator as an aid to fiberoptic tracheal intubation. The fiberoptic scope has been passed through the oral airway intubator into the trachea and the endotracheal tube has been passed over the fiberoptic scope. The fiberoptic scope then is removed, and the airway intubator is either left in place as a bite block or removed over the endotracheal tube (prior to attachment of the endotracheal tube adaptor). Reproduced with permission from reference 12.

patient's feet and head, at 6 and 12 o'clock, respectively. This orientation of the fiberoptic bronchoscope allows movement of the tip to be in an anterior-posterior axis. The fiberoptic bronchoscope is then introduced and advanced through the Airway Intubator, through the vocal cords, and on into the trachea. This trip is made relatively easy by the airway intubator because it is easy to distinguish the smooth, pink surface of the Airway Intubator on the posterior side from the rough, papillary, silver surface of the tongue on the anterior side, and when the fiberoptic bronchoscope emerges from the end of the Airway Intubator, the epiglottis is usually in view and often the vocal cords can already be seen in the distance. The rest of the trip into the trachea requires the intubationist to dip posteriorly around the epiglottis, advance a little bit, come back anteriorly until the vocal cords are in the center of the field, and then maintain the vocal cords in the center of the field as the vocal cords are approached. Once the tip of the fiberoptic bronchoscope is positioned well into the trachea, but above the carina, it is used as a guide over which the endotracheal tube is advanced (Fig. 3) (12). The fiberoptic bronchoscope is used to verify correct positioning of the endotracheal tube before it is removed. The oral Airway Intubator is either removed over the endotracheal tube (and then the endotracheal tube adaptor inserted) or is left in place to be used as a bite block (endotracheal tube adaptor inserted right away). General anesthesia is then induced intravenously.

B. Nasal Fiberoptic Intubation

A well lubricated nasotracheal tube is passed to approximately the 16-17 cm mark through the nose into the pharynx (Fig. 4). The nasotracheal tube should not be so deep as to prevent any manipulation of the tip of the fiberoptic bronchoscope, either anteriorly (if the tip of the tube is facing too posteriorly and towards the esophagus) or posteriorly (if the tip of the tube is facing too anteriorly and towards the vallecula), or be so proximal as to require the anesthesiologist to negotiate un-aided a long distance of the upper airway with the fiberoptic bronchoscope. Once the trachea, down to the carina, has been cannulated by the fiberoptic bronchoscope, the nasotracheal tube is passed over the fiberoptic bronchoscope stylet into the trachea, the fiberoptic bronchoscope is removed, the adaptor to the nasotracheal tube is inserted, the patient is connected to the breathing circuit and general anesthesia is induced.

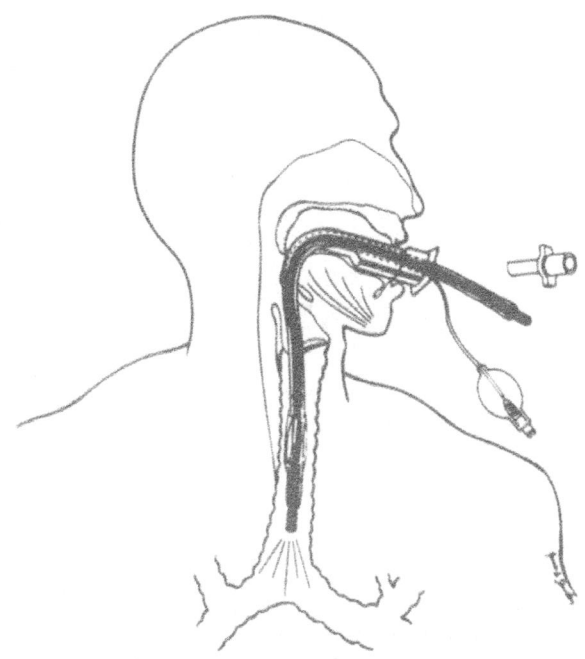

Figure 4. Fiberoptic nasotracheal intubation. The nasotracheal tube is passed to the 16-17 cm mark. The fiberoptic bronchoscope is passed through the nasotracheal tube into the trachea, and the nasotracheal tube is pushed in over the fiberoptic bronchoscope stylet.

III. RETROGRADE TECHNIQUE (RELATIVELY BLOODY, EMERGENT PROBLEM)

If the patient is awake, the skin and subcutaneous tissue overlying the cricothyroid membrane should be infiltrated with local anesthetic. The basic technique consists of puncturing the cricothyroid membrane with a needle pointed at approximately 30° cephalad from a line perpendicular to the trachea at the level of the cricothyroid membrane. A long, flexible, wire guide or some type of long, thin, hollow catheter (see below) should then be passed through the needle into the pharynx. The mouth is then opened and the wire or catheter is drawn out of the mouth with the fingers or by a clamp (Fig. 5) (13,14). Occasionally the wire or catheter will

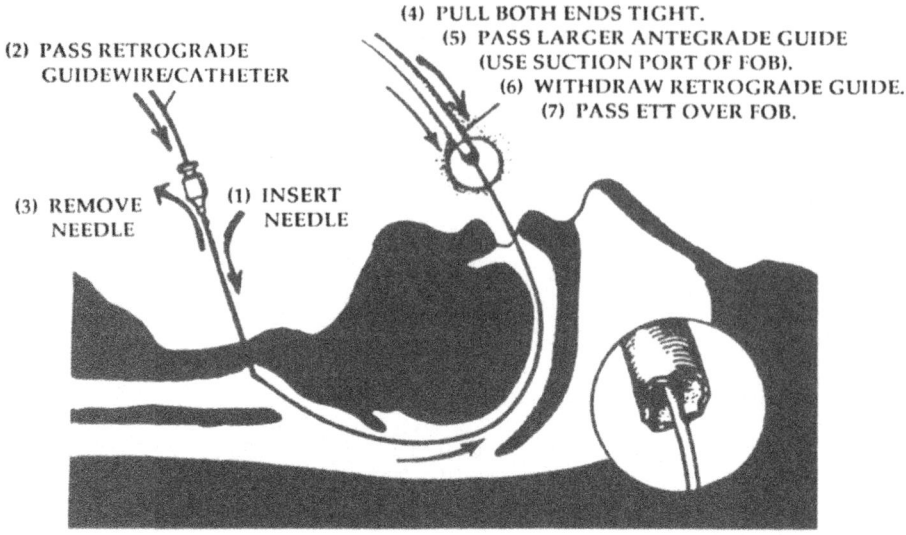

(2) PASS RETROGRADE GUIDEWIRE/CATHETER

(4) PULL BOTH ENDS TIGHT.
(5) PASS LARGER ANTEGRADE GUIDE (USE SUCTION PORT OF FOB).
(6) WITHDRAW RETROGRADE GUIDE.
(7) PASS ETT OVER FOB.

(3) REMOVE NEEDLE

(1) INSERT NEEDLE

Figure 5. Retrograde intubation technique. A needle punctures the cricothyroid membrane so that either a flexible guidewire or catheter is passed retrograde into the pharynx. The wire or catheter is usually retrieved from the mouth. If the endotracheal tube will not pass over the retrograde wire/catheter after it has been pulled tight at both ends, then the outside diameter of the retrograde wire/catheter can be enlarged by antegrade passage of many types of catheters over the retrograde wire/catheter, including a fiberoptic bronchoscope. When a fiberoptic bronchoscope is used, the guidewire must be passed through the distal suction port out the proximal control head; the fiberoptic bronchoscope is then threaded over the wire, under direct vision, into the trachea, the guidewire is released while the trachea (cartilaginous rings, posterior membrane, carina) continues to be visualized, and then the endotracheal is inserted over the fiberoptic bronchoscope stylet.

spontaneously come out the mouth and rarely out of the nose. If the airway is bloody, then a catheter should be used (such as a CVP, epidural or PA catheter), because air can be ejected through the hub of the catheter by syringe so that the tip of the catheter in the pharynx can be more easily identified by locating the emerging and surrounding bubbles of air (forms a rosette). After pulling both ends of the guidewire or catheter stylet taut, the ET tube should be passed over the retrograde guidewire/catheter into the trachea. The endotracheal tube usually enters the trachea, but may not because the tip of the bevel impinges on the right vocal cord at 3 o'clock (or perhaps anteriorly on the epiglottis/vallecula). Rotating the tube 90° counter-clockwise, so that tip of the bevel is at 12 o'clock, usually allows the ET tube to slip into the trachea. If the ET tube still will not go over (follow) the retrograde guidewire/catheter into the trachea, then the outside diameter of the retrograde wire/catheter can be enlarged by passing some type of slightly larger catheter, antegrade, over the wire, such as a nasogastric tube, suction catheter, the plastic sheath that houses guidewires in unopened packages, CVP catheter, epidural catheter, or fiberoptic bronchoscope (wire passed up the suction port of the fiberoptic bronchoscope; the author's best choice) (Fig. 5). The bigger the outside diameter of the stylet in relation to the inside diameter of the endotracheal tube, the greater the chance the endotracheal tube will follow the stylet into the trachea (thus, the rationale for enlarging the outside diameter of a retrograde wire with an antegrade catheter). In other words, the guide is enlarged by a one-step Seldinger-type technique. The advantages of a fiberoptic bronchoscope that make it uniquely suited to be an antegrade guide (over the initial retrograde guide) are 1) the central position of the suction port (fiberoptic bronchoscope cannot railroad or ricochet very far off the retrograde guide in any one direction); 2) the small internal diameter of the fiberoptic bronchoscope is very nearly equal to the outside diameter of the retrograde guide (fiberoptic bronchoscope cannot railroad or ricochet very far off the retrograde guide in any one direction): 3) the outside diameter of the fiberoptic bronchoscope makes it a large sturdy guide for the endotracheal tube and 4) the intubationist can directly visualize the entrance into and continued presence of the fiberoptic bronchoscope in the trachea.

REFERENCES

1. Fink RB: The Human Larynx—A Functional Study. New York, Raven Press, 1975
2. Rogers S, Benumof JL: New and easy fiberoptic endoscopy-aided tracheal intubation. Anesthesiology 59:569-72, 1983
3. Siverajan M, Fink RB: The position and the state of the larynx during general anesthesia and muscle paralysis Anesthesiology 72.439-42, 1990
4. Benumof JL, Scheller MS: The importance of transtracheal jet ventilation in the management of the difficult airway. Anesthesiology 72:828-33, 1990
5. McLellan KJ, Gordon P, Khawaja S: Percutaneous transtracheal high frequency jet ventilation as an aid to difficult intubation. Can Anaesth Soc J. 35:404-5, 1988

6. Baraka A: Transtracheal jet ventilation during fiberoptic intubation under general anesthesia. Anesth Analg 65:1091-92, 1986

7. Benumof JL: Anesthesia for Thoracic Surgery. Philadelphia, WB Saunders, 1987, p. 331

8. Woods AM, Lander CJ: Abolition of gagging and the hemodynamic response to awake laryngoscopy. Anesthesiology 67:A220, 1987

9. Barton S, Williams JD: Glossopharyngeal nerve block. Arch Otolaryngol 93:186-88, 1971

10. Cooper M, Watson RL: An improved regional anesthetic technique for perioral endoscopy. Anesthesiology 43:372-4, 1975

11. Williams RT, Maltby JR: Airway intubator. Anesth Analg 61:309, 1982

12. Rogers SN, Benumof JL: New and easy techniques for fiberoptic endoscopy-aided tracheal intubation. Anesthesiology 59:569-72, 1983

13. King HK, Wang LF, Khan AK: Translaryngeal guided intubation for difficult intubation. Crit Care Med 15:869-71, 1987

14. Freund PA, Rooke A, Schwind H: Retrograde intubation with a modified Eschman stylet. Anesth Analg 67:596-606, 1988

MANAGEMENT OF THE DIFFICULT AIRWAY PART III: THE ANESTHETIZED PATIENT WHOSE TRACHEA IS DIFFICULT TO INTUBATE, TRANSTRACHEAL JET VENTILATION, THE DIFFICULT EXTUBATION AND JET STYLETS

J. L. Benumof

I. THE ANESTHETIZED PATIENT WHO IS DIFFICULT TO INTUBATE

There are four general situations in which an anesthesiologist will be required to intubate an unconscious or generally anesthetized patient who has a very difficult airway. First, the patient may already be unconscious (e.g., posttrauma) or generally anesthetized (e.g., drug overdose). Second, the patient may absolutely refuse to be intubated awake (e.g., an intoxicated combative patient). Third, and perhaps the largest category, the anesthesiologist failed to recognize intubation difficulty on the preoperative evaluation. Fourth, and perhaps a subset of number 2 above, pediatric patients older than several months usually require general anesthesia for ETT intubation irrespective of the findings on preoperative airway evaluation. Of course, even in situations 1, 2, and 4 above, the preoperative airway evaluation is very important because the findings may still dictate the choice of ETT intubation technique.

All of the ETT intubation techniques that were described for the awake patient can be used in the unconscious or generally anesthetized patient without modification. However, conventional and fiberoptic laryngoscopy may be slightly more difficult in the paralyzed anesthetized patient compared to the awake patient because the larynx may move to a more anterior position (1) and the upper airway structures may coalesce into a horizontal plane instead of separating out in a vertical plane (2,3).

In the generally anesthetized patient who has proven to be difficult to intubate, it is of paramount importance to maintain gas exchange between intubation attempts by mask ventilation and during intubation

179

T. H. Stanley and R. J. Sperry (eds.), Anesthesia and the Lung 1992, 179–191.
© 1992 *Kluwer Academic Publishers.*

attempts whenever possible. Ventilation by mask must be interrupted when intubation is by conventional laryngoscopy and when the illuminating stylet is used. With a retrograde technique it is ordinarily necessary to interrupt ventilation only when bringing the retrograde guide out of the mouth and when the antegrade guide (including a fiberoptic bronchoscope) and/or ETT is being passed over the retrograde guide. Ventilation of the anesthetized patient may be maintained during a nasal fiberoptic intubation by placing a ETT adaptor into an oral airway (Nosworthy chimney) (4), or Airway Intubator (5), or soft nasopharyngeal airway in the other naries and connecting the ETT adaptor to the anesthesia circle system.

Positive pressure ventilation may be continuously maintained during fiberoptic endoscopy-aided orotracheal intubation by using an anesthesia mask that has a special fiberoptic instrument port that is covered by a self-sealing diaphragm (instead of the standard anesthesia mask) as well as using an airway intubator (instead of the standard oropharyngeal airway) (3,6). While a positive pressure seal is continuously maintained with the anesthesia mask with fiberoptic diaphragm, the fiberoptic instrument is passed through the self-sealing port, the airway intubator and into the trachea. The ETT is pushed over the fiberoptic stylet (Fig. 1). Since ventilation can be continuously maintained around the fiberoptic instrument throughout this intubation procedure, it is the author's choice in the anesthetized patient who cannot be intubated conventionally.

It is extremely important to realize that the amount of laryngeal edema and/or bleeding will very likely increase after every intubation attempt; although laryngeal edema and bleeding can occur with any intubation method it is most common after use of a laryngoscope or retraction blade. Consequently, if there does not appear to be anything really new or different that can be atraumatically and quickly tried (better sniff position, new blade, new technique, etc.) after a few failed intubation attempts, and ventilation by mask can still be maintained, it would be prudent at this point to cease attempting to intubate the patient and either awaken the patient, do the case by mask or perform a tracheostomy or cricothyrotomy before the ability to ventilate the patient by mask is lost (see Part I, Fig. 2). In fact, the most common scenario in the respiratory catastrophes in the ASA Closed Claim Study was the development of progressive difficulty in

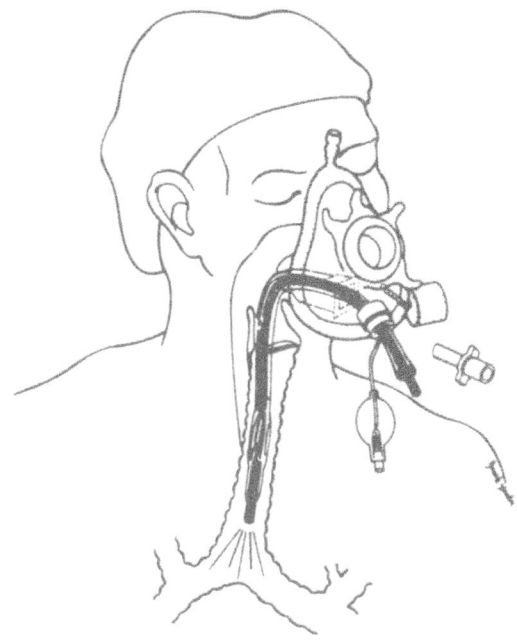

Figure 1. Schematic diagram showing the use of the anesthesia mask with diaphragm and oral Airway Intubator as aids to fiberoptic tracheal intubation in an anesthetized (and paralyzed) patient. The procedure is the same as in Figure 3, in Part II except that the fiberoptic scope and endotracheal tube have been introduced through the diaphragm in the anesthesia mask. After the endotracheal tube is in place, the fiberoptic scope is removed from within the endotracheal tube and the anesthesia mask with diaphragm is removed over the endotracheal tube (before the endotracheal tube adaptor is connected). Removal of the oral airway intubator is optional as in Figure 3 in Part II. Reproduced with permission from reference 3.

ventilating by mask in between persistent and prolonged failed intubation attempts that ultimately resulted in the inability to ventilate by mask and provide gas exchange (7). If the surgical procedure does not have to be performed, awakening the patient and doing the intubation another day will allow for better planning (e.g., change in technique). Still many other cases may be done (and may have to be done) with mask ventilation (e.g., Caesarian section) if mask ventilation remains reasonably easy. Finally, some cases, if they have to be done that day, will have to have the trachea intubated by tracheostomy or cricothyrotomy (e.g., thoracotomy, intracranial/head/neck cases and use of the prone position).

182

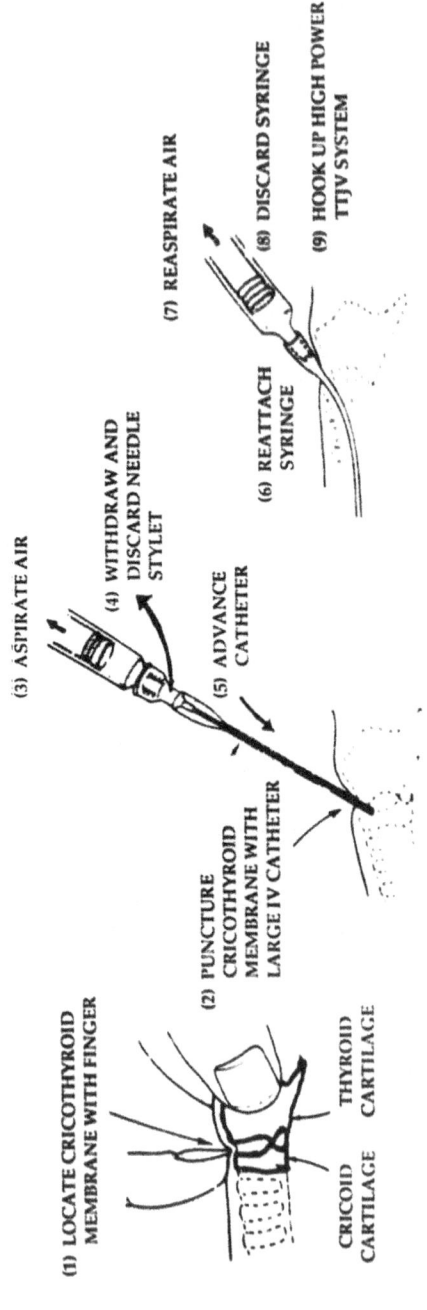

Figure 2. Cricothyroid membrane puncture with an IV catheter was accomplished by: 1) stabilizing the trachea and locating the cricothyroid membrane by finger palpation; 2) puncture of cricothyroid membrane with an IV catheter; 3) aspirating for air to assure intratracheal position and then 4) removing the needle and syringe and 5) advancing the catheter; 6) reattaching a syringe to the catheter; 7) re-aspirating air to confirm proper position; 8) discarding syringe and 9) hooking up to a high powered O₂ source for TTJV. Modified with permission from reference 9.

II. THE LOST AIRWAY AND TRANSTRACHEAL
JET VENTILATION (TTJV)

The cannot ventilate via mask, cannot intubate situation has been responsible for a previously irreducible 1-28% of all deaths associated with anesthesia (7). Thus, the incidence of cannot ventilate by mask, cannot intubate has ranged 0.01-2.0/10,000 anesthetics (7).

A. TRANSTRACHEAL JET VENTILATION

There is widespread agreement in the literature that percutaneous transtracheal jet ventilation (TTJV) using a large intravenous catheter inserted through the cricothyroid membrane is a very simple, relatively safe, extremely effective treatment of choice for the desperate cannot ventilate via mask, cannot intubate situation (7). To initiate this treatment an intravenous (IV) catheter is inserted through the cricothyroid membrane pointing at an angle, 30° caudad to a line perpendicular to the trachea (Fig. 2) (8,9). After the IV catheter enters the trachea (identified by aspiration of air by a 20 ml syringe attached to the IV catheter), the catheter is fully advanced caudally in the trachea while the needle stylet is removed (just as is done with inserting the same catheter in a peripheral vein) (Fig. 2) (8,9). Whatever TTJV system is attached to the hub of the IV catheter (see next paragraph for acceptable systems), it is important to stress that the O_2 source must be high power (near 50 PSI) and connected to the IV catheter by noncompliant tubing; it is not possible to adequately ventilate a patient through an IV catheter manually by squeezing an Ambu or reservoir bag, or by using a conventional ventilator, or if there is corrugated compliant tubing in the system. Another way of making the same point is to realize that one PSI equals 68.4 cm H_2O and 50 PSI equals 3,420 cm H_2O; 50 psi is the only way to get an adequate tidal volume through an IV catheter in a short period of time. Equally important, it should be understood that the only way that the jetted inspired gas can be exhaled is through the natural airway and attempts to maintain the natural airway must be continued. The chest must be carefully observed to rise and fall after each jet (just as with any other type of IPPB).

Many systems have been suggested for TTJV and, in particular, a great deal has been written about how to connect the hub of a transtracheal IV catheter to a ventilatory source. Distillation of this literature reveals that there are three basic acceptable TTJV systems that work reliably and can be easily and inexpensively assembled from readily available materials. The first acceptable TTJV system consists of a jet injector (blow gun) powered by a regulated (Table 1, reproduced with permission from reference 7) or unregulated central wall oxygen pressure. The advantage of using wall pressure to power the jet injector (provided the system is already plugged in) is the guaranteed immediate availability of a pre-assembled, reliable, tightly jointed system to attach to the transtracheal IV catheter. The advantage of a regulated wall pressure is the ability to minimize barotrauma, especially in pediatric patients. The second TTJV system consists of a jet injector powered by an oxygen tank regulator. Tank regulators may be high flow or low flow. A high flow O_2 tank regulator may be set at 50 psi and will deliver O_2 at the same flow rate as wall pressure. A low flow regulator (commonly on O_2 transport tanks) will provide adequate jet ventilation tidal volumes if an I:E=1:1 is used, where a unit of time=one second (i.e., a respiratory rate of 30 breath/min) (10). The advantage of a tank powered system is that it is mobile and can be used in anesthetizing locations that do not have a central (wall) source of high pressure oxygen. However, for this system to be effective, it must be standing by, or brought to these anesthetizing locations prior to the induction of anesthesia. The third TTJV system utilizes the anesthesia machine flush valve as the jet injector. However, only the Dräger and not an Ohmeda machine can be used in this way; the former provides 45 L/min whereas the latter provides only 7-8 L/min (11). The Dräger anesthesia machine flush valve can, of course, be powered either by a wall or tank high pressure oxygen source. The fresh gas outlet of the Dräger anesthesia machine (now an industry wide standard 15 mm male outlet) is connected to a noncompliant oxygen supply tubing by a standard 15 mm endotracheal tube adaptor, which fits a 4 or 5 mm endotracheal tube (see Table 2, reproduced with permission from reference 7). The noncompliant oxygen supply tubing allows for bypass of the very compliant reservoir bag and corrugated tubing of the anesthesia circle system. This third TTJV system is completed by connecting the oxygen supply tubing to the TTJV

Table 1. Transtracheal jet ventilation systems using regulated wall O_2 pressure.

Transtracheal Jet Ventilation (TTJV) Systems	Component-to-Component Schematic	Part	Company	Model Number
TTJV using jet injector powered by regulated central wall O_2 pressure	Wall O_2 pressure [1]	[1] Chemetron wall O_2 quick disconnect + 1/4" OD hose barb	Tri-Anim	11-01-0003
	[2] O_2 hose	[2] Chemetron O_2 hose	Tri-Anim	15-11-0001
	[3]	[3] 1/4" ID hose barb + 1/8" NPT adapter	Western Enterpr.	MH-7
	[4] Regular	[4] Miniregulator gauge 0-50 psi	Bird Bird	2322 6765
	[5]	[5] 1/8" NPT male reducing adapter + 1/4" NPT female adapter	Western Enterpr.	MA-9
	[6] Air hose	[6] Air hose 25'	Lawson or Sears	81070 or 9HT16224
	[7] Jet injector	[7] Jet injector	Lawson or Sears	11903 or 9HT16235
	[8]	[8] 1/8" NPT male adapter + 1/4" ID hose barb	Western Enterpr.	MH-7
	[9] O_2 tubing	[9] Tygon tubing R-3603	Cole-Parmer	6408-50
	[10]	[10] 1/4" hose barb + male luer lok	Becton-Dickinson	9067
	[11] TTJV Catheter	[11] Intravenous catheter with standard hub		

Table 2. Transtrachael jet ventilating systems using anesthesia machine fresh gas outlet and flush valve.

Transtracheal Jet Ventilation (TTJV) Systems	Component-to-Component Schematic	Part	Company	Model No.
TTJV using anesthesia machine fresh gas outlet and flush valveTTJV using anesthesia machine fresh gas outlet and flush valve	1 Anesthesia machine fresh gas outlet 2 O_2 Supply tubing 3 4 TTJV Catheter	1 15-mm ET tube adapter for 4-mm ID ET tube	Many companies	
		2 O_2 supply tubing	Many companies	
		3 1/4" hose barb male luer lok or 3 cut-off 1-ml syringe	Becton-Dickinson	9067
		4 Intravenous catheter with standard hub		

Table 2). catheter; although this may be accomplished in many ways, our permanent TTJV sets have a bonded Luer lock/hose barb connector (Left #3. As a quick makeshift alternative, the TTJV catheter/O_2 supply tubing connection can be accomplished by cutting the barrel of a 1 ml syringe with scissors and inserting the cut end of the barrel into the oxygen supply tubing, and the other uncut standard male end into the standard female intravenous catheter hub (Right #3, Table 2). The advantage of this third TTJV system is that it can be preassembled and used wherever there is a Dräger anesthesia machine but, of course, to be effective it must be ready to go at all times.

B. Conclusions Concerning the Management of the Difficult Airway Algorithm

Difficulty in managing the airway is the single most important cause of anesthesia-related major morbidity and mortality. Successful management of a difficult airway begins with recognizing that an airway may be difficult and every anesthesiologist should examine every patient for degree of mouth opening and structures visible upon mouth opening, how large the mandibular space is, and the ability of the patient assume the sniff position. If an intubation and/or ventilation by mask is considered to have a good chance of being difficult, then the airway should be secured while the patient is still awake. In order for an awake intubation to be successful, it is absolutely essential that the patient be properly prepared; otherwise, the anesthesiologist will simply fulfill a self-defeating prophecy. Once the patient is properly prepared, it is likely that any one of a number of ETT intubation techniques will be successful. If the patient is anesthetized and/or paralyzed and intubation is found to be difficult, many repeated attempts at intubation should be avoided because the ability to ventilate by mask may be lost due to the progressive development of laryngeal edema and hemorrhage. After several attempts at intubation, it may be best to either awaken the patient, do a semi-elective tracheostomy, or do the case by mask ventilation. In the event that the ability to ventilate by mask is lost and the patient still cannot be ventilated, transtracheal jet ventilation should be instituted immediately.

III. THE DIFFICULT EXTUBATION AND JET STYLETS

Recently the concept and use of a jet stylet during extubation of a patient who will likely be very difficult to ventilate by mask and/or reintubate has been described (12-14). A jet stylet is a small internal diameter semi-rigid hollow catheter (such as a commercial tube changer), that is inserted into an in-situ endotracheal tube (ETT). After the ETT is withdrawn over the jet stylet, the hollow catheter can be used for jet ventilation using an appropriately sized IV catheter (preferred) (7) or a 2-3 mm ETT adaptor (i.e., the jet function) or as an intratracheal stylet for reintubation (i.e., the stylet function). The jet function often allows additional time to assess the need for the reintubation stylet function.

A hollow catheter that makes a good jet stylet is a tube exchanger. Tube exchangers may be adapted for jet ventilation by wedging an appropriately sized IV catheter into the proximal end of a tube exchanger or by placing a short length of an appropriately sized endotracheal tube ETT connected to a female Luer lock-barbed cone adaptor over the proximal end of the tube exchanger (14). The 50 psi flow rate through all sized tube exchangers is adequate for jet ventilation (14).

When utilizing the reintubation stylet function, it has heretofore been thought that after a new ETT has been inserted over the jet stylet, the jet stylet would have to be removed in order to allow connection of the new ETT to the breathing circuit and confirmation tracheal placement of the ETT (by capnography, breath sounds, etc.). However, removing the jet stylet to confirm proper ETT placement means that both the jet and stylet functions are now lost and in cases where the ETT is not in the trachea, a cannot ventilate by mask, cannot intubate situation may develop.

There are two different methods for preserving the intratracheal location of the stylet while concurrently confirming intratracheal placement of the reintubation ETT (15). First, if the tube exchanger is inserted through a self-sealing diaphragm in the elbow connector to the ETT (i.e., the commonly available elbow connector used for fiberoptic bronchoscopy), then ventilation may be maintained and confirmation of the ETT position may be made while the tube exchanger remains in the ETT (Fig. 3).

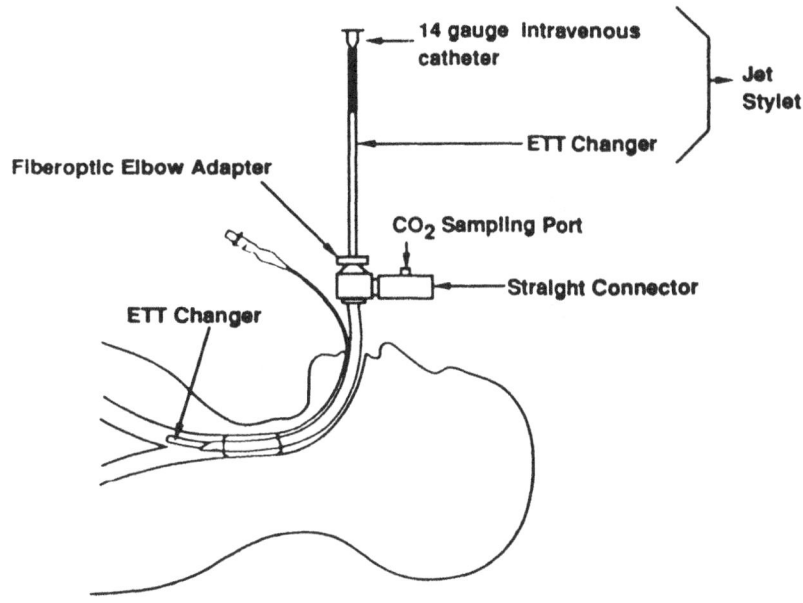

Figure 3. Schematic diagram of the method to preserve the intratracheal location of the endotracheal tube (ETT) changer during confirmation of intratracheal placement of ETT. The ETT changer is passed through a self-sealing diaphragm in a fiberoptic elbow adaptor. With this method, positive pressure ventilation and CO_2 sampling may be around the ETT changer but within the ETT.

Second, an alternative method of preserving the intratracheal location of the jet stylet while the position of the new ETT is confirmed would be to use a straight connector to the Y piece of an anesthesia circle system and then thread the ETT changer retrograde through the straight connector into either the inspiratory or expiratory limb of the circle system (Fig. 4). This is a perfectly viable option in the OR when a bronchoscopy elbow connector is not available; however, the method is a little more difficult to use since the proximal end of the ETT changer may intermittently hang up on the corrugations of the anesthesia circle tubing.

Finally, a fiberoptic bronchoscope (FOB) may be effectively used as a jet stylet (16). In addition to allowing for jet ventilation (via the suction port) and serving as a reintubation stylet, the FOB provides the additional advantages of allowing for suctioning of the airway, continuously insufflating oxygen, and visualization of the entire airway during withdrawal of the FOB.

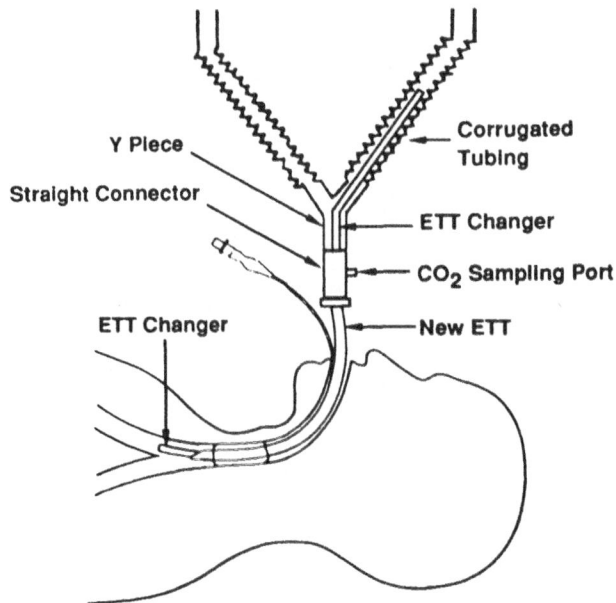

Figure 4. Schematic diagram of method to preserve the intratracheal location of the endotracheal tube (ETT) changer during confirmation of intratracheal placement of ETT. The ETT changer is passed up one of the corrugated tubing limbs of the anesthesia circle system. With this method, positive pressure ventilation and CO_2 sampling may be around the ETT changer but within the ETT.

The FOB extubation method for patients for whom there is a high degree of suspicion of airway damage/edema involves a controlled, gradual, but reversible withdrawal from the airway. First, an airleak around the deflated ETT cuff is confirmed for a few minutes of cuff deflation; the airleak rules out the possibility that a reactive hyperemia at the cuff level could cause airway swelling to at least the outside diameter of the ETT. Next, the ETT is removed over an FOB and the ability of the patient to easily breathe around the FOB for a few minutes is ascertained; the ability to easily breathe around the FOB rules out the possibility that the airway, at any level, has significantly narrowed around the outside diameter of the FOB. During this period the patient may be jet ventilated to any level desired. During this period of breathing around the FOB, oxygen can just as easily be continuously insufflated down the suction port of the FOB. Finally, the fiberoptic bronchoscope allows for diagnostic evaluation of the larynx upon exiting the trachea. We suggest that this extubation method be used in patients in whom access to the upper airway is limited (e.g., by halo traction) and in whom the risk of airway edema is increased (e.g., patients who have undergone an anterior approach to repair a cervical fracture).

REFERENCES

1. Sivarajan M, Fink RB: The position and the state of the larynx during general anesthesia and muscle paralysis. Anesthesiology 72: 439-442, 1990
2. Fink RB: The Human Larynx - A Functional Study. New York, Raven Press, 1975
3. Rogers S, Benumof JL: New and easy fibreoptic endoscopy-aided tracheal intubation. Anesthesiology 59:569-572, 1983
4. Coe PA, King TA, Towey RM: Teaching guided fiberoptic nasotracheal intubation. Anaesthesia 43:410-413, 1988
5. Williams RT, Maltby JR: Airway intubator. Anesth Analg 61:309, 1982
6. Patil V, Stehling LC, Zauder HL: Mechanical aids for a fiberoptic endoscopy. Anesthesiology 57:69-70, 1982
7. Benumof JL, Scheller MS: The Importance of transtracheal jet ventilation in the management of the difficult airway. Anesthesiology 71:769-778, 1989
8. Sharoff PK, Skerman JH, Benumof JL: Transtracheal ventilation. Chapter 6. In Clinical Procedures in Anesthesia and Intensive Care. Benumof JL (ed). Philadelphia, JB Lippincott (in press, 1990)
9. Cote' CJ, Eavey RD, Todres ID, Jones DE: Cricothyroid membrane puncture: Oxygenation and ventilation in a dog model using an intravenous catheter. Crit Care 16:616, 1988
10. Gaughan S, Ozaki G, Benumof JL: Can a low flow O_2 regulator to be used for transtracheal jet ventilation? Anesthesiology (in Press)
11. Gaughan S, Ozaki GT, Benumof JL: The Dräger but not the Ohmeda anesthesia machine may be used for transtracheal jet ventilation. Anesthesiology (in Press)
12. Bedger RC, Chang JL: A jet-stylet endotracheal catheter for difficult airway management. Anesthesiology 66:221-223, 1987
13. Benumof JL, Gaughan S, Ozaki GT: Adapting a jet stylet for jet ventilation. Anesthesiology (in press)
14. Gaughan S, Benumof JL, Ozaki GT: Quantitating the jet function of a jet stylet. Anesthesiology (in press)
15. Goskowicz R, Gaughan S, Ozaki GT: It is not necessary to remove a jet stylet in order to confirm endotracheal tube position. J Clin Anes (in press)
16. Wheeler S, Fontenot R, Gaughan S: Use of a fiberoptic bronchoscope as a jet stylet. Anesthesiology Review (in press)

INFLUENCE OF ANESTHETICS ON PULMONARY GAS EXCHANGE

B. E. Marshall and C. Marshall

INTRODUCTION

During general anesthesia the arterial oxygen tension (P_aO_2) is often less than expected. This was first emphasized by Bendixen et al. (1) and research into the causes of this observation continue to this day. This work has led to a systematic understanding of the physiologic and patho-physiologic principles involved (2) and the purpose of these three essays is to summarize some aspects of these concepts.

CAUSES OF REDUCED ARTERIAL OXYGEN TENSION

The ability to monitor continuously the inspired and expired gas concentrations and the arterial oxygen saturation has reduced the time delay in recognizing that a problem has developed. It is, therefore, essential to have a systematic approach to diagnosis (3).

If the oxygen saturation is reduced, inspired oxygen (P_IO_2) should be determined and adjusted if necessary.

If P_IO_2 is adequate, then the ventilation and the end-tidal carbon dioxide tension should be evaluated. If the end-tidal PCO_2 is increased, then ventilation is inadequate and if PCO_2 is near zero and/or not changing, then the ventilation may be disconnected or the airway obstructed or misplaced. These are all causes of a decreased alveolar oxygen tension (PAO_2).

If the inspired and alveolar oxygen tensions are satisfactory, then the cause of denaturation is an increased alveolar to arterial oxygen tension difference ($P[A-a]O_2$) for which there are two general causes. The first

193

T. H. Stanley and R. J. Sperry (eds.), Anesthesia and the Lung 1992, 193–202.

is extrapulmonary, primarily a decreased venous oxygen tension. This is due to the cardiac output becoming less than that required for the existing oxygen consumption. Impairment of the tida variation of expired carbon dioxide is suggestive of this mechanism.

The second group of causes of an increased $P(A-a)O_2$ are intrapulmonary ones. These are subdivided into increased shunts ($\dot{Q}s/\dot{Q}_T$) and increased spread of ventilation/perfusion $\dot{V}A/\dot{Q}C$ ratios.

The diagnosis and treatment of the factors that lead to decreased P_IO_2 or PAO_2 is generally straightforward. For the causes of $P(A-a)O_2$ it is necessary to measure the arterial and mixed venous blood gas tension because this allows more precise characterization of the extent of the abnormality and permits identification of the extrapulmonary component. The patient with increased $P(A-a)O_2$ after all these causes and preexisting disease have been excluded are the ones of special interest because in them it is the general anesthetic that results in impaired intrapulmonary gas exchange. Much research has, therefore, been directed at discovering the basis for this impairment.

VENTILATION/PERFUSION

Each of the 300 million alveoli in the human lung are capable of receiving gas and blood. If all of these receive the same proportion of both, the distribution of ventilation/perfusion ratios ($\dot{V}A/\dot{Q}C$) would be homogeneous and no impairment of oxygen exchange would be due to this cause.

However, gravitational (Fig. 1) and non-gravitational factors result in changes in the distribution of regional ventilation and blood flow so that the distribution of $\dot{V}A/\dot{Q}C$ is not homogeneous (4). Some alveoli have greater oxygen tensions than others and the alveoli with the lower oxygen tensions are the ones with the greater blood flow. The latter, together with the sigmoid shape of the oxygen/hemoglobin dissociation curve, causes the arterial oxygen tension resulting when the blood from all the alveolar are mixed together to be less than the oxygen tension resulting when the gas from all the alveolar are mixed together. The greater the inhomogeneity of $\dot{V}A/\dot{Q}C$, the greater the $P(A-a)O_2$. This is a predominant cause of hypoxemia in many chronic lung diseases.

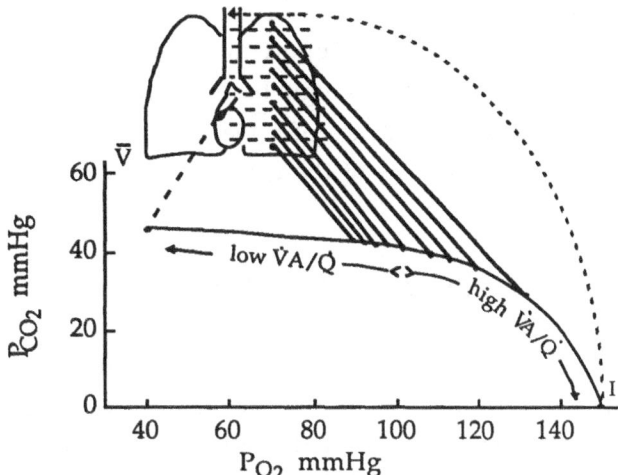

Figure 1. Oxygen-carbon dioxide diagram showing how the change in ventilation-perfusion ratio up the lung determines the regional composition of alveolar gas. The lung is divided into 9 imaginary horizontal slices each of which has its own position on the ventilation-perfusion ratio line. It can be seen that the alveolar PO_2 will increase up the lung in so far as the points move horizontally to the right, and that the alveolar PCO_2 will fall as the points move vertically downwards. Dashed lines show the composition of mixed venous (pulmonary arterial) blood and inspired (tracheal) gas. (From West JB with permission).

Increased abnormality of the distribution of $\dot{V}A/\dot{Q}C$ was, therefore, assumed to be a likely basis for the impaired oxygenation during anesthesia. The earliest and most frequent emphasis for research has been measurement of airway and chest wall mechanics. For all general anesthetics similar changes result on induction whether with inhalational or injectable agents. These changes include reduction of functional residual capacity, small airway closure, reduced lung compliance and more subtle changes in the relationship of the lung to the chest wall and diaphragm (5). However impaired arterial oxygenation is more frequently associated with inhalational rather than injectable agents so changes in lung mechanics could not be a significant explanation (6,7).

The multiple inert gas technique (8) allows the $\dot{V}A/\dot{Q}C$ distribution to be estimated. This technique has been applied to human patients and volunteers. (9,10,11) The results have shown subtle changes in healthy volunteers and animals receiving injectable anesthetics with more substantial changes in patients and animals receiving inhalational anesthetics. In general, the blood flow distribution is shifted to the lower $\dot{V}A/\dot{Q}C$ regions and shunts appear and are increased.

These observations do not support the concept of increased spread of $\dot{V}A/\dot{Q}C$ ratios as the pathophysiologic basis for hypoxemia during anesthesia, rather they provide evidence of a biased increase of blood flow to the least well ventilated regions of the lung when inhalational anesthesia are administered.

SHUNTS ATELECTASIS

Pulmonary shunts result from blood flow passing from the left to the right heart without undergoing alveolar gas exchange. Some fraction is due to bronchial blood flow and thebesian vein drainage but, in the absence of congenital heart disease, the usual cause of pulmonary shunt is blood flow to alveoli that receive little or no ventilation or alveoli that are collapsed (atelectasis).

In the original description of the hypoxemia associated with anesthesia Bendixen et al. (1) suggested atelectasis as the cause but because they were unable to demonstrate the site by roentgenography they suggested that the atelectasis was distributed or miliary. Recently Hedenstierna and his colleagues (12) in a series of studies have demonstrated with CAT scanning that indeed general anesthesia is associated with dependent atelectasis. This, and the previous work with multiple inert gases therefore demonstrated that general anesthesia is associated with atelectasis and increased blood flow to low $\dot{V}A/\dot{Q}C$ regions without greatly influencing the remaining distribution of the $\dot{V}A/\dot{Q}C$ ratios (Fig. 2).

However while this may be the necessary prerequisite cause some additional cause is required to explain the predominant association of impaired oxygenation with inhalational anesthetic agents.

HYPOXIC PULMONARY VASOCONSTRICTION

When atelectasis is deliberately introduced in a lung segment the blood flow to that region decreases. Originally this observation was thought to be due to mechanical effects that cause wrinkling of the blood vessels, but more recent studies have shown that there is no mechanical

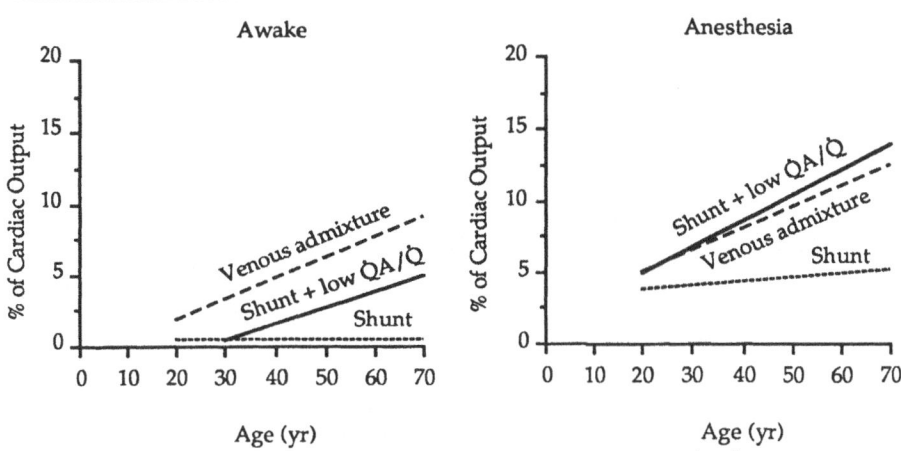

Figure 2. The effects of age and anesthesia on pulmonary shunt and V̇A/Q̇C abnormalities. The upper panel, in the awake state the multiple inert gas techniques reveals very little pulmonary shunt at any age but perfusion to regions of very low V̇A/Q̇C ratio and the increased spread of V̇A/Q̇C ratio (included in venous admixture) are both greater with increasing age. The lower panel, during anesthesia, demonstrates predominant increases in perfusion to the regions of pulmonary shunt and low V̇A/Q̇C ratio at all ages. The data are summarized from the work of Hedenstierna and his colleagues with permission.

effect (13,14) and the entire reduction of blood flow is due to active vaso-constriction resulting from hypoxic pulmonary vasoconstriction (HPV).

The HPV response was first demonstrated by ventilation of lungs with hypoxic gas mixture and alveolar oxygen was thought to be the stimulus but mixed venous and arterial oxygen tensions have now been shown to contribute and the site of action for the hypoxia is the pulmonary vascular smooth muscle cell itself.

For an atelectatic lung the "alveolar" oxygen tension is the same as the mixed venous and therefore the stimulus for HPV is the mixed venous oxygen tension. This tension is normally 40 mmHg, and less during hypoxemia, and this is a powerful and near maximal stimulus for HPV. One of the striking pieces of evidence against the mechanical effect of atelectasis is the observation that the blood flow to an atelectatic lung returns to normal if its mixed venous oxygen tension is increased to 100 mmHg (Fig. 3).

The special interest of HPV for anesthesiologists was emphasized by the reports by Bjertmaes et al. (15), in Norway, Sykes et al. (16) in England and Benumof et al. (17) in the USA that inhalational agents inhibit HPV in a dose-related manner while injectable agents do not. Results both in *vivo* and *in vitro* and in experimental animals and man are now consistent with this conclusion (Fig. 4).

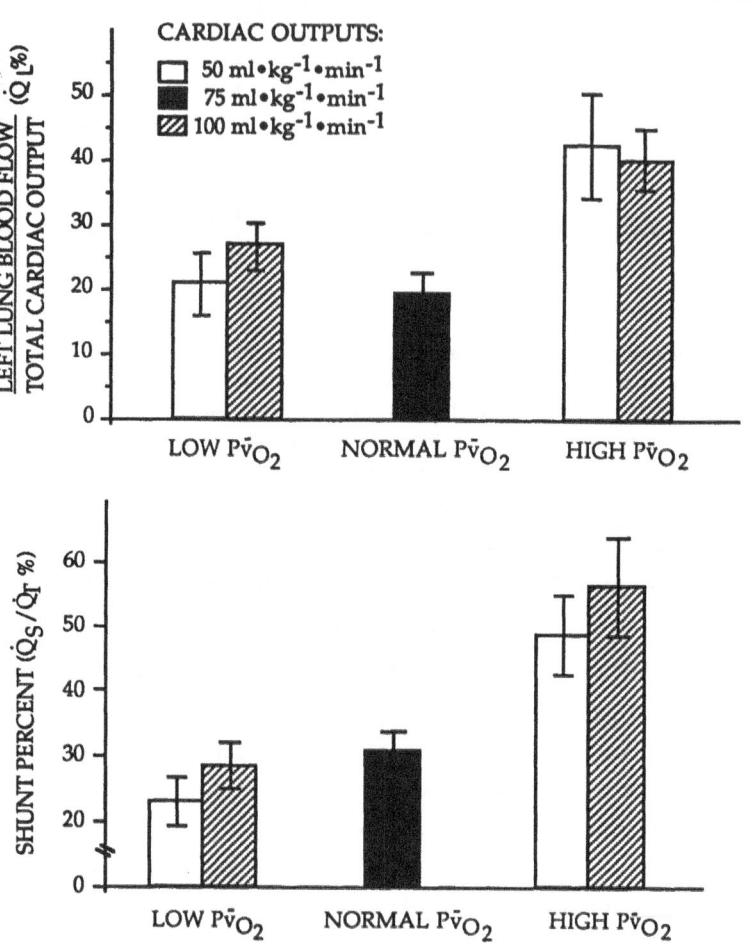

Figure 3. Effects of $P\bar{v}O_2$ on left-lung blood flow as percentage of total blood flow ($\dot{Q}_L\%$) and shunt per cent ($\dot{Q}_S/\dot{Q}_T\%$) during the left-lung atelectasis. Data from three cardiac outputs (CO) are represented. Cardiac output did not influence either $\dot{Q}_L\%$ or $\dot{Q}_S/\dot{Q}_T\%$. *Upper panel:* $\dot{Q}_L\%$ was 19-25% when $P\bar{v}O_2$ was low or normal. When $P\bar{v}O_2$ was raised to greater than 100 mmHg, $\dot{Q}_L\%$ was increased significantly to 40%, nearly the flow expected for normoxic ventilated left lung. *Lower panel:* $\dot{Q}_S/\dot{Q}_T\%$ was significantly greater when $P\bar{v}O_2$ was high than when it was normal or low.

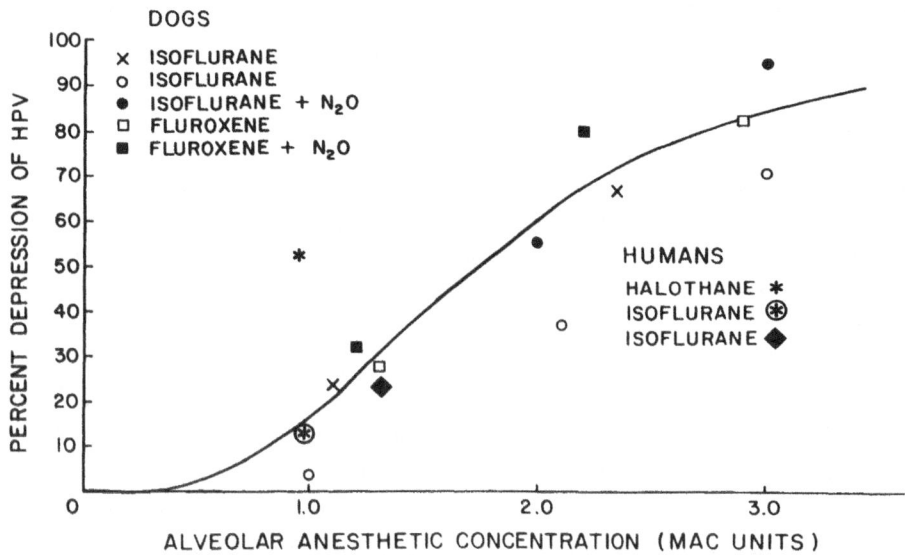

Figure 4. Depression of HPV by Inhalational Anesthetics in Vivo. Studies were of dogs in which the anesthetic was administered only to hypoxic lung segments. Both isoflurane and fluroxene were associated with dose-related depression of HPV, summarized as a sigmoid in the equation. The crosses are for isoflurane, while the open circles and squares refer to isoflurane and fluroxene, respectively, and the closed circles and squares are the same agents in the presence of nitrous oxide. Studies in human subjects are also shown for comparison as indicated.

ONE-LUNG ANESTHESIA

One-lung ventilation during anesthesia for thoracic procedures provides a special opportunity to observe the influence of anesthetic agents on atelectatic lung blood flow and oxygenation. These studies were shown in the previous paragraphs to be consistent with the mean effect expected in experimental animals and man. However, examination of the clinical results in more detail reveals (Table 1) that the important effects are identified better by the variability than by the means. In human subjects these data suggest that halothane more severely impairs HPV while isoflurane imposes more variability, but with either hypoxemia (P_aO_2 less 60 mmHg or 100% oxygen) is to be expected in 10 to 20% of patients (Fig. 5).

Table 1. Intraoperative arterial oxygen tension (mmHg) (mean ± SD).

| Study | Ref. no. | Ventilation | |
		Two-lung	One-lung
Torda et al. (1974)	(27)	377 (472-282)	111 (165-57)
Kerr et al. (1974)	(30)	452 (562-342)	248 (499-47)
Capan et al. (1980)	(28)	376 (469-283)	155 (238-72)
Katz et al. (1982)	(29)	421 (471-372)	210 (334-86)
		437 (524-350)	234 (336-132)
Rogers et al. (1985)	(31)	445 (520-370)	278 (400-156)
Benumof (1987)	(26)	442 (500-384)	232 (329-135)
		484 (533-435)	116 (117-55)

The resemblance between these figures obtained in vivo and results obtained in vitro are so striking as to suggest that halothane and isoflurane exert different modulatory influences on the pulmonary circulation and preliminary evidence implicates the endothelium is the source.

There are other causes of variability during thoracic procedures that can have important influences on HPV. Temperature, Sex, PCO_2, pH, age, disease, trauma and concomitant drugs are some of these secondary variables.

CONCLUSION

General anesthesia is associated with dependent atelectasis in all animals. The blood flow to atelectatic regions is normally reduced by hypoxic pulmonary vasoconstriction so that shunt and low $\dot{V}A/\dot{Q}C$ blood flow is only modestly increased. However inhalational anesthetics, but not injectable anesthetics, inhibit HPV in a dose related manner and this together with the other known modulators of HPV accounts for the occurrence of unexpected hypoxemia during anesthesia with general anesthetic agents.

Acknowledgement

This work was supported in part by NIGMS Grant RO1-GM29628 for NIH.

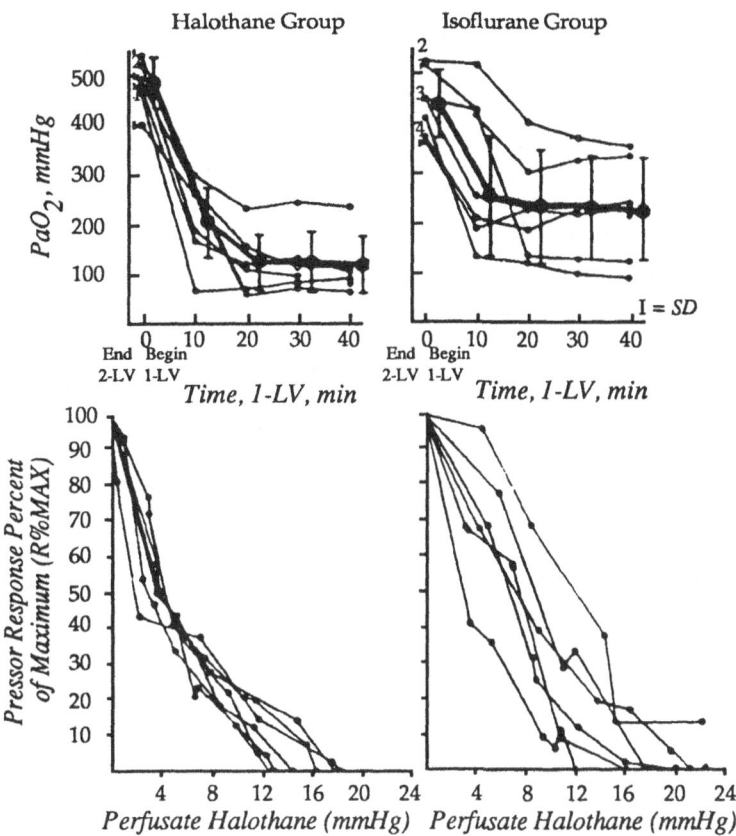

Figure 5. The upper panels demonstrate the changes in P_aO_2 that follow the introduction of one-lung anesthesia (1-LV) with either halothane or isoflurane in human subjects (26). The data suggests that the mean P_aO_2 is lower but the variability is less in the presence of halothane than with isoflurane. This conclusion is consistent with the results of the lower panels for rat lungs ventilated and perfused *in vitro*, where again the difference in variability between the two agents is particularly evident.

REFERENCES

1. Bendixen HH, Hedley-Whyte J, Laver MB: Impaired oxygenation in surgical patients during general anesthesia with controlled ventilation. N Engl J Med 269:991-9, 1963
2. Nunn JF: Applied Respiratory Physiology. 3rd Edition. London, Butterworth, 1987
3. Marshal BE, Wyche MQ: Hypoxemia during and after anesthesia. Anesthesiology 37:178-209, 1972

4. West JB: Ventilation/blood flow and gas exchange. 3rd Edition. Philadelphia, FA Davis, 1983
5. Render K: Anesthesia and the mechanics of respiration. Effects of Anesthesia, Covino BG, Fozzard HA, Render K, Strichartz G (eds.). Bethesda, American Physiological Society, 1985
6. Marshall BE, Hoffmand A, Neufeld GR et al: Influence of induction agent on pulmonary venous admixture during halothane: oxygen anaesthesia with controlled respiration in man. Can Anaesth Soc J 21:461-6, 1974
7. Dueck R, Rathburn M, Harrison WK: Canine V/Q distribution responses to inhalational anesthesia and mechanical ventilation. Anesthesiology 55:127-37, 1981
8. West JB, Wagner PD: Ventilation-perfusion relationships. The Lung Scientific Basis. Vol. 2. Crystal RQ, West JB, Barnes JP, Cherniack NS, Weibel ER (eds.) New York, Reven Press, pp. 1289-1305, 1991
9. Render K, Knopp TJ, Sessler AD, Didier EP: Ventilation-perfusion relationship in young healthy awake and anesthetized-paralyzed man. J Appl Physiol, 47:745-53, 1979
10. Bindslev L, Santesson J, Hedenstierna G: Distribution of inspired gas to each lung in anesthetized human subjects. Acta Anaesthesiol Scand, 25:297-302, 1981
11. Dueck R, Young I, Clausen J, Wagner PD: Altered distribution of pulmonary ventilation and blood flow following induction of inhalational anesthesia. Anesthesiology, 52:113- 25, 1980
12. Klingstedt C, Hedenstierna G, Lindquist H, Strandberg A, Tokics L, Brismar B: The influence of body position and differential ventilation on lung dimension and atelectasis formation in anesthetized man. Acta Anaesthesiol Scand 34:315-22, 1990
13. Miller FL, Chen L, Malmkvist G et al: Mechanical factors do not influence blood flow distribution in atelectasis. Anesthesiology 70:481-8, 1989
14. Domino KB, Wetstein L, Glasser SA et al: Influence of P_VO_2 on blood flow to atelectatic lung. Anesthesiology 59:428-34, 1983
15. Sykes MK, Loh L, Seed RF et al: The effect of inhalational anesthetics on hypoxic pulmonary vasoconstriction and pulmonary vascular resistance in the perfused lungs of dogs and cats. Br J Anaesth 44:776-88, 1972
16. Bjertnaes LJ: Hypoxia-induced vasoconstriction in isolated perfused lungs exposed to injectable or inhalation anesthetics. Acta Anaesthesiol Scand 21:133-47, 1977
17. Benumof JL, Wahrenbrock EA: Local effects of anesthesia on regional hypoxic pulmonary vasoconstriction. Anesthesiology 43:525-32, 1975

ASSESSMENT OF RESPIRATORY MECHANICS DURING MECHANICAL VENTILATION

J. Milic-Emili and N. T. Eissa

INTRODUCTION

There have been relatively few systematic measurements of respiratory mechanics in mechanically ventilated humans, probably reflecting the notion that under these conditions respiratory mechanics data are difficult to obtain. In reality, during mechanical ventilation a detailed analysis of respiratory mechanics can be readily performed. In this article, we will focus on the technique of rapid airway occlusion during constant-flow inflation because it can be used with commercial ventilators (e.g., Siemens Servo 900C). Such ventilators are versatile and have built-in devices for measuring flow and pressure.

TECHNIQUE OF RAPID AIRWAY OCCLUSION DURING CONSTANT-FLOW INFLATION

This technique is essentially a combination of two basic approaches for measuring flow resistance described in 1927 by von Neergaard and Wirz (1), namely the *interrupter* and the *elastic subtraction* methods. If airway pressure (Pao) is measured, this technique allows assessment of (a) static and dynamic elastance of the total respiratory system, and (b) of overall respiratory resistance (Rrs) which can be partitioned into its airway and tissue (viscoelastic) components (2). If esophageal pressure is measured as well, the respiratory system's mechanics can be partitioned into the pulmonary and chest wall components (3,4).

T. H. Stanley and R. J. Sperry (eds.), Anesthesia and the Lung 1992, 203–208.
© 1992 *Kluwer Academic Publishers.*

PRINCIPLES AND MEASUREMENT

Sudden end-inspiratory airway occlusion during constant-flow inflation is associated with an immediate drop in airway pressure from a maximal value (Pmax) to P1, followed by a gradual decay in pressure to an apparent plateau (P plateau) which reflects the static end-inspiratory elastic recoil pressure of the total respiratory system (Pst,rs). Dividing Pmax-P plateau by the flow ($\dot{V}$) immediately preceding the occlusion yields the overall respiratory system's flow resistance (Rrs):

$$Rrs = (Pmax - P\ plateau)/\dot{V} \qquad (1)$$

Since P plateau = Pst,rs, this resistance corresponds to the elastic subtraction method of von Neergaard and Wirz (1).

Dividing Pmax-P1 by the flow immediately preceding the occlusion yields a resistance which corresponds to the interrupter method of von Neergaard and Wirz (1). This has been labelled interrupter (Rint) (5) or minimal (Rmin) (2,3,6) resistance:

$$Rrs,int = (Pmax-P1)/\dot{V} \qquad (2)$$

The resistance of the endotracheal tube and ventilator tubings (plus equipment if any) between the subject's trachea and the site of measurement of airway pressure needs to be subtracted (7) to obtain the Rrs (Eq. 1) and Rrs,int (Eq. 2) of the subject. Alternately, tracheal pressure can be measured directly (8).

The significance of Rrs,int has been recently clarified both in theory (6) and experimentally (3,5). In humans it essentially reflects airway resistance. Indeed, in experiments on open-chested dogs in which alveolar pressure was measured directly using the alveolar capsule technique of Fredberg et al. (9) and Bates et al. (5) have shown that the immediate change in transpulmonary pressure following airway occlusion was a virtually identical to the pre- interruption pressure drop between the trachea and alveoli, indicating that the transpulmonary component of Pmax-P1 reflects only the flow resistance of the airways. This implies that the pulmonary tissues do not contribute to Pmax-P1. Unlike dogs (4), cats (10) and guinea pigs (11), in humans there is no appreciable immediate drop in esophageal pressure following airway occlusion (3), indicating that Rrs,int (Eq. 2) reflects essentially airway resistance (Raw).

The difference between Rrs and Rrs,int, i.e., ΔRrs, reflects the slow post-occlusion decay in airway pressure [ΔRrs = (P1 - P plateau)/$\dot{V}$]. This may be due to "pendelluft" within the lung (6,12), or viscoelastic phenomena within the pulmonary and chest wall tissues (2-5,13,14). If there are time constant inequalities within the lung during inflation, the alveolar pressure will be higher in the lung regions with short time constant relative to the alveoli with long time constant. In this case, during occlusion at end-inspiration there will be static readjustment of regional dynamic volume and pressure differences resulting in a decay in post-occlusion pressure, a phenomenon termed "pendelluft" (6,12). In normal lungs the contribution of "pendelluft" to ΔRrs is probably negligible but may become prominent in ICU patients with chronic obstructive pulmonary disease (15,16). In normal subjects, ΔRrs is probably due mainly to viscoelastic behavior of the pulmonary (9) and chest wall tissues (2,3,13,14). At normal resting flow rates, ΔRrs is the major component of Rrs (2,3).

In the absence of intrinsic PEEP (PEEPi) (17-19), the static elastance of the total respiratory system (Est,rs) can be computed by dividing the end-inspiratory Pst,rs (Pst,rs = P plateau) by the corresponding inflation volume ($\Delta\dot{V}$). If PEEP and/or PEEPi are present, Est,rs is given by (17):

$$Est,rs = (Pst,rs - PEEP - PEEPi)/\Delta\dot{V} \qquad (3)$$

PEEPi can be determined by occluding the airway at end-expiration until a plateau in Pao is obtained (17-19).

Dynamic respiratory system elastance (Edyn,rs) is obtained by dividing the difference in Pao between points of zero flow and the tidal volume delivered by the ventilator. In the absence of PEEPi, Edyn,rs is given by (4):

$$Edyn,rs = (P1 - PEEP)/\Delta\dot{V} \qquad (4)$$

where P1 is the airway pressure immediately following end- inspiratory airway occlusion. If PEEPi is present, the airway pressure at the onset of inspiratory flow should be subtracted from P1 (15).

The technique of rapid airway occlusion during constant-flow inflation thus allows a detailed assessment of respiratory mechanics. This topic has been previously reviewed in detail (20).

FLOW AND VOLUME DEPENDENCE OF RESISTANCE

The relationship between respiratory system resistance and flow is commonly described in terms of Rohrer's equation: $Rrs = K_1 + K_2\dot{V}$ (21). As a result, a basic tenet of respiratory mechanics is that Rrs <u>increases</u> with $\dot{V}$. However, results on anesthetized-paralyzed animals (4,10) and humans (2,3) indicate that this is true only in terms of Rrs,int which in humans essentially reflects airway resistance (Raw):

$$Rrs,int = Raw = K_1 + K_2\dot{V} \qquad (5)$$

In contrast, Rrs at fixed inflation volume actually decreases with flow. This is also true in patients with chronic obstructive pulmonary disease (COPD) and adult respiratory distress syndrome (ARDS) (22).

The decrease of Rrs with increasing $\dot{V}$ is due to the fact that ΔRrs (i.e., the so-called tissue resistance) declines with increasing $\dot{V}$. The nature of this phenomenon is not fully understood. Barnas et al. (13,14) attributed it to "plastoelastic, linear viscoelastic" behavior of the respiratory system, as originally proposed by Hildebrandt (23). D'Angelo et al. (2,3) and Bates et al. (24) believe that it is mainly due to the viscoelastic compartment within the pulmonary and chest wall tissues which has a long time constant. "Pendelluft" should also result in a decrease of $\dot{V}$Rrs with increasing flow (12). However, in normal subjects "pendelluft" probably plays a relatively small role. In patients with abnormalities of pulmonary mechanics its role may become important.

Another basic tenet of respiratory mechanics is that flow resistance of the respiratory system *decreases* with increasing lung volume. Using the body plethysmographic technique, Briscoe and Dubois (25) have shown that airway resistance decreases with increasing lung volume. This, as expected is also true in terms of Rrs,int (2-4,10). By contrast, Rrs increases with increasing lung volume in anesthetized cats (10), dogs (4) and humans (2,3), as well as patients with ARDS (22).

The marked flow, volume, and time dependence of Rrs,int, Rrs and ΔRrs implies that, for meaningful comparison, measurements of resistance should be standardized. Such standardization has not been made in previous studies on ICU patients (15,16).

TECHNICAL CONSIDERATIONS

The technical requirements for accurate measurement of resistance using the technique of rapid airway occlusion during constant-flow inflation (RAO method) have been previously discussed in detail (2-4,10,26,27). The most important requirement is to have a valve with a very fast occlusion time (less than 10 ms) otherwise corrections have to be made (2-4,26).

REFERENCES

1. Neergaard K, von, Wirz K: Die Messung der Strömungswiderstand in der Atemwege des Menschen insbesondere bei Asthma und Emphysema. Z Klin Med 105:51-82, 1927
2. D'Angelo E, Calderini E, Torri G, et al: Respiratory mechanics in anesthetized paralyzed humans: effects of flow, volume and time. J Appl Physiol 67:1556-64, 1989
3. D'Angelo E, Robatto FM, Calderini E, et al: Pulmonary and chest wall mechanics in anesthetized paralyzed humans. J Appl Physiol 70:2602-10, 1991
4. Similowski T, Levy P, Corbeil C, et al: Viscoelastic behaviour of lung and chest wall in dogs determined by flow interruption. J Appl Physiol 67:2219-29, 1989
5. Bates JHT, Ludwig MS, Sly PD, et al: Interrupter resistance elucidated by alveolar pressure measurement in open-chest normal dogs. J Appl Physiol 64:408-14, 1988
6. Bates JHT, Rossi A, Milic-Emili J: Analysis of the behaviour of the respiratory system with constant inspiratory flow. J Appl Physiol 58:1840-8, 1985
7. Behrakis PK, Higgs BC, Baydur A, et al: Respiratory mechanics during halothane anesthesia and anesthesia-paralysis in humans. J Appl Physiol 55:1085-92, 1983
8. Don HF, Robson JG: The mechanics of the respiratory system during anesthesia: The effect of atropine and carbon dioxide. Anesthesiology 26:168-78, 1965
9. Fredberg JJ, Ingram RH, Castille RG, et al: Nonhomogeneity of lung response to inhaled histamine assessed with alveolar capsules. J Appl Physiol 58:1914-22, 1985
10. Kochi T, Okubo S, Zin WA, Milic-Emili J: Flow and volume dependence of pulmonary mechanics in anesthetized cats. J Appl Physiol 64:2636-46, 1988
11. Martins MA, Saldiva PHN, Caldeira MPR, et al: Respiratory system, lung, and chest wall mechanics in guinea pigs. Brazilian J Med Biol Res 21:353-63, 1988
12. Otis AB, McKerrow CB, Bartlett RA, et al: Mechanical factors in distribution of pulmonary ventilation. J Appl Physiol 8:427-43, 1956

13. Barnas GM, Yoshino K, Loring SH, Mead J: Impedance and relative displacements of the relaxed chest wall up to 4 Hz. J Appl Physiol 62:71-81, 1987

14. Barnas GM, Yoshino K, Stamenovic D, et al: Chest wall impedance partitioned into rib cage and diaphragm-abdominal pathways. J Appl Physiol 66:350-9, 1989

15. Rossi A, Gottfried SB, Higgs BD, et al: Respiratory mechanics in mechanically ventilated patients. J Appl Physiol 58:1849-58, 1985

16. Broseghini C, Brandolese R, Poggi R, et al: Respiratory mechanics during the first day of mechanical ventilation in patients with pulmonary edema and chronic airway obstruction. Am Rev Respir Dis 138:355-61, 1988

17. Rossi A, Gottfried SB, Zocchi L, et al: Measurement of static compliance of the total respiratory system in patients with acute respiratory failure during mechanical ventilation. Am Rev Respir Dis 131:672-7, 1985

18. Jonson B, Nördstrom L, Olsson SG, Akerback D: Monitoring of ventilation and lung mechanics during automatic ventilation. A new device. Bull Eur Physiopathol Respir 11:729-43, 1975

19. Pepe PE, Marini JJ: Occult positive end-expiratory pressure in mechanically ventilated patients with airflow obstruction. Am Rev Respir Dis 126:166-70, 1982

20. Milic-Emili J, Robatto FM, Bates JHT: Respiratory mechanics in anesthesia. Br J Anaesthesia 65:4-12, 1990

21. Mead J, Agostoni E: Dynamics of Breathing, Handbook of Physiology. Vol. 1. Macklem PT, Mead J (eds). Am Physiol Soc, Washington, DC, sect. 3, chapt. 14, 1964, pp. 411

22. Eissa NT, Ranieri VM, Corbeil C, et al: Analysis of behavior of the respiratory system in ARDS patients: effects of flow, volume, and time. J Appl Physiol 70:2719-29, 1991

23. Hildebrandt J: Pressure-volume data of cat lung interpreted by a plastoelastic linear viscoelastic model. J Appl Physiol 28:365-72, 1970

24. Bates JHT, Baconnier P, Milic-Emili J: A theoretical analysis of the interrupter technique for measuring respiratory mechanics. J Appl Physiol 64:2204-14, 1988

25. Briscoe WA, Dubois AB: The relationship between airway resistance, airway conductance and lung volume in subjects of different age and body size. J Clin Invest 37:1279-85, 1958

26. Bates JHT, Hunter I, Sly PD, et al: The effect of closure time on the determination of respiratory resistance by flow interruption. Med Biol Eng Comput 25:136-40, 1987

27. Sly PD, Bates JHT, Milic-Emili J: Measurement of respiratory mechanics using the Siemens Servo Ventilator 900C. Ped Pulm 3:400-5, 1987

PHYSIOLOGIC EFFECTS OF RAISED AIRWAY PRESSURE

J. B. Downs

Clinicians frequently adopt an empirical approach to the respiratory care of patients with pulmonary failure. As a result, only the symptomatology is treated, which often fails to restore normal pulmonary function. Now, more than at any other time in the past, it is possible to direct care towards specific pulmonary derangements and accurately evaluate the effects of therapy. The following pages will emphasize a goal-oriented approach to the treatment of patients requiring respiratory support, through appropriate adjustment of mechanical ventilation, inspired oxygen and airway pressure. Because therapeutic interventions may have variable physiologic consequences and rational application of therapies requires an understanding of such effects, applied cardiopulmonary physiology also will be reviewed.

PHYSIOLOGIC CONSIDERATIONS

Ventilation

Inspiration will occur whenever a pressure differential is created between the upper airway and the alveoli. During spontaneous inspiration, diaphragmatic contraction occurs, thereby decreasing intrapleural pressure and creating a pressure differential. During mechanical ventilation, inspiration occurs when positive pressure is applied to the distal airway, which produces the pressure differential. In either case, the distending, or transpulmonary, pressure (airway pressure [Paw] minus intrapleural pressure [Ppl]) is increased. The magnitude of change in transpulmonary pressure and the time during which the change occurs determine both tidal volume and inspiratory gas flow (5). For a given

209

T. H. Stanley and R. J. Sperry (eds.), Anesthesia and the Lung 1992, 209–241.
© 1992 Kluwer Academic Publishers.

tidal volume (VT), the required transpulmonary prepressure depends on the resistance of the respiratory system to deformation which is determined by the intrinsic elasticity of the system and resistance of the airways to gas flow.

Resistance of the respiratory system to deformation can be quantified by determining compliance, which is the change in volume divided by the change in pressure. Individual lung (CL) and thorax (CT) compliances determine lung-thorax compliance (CLT) (6). These relationships are expressed by the following equations (7):

$$\frac{1}{CLT} = \frac{1}{CL} + \frac{1}{CT} \quad \text{where:}$$

$$CLT = \frac{VT}{\Delta Paw}$$

$$CL = \frac{VT}{\Delta PL} = \frac{VT}{\Delta Paw - \Delta Ppl}$$

$$CT = \frac{VT}{\Delta Ppl}$$

$$CT = \frac{VT}{DPpl}$$

An understanding of these equations is helpful in clinical practice. Lung-thorax compliance usually is decreased in patients who have acute lung injury. The decrease may result from a decremental change in lung and/or thorax compliance. To determine the contribution of each would require measurement of intrapleural pressure, a difficult procedure clinically. Attempts to estimate intrapleural pressure by measuring esophageal pressure are very error-prone and, therefore, may not be useful in determining compliance. Resistance to gas flow increases when laminar flow becomes turbulent, or if airway diameter decreases (8). For a given tidal volume, an increased flow resistance may require a greater change in transpulmonary pressure because gas flow is related to the product of resistance and transpulmonary pressure. Thus, if there is a decrease in intrinsic elasticity, as may occur following lung injury, or an increase in resistance to gas flow, or both, the change in transpulmonary pressure required for spontaneous breathing may become extreme. Since an increased change in transpulmonary pressure requires greater diaphragmatic contraction, the work of breathing also will increase. These considerations will be discussed later.

The change in transpulmonary pressure required to produce a given tidal volume is similar whether it is generated by spontaneous breathing or mechanical ventilation. However, the distribution of inspired gas varies. Bynum, Rehder, and their coworkers have shown that mechanical ventilation alters the anatomical distribution of inspired gas (9,10). They found that gas is delivered preferentially to dependent lung regions during spontaneous ventilation. After mechanical ventilation is instituted, gas is distributed primarily to superior lung regions. This redistribution of inspired gas appears to be unrelated to the rate of gas flow (11).

Froese and her colleagues offered an explanation for these observations (12). With fluoroscopy, they observed that posterior regions of the diaphragm have the greatest motion during spontaneous breathing in supine individuals, presumably because of the smaller radius of curvature of that portion of the diaphragm. Hence, the distribution of inspired gas should be greatest to the posterior dependent lung fields. During mechanical ventilation, diaphragmatic motion is limited in the dependent regions and greatest superiorly. Therefore, gas distribution occurs preferentially in the superior lung regions. This anatomical alteration of gas distribution explains the previously observed increase in physiological dead space volume during mechanical ventilation.

Physiological dead space volume is the portion of each inhaled breath that does not participate in gas exchange. Both anatomical and alveolar compartments contribute to the total physiological dead space (13). The calculated dead space of patients requiring ventilatory support was found to decrease linearly when mechanical ventilator rates gradually were changed from 20 to 0 breaths per minute (14,15). When patients began to breathe spontaneously, average dead space decreased 50%, despite a ventilator rate between nine and six breaths per minute. Physiological dead space continued to decrease linearly as spontaneous ventilation became more effective and the ventilator rate was reduced to zero breaths per minute. When patients breathed spontaneously without mechanical ventilation, dead space volume returned to predicted normal values. To account for the increase in physiologic dead space when spontaneous respiration ceases, a maldistribution of inspired gas, pulmonary perfusion, or both, must occur during mechanical ventilation. Thus, mechanical ventilation actually induces a mismatching of ventilation and perfusion.

Maintenance of normal alveolar minute ventilation may be difficult during mechanical ventilation and decreased P_aCO_2 is common. During mechanical ventilation, normal alveolar minute ventilation and P_aCO_2 usually can be achieved with a tidal volume of 12 to 15 ml/kg and a respiratory rate of 7.5 breaths/minute (16). With such settings, patients usually will attempt to breathe spontaneously, making control of ventilation difficult. To suppress such spontaneous efforts, alveolar ventilation must be such that P_aCO_2 is below the apneic threshold, thereby abolishing the carbon dioxide respiratory drive. This usually occurs when P_aCO_2 is 30 to 32 torr, a level which may result in respiratory alkalemia and associated undesirable side effects. To provide a more normal alveolar ventilation and to avoid these effects in patients receiving mechanical ventilation, the respiratory response to carbon dioxide may be altered and the apneic threshold increased with sedatives or narcotics. Alternatively, some clinicians have administered muscle relaxants. Attempts to achieve normal P_aCO_2 by adding mechanical dead space or exogenous carbon dioxide are successful only if the apneic threshold is elevated sufficiently.

Assisted mechanical ventilation once was thought to avoid such problems. However, if the ventilator is set to cycle with minimal patient effort, mechanical cycling will result whenever the patient attempts to breathe, which he will do whenever the P_aCO_2 exceeds the apneic threshold. Therefore, it is not surprising that assisted ventilation commonly produces respiratory alkalemia. This has been confirmed by Llewellyn and Swyer (17) and Downs and colleagues (18), who found that controlled and properly adjusted assisted mechanical ventilation produce equivalent P_aCO_2 values.

Intermittent mandatory ventilation, IMV, can avoid many of these problems. Intermittent mandatory ventilation will permit unrestricted, unassisted spontaneous ventilation to occur between mechanical breaths which are applied at a rate just sufficient to prevent respiratory acidemia. By maintaining spontaneous ventilation, alterations in inspired gas distribution and physiologic dead space volume are minimized. In addition, it is possible to maintain normal alveolar minute ventilation without sedatives, muscle relaxants, addition of dead space, carbon dioxide, or any combination of these (19). A person breathing spontaneously will attempt to maintain normal ventilation by changes of tidal volume and respiratory rate, depending upon respiratory system compliance, airway resistance, P_aCO_2, and carbon dioxide production (20,21). If a patient is unable to support adequate ventilation, the IMV rate can be adjusted to deliver the required amount of mechanical augmentation needed to normalize alveolar ventilation. Thus, respiratory acidemia and alkalemia can be minimized with IMV. As spontaneous ventilation improves, IMV can be decreased progressively until spontaneous breathing alone can maintain a normal alveolar ventilation.

Recently, several manufacturers of mechanical ventilators have offered an option described as a "pressure assist" mode. An inspiratory effort by the patient will initiate a variable flow of gas to cause a predetermined airway pressure to be maintained throughout the patient's effort. When inspiratory effort wanes, flow will decrease. When the patient begins to exhale, pressure will decrease to allow passive exhalation. Introduced in an effort to decrease work of breathing with demand valve IMV systems, pressure-support has been recognized as a true assist mode, unlike patient-triggered mechanical ventilation mentioned previously. The degree of assistance offered by pressure-support depends on the level of airway pressure selected by the clinician, but may vary from minimal to complete ventilatory assistance.

Many criteria have been proposed to evaluate a patient's ability and drive to breathe spontaneously (22). Since patients may require different levels of P_aCO_2 to maintain normal arterial pH, the latter usually is a superior criterion of ventilatory adequacy. Therefore, this measurement is used to evaluate the adequacy of mechanical and spontaneous ventilation in patients receiving IMV (19,22)

In summary, institution of mechanical ventilation and loss of spontaneous efforts can alter normal respiratory physiology. Changes include altered intrapulmonary gas distribution, increased physiologic dead space, and difficulty in maintaining normal alveolar ventilation. IMV allows spontaneous breathing to persist during mechanical ventilation, which will assure more normal distribution of inspired gas, reduction of physiological dead space and improved matching of ventilation and perfusion.

In addition, a normal alveolar ventilation and arterial pH are more easily obtained.

Hemodynamic Responses

The respiratory system affects cardiovascular function primarily by variation in venous blood return and pulmonary vascular resistance. Return of venous blood to thoracic veins greatly depends upon the extrathoracic-intrathoracic intravascular pressure gradient. This gradient is determined largely by intrapleural pressure, which normally is sub-ambient because of two opposing forces: lung recoil and retraction of the thorax (6). Any change in these forces alters intrapleural pressure and the intravascular pressure gradient. Intrapleural pressure will increase following loss of spontaneous breathing, disruption of the chest wall, or application of positive airway pressure, thereby decreasing the extrathoracic-intrathoracic pressure gradient, venous inflow, and cardiac output. Intrapleural pressure is decreased by spontaneous inspiration, thereby increasing the pressure gradient, thoracic venous blood inflow and cardiac output. The increase in intrapleural pressure following application of positive airway pressure depends upon how much of the airway pressure is transmitted to the intrapleural space. Transmission of airway pressure is determined by lung and thorax compliances and can be determined from the following equations (7):

$$CL \; = \; \frac{VT}{\Delta PL} \; = \; \frac{VT}{\Delta Paw - \Delta Ppl}$$

$$CL \; = \; \frac{VT}{\Delta Ppl}$$

Whenever lung volume changes, there must be an equivalent alteration in the volume of the thorax. Therefore:

$$VT = CL(\Delta Paw - \Delta Ppl) = CT\Delta Ppl$$

The fractional transmission of airway pressure to the intrapleural space ($\Delta Ppl/\Delta Paw$) can be determined:

$$C_L\Delta Paw = (C_T+C_L)\Delta Ppl$$

$$\frac{\Delta Ppl}{\Delta Paw} = \frac{C_L}{C_T + C_L}$$

When lung and thorax compliances are equal, 50% of a change in airway pressure is transmitted to the intrapleural space. If lung compliance decreases, fractional transmission is less than 50%. A decrease in thorax compliance increases pressure transmission. These relationships can explain some frequent clinical observations.

Patients with acute respiratory failure often tolerate high levels of positive end-expiratory pressure (PEEP) without deleterious cardiovascular consequences. This reflects decreased airway pressure transmission secondary to decreased lung compliance. Patients who have abdominal distention, or who have decreased lung volume following operative procedures, often have reduced thorax compliance and increased airway pressure transmission. Thorax compliance is decreased, and lung compliance is increased in patients with chronic obstructive lung disease. As we would predict on a basis of increased transmission of the positive airway pressure to the intrapleural space, such patients often are intolerant of mechanical ventilation and PEEP, which may cause significant decline in cardiac output. Thus, many clinical conditions can affect transmission of positive airway pressure and the resulting hemodynamic responses. Such conditions should be considered when assessing the effects of ventilatory support on cardiopulmonary function. Measurements of thoracic vascular pressures frequently are used to evaluate cardiac filling and function. When airway pressure increases, all or part of the change in intrapleural pressure will be transmitted to the lumen of the intrathoracic vessels (23). Thus, evaluation of cardiac function may be difficult without accurate estimation of true intravascular filling pressure (23,24,25). Intravascular filling pressure is determined by subtraction of the intrapleural from the intravascular pressure. Therefore, precise knowledge of the intrapleural pressure may be valuable. At present, the measurement of intrapleural pressure is difficult and requires the placement of a catheter into the pleural space (25). Attempts to estimate intrapleural pressure with an esophageal balloon have been made, but interpretation of esophageal pressure is difficult because great pressure variations occur within the esophagus (26). In addition, when esophageal pressure exceeds atmospheric pressure, compliance of the esophageal balloon may limit accuracy of the measurement (27). Such inaccuracy may influence calculated filling pressures and lead to significant error.

Expiratory intrapleural pressure varies little with different respiratory patterns, as long as expiratory airway pressure is similar. Therefore, the most important determinant of mean airway, intrapleural and vascular filling pressures is the inspiratory airway pressure pattern. During mechanical inspiration, filling pressures will decrease, since airway and intrapleural pressures are increased. When filling pressure, or preload, is lowered, cardiac output likely will decrease. This is not the case during spontaneous breathing, even with PEEP. During spontaneous exhalation, intrapleural and filling pressures are equivalent to those recorded during mechanical ventilation with the same PEEP level. However, during inspiration, intrapleural pressure decreases, increasing cardiac filling. The effect of spontaneous inspiration on filling pressure of the heart and cardiac output depends on the change in airway pressure. Continuous positive airway pressure (CPAP) is produced by gas flowing through a circuit terminated by a threshold resistor valve. Airway pressure is increased throughout the spontaneous respiratory cycle and inspiratory airway pressure should not decrease significantly (28). If the airway is not pressurized throughout the respiratory cycle, inspiratory airway pressure will decrease toward ambient during breathing with PEEP. The resultant higher mean airway and intrapleural pressure with CPAP may decrease thoracic venous inflow of blood and cardiac output. Weinstein and coworkers found no difference between CPAP and spontaneous ventilation with PEEP (29). However, they insured that filling pressure was normal, or elevated, during CPAP. Other studies have reported that venous return is affected most by controlled mechanical ventilation and PEEP, less by CPAP, and least by spontaneous respiration with PEEP and ambient inspiratory airway pressure (24,28,30,31).

Principal respiratory factors affecting pulmonary vascular resistance and pulmonary blood flow and its distribution, are airway pressure and lung volume. When expiratory lung volume, functional residual capacity (FRC), is normal, pulmonary vascular resistance is minimal (32). Changes in lung volume above or below normal FRC increase pulmonary vascular resistance. Therefore, normal FRC should be maintained whenever possible. Even though FRC may be independent of the inspiratory airway pressure pattern, the mode of inspiration can affect pulmonary vascular resistance. During mechanical inspiration with large tidal volumes, pulmonary vascular resistance may increase as some alveoli become overdistended. Resistance may be increased further by PEEP since compliant lung areas are enlarged further. Increased pulmonary vascular resistance and decreased venous return from elevated intrapleural pressure additively can depress cardiac output. This may account for reports that mechanical ventilation with PEEP greater than 11 torr frequently depresses cardiac output (33,34). In contrast, cardiac output is not adversely affected with 11 torr PEEP when spontaneous ventilation is maintained (35). In fact, the cardiac output of patients treated for respiratory failure with IMV was unaffected by PEEP at an average level of 22 torr (35). The deleterious effects of PEEP on venous return, cardiac output, and pulmonary vascular resistance appear to be minimized by maintaining spontaneous respiration and a lower mechanical cycling frequency.

It has been suggested that nonsynchronous application of mechanical ventilation to spontaneously breathing patients may cause cardiovascular depression (36). Recently, IMV synchronized with spontaneous breaths (SIMV) and nonsynchronous IMV were compared (37). Mean airway pressure was an average of 0.5 torr lower during SIMV, but there were no differences in intrapleural pressure, cardiac output, or stroke volume. From these results one can conclude that SIMV offers little advantage when compared to IMV, and may be a disadvantage due to the extra cost for that capability.

Application of positive airway pressure during spontaneous breathing may benefit some patients with compromised myocardial function. Patients who breathed spontaneously with 11 torr PEEP after operation for coronary revascularization had increased stroke index and cardiac output (28). It is possible that PEEP may affect several of the determinants of cardiac output. Intrapleural pressure, increased by PEEP, could augment ventricular contraction during exhalation. The external compression may serve to "unload" the left ventricle. Because intrapleural pressure is lower during spontaneous inspiration, left ventricular filling pressure may increase.

Positive airway pressure has been reported to depress renal function, presumably secondary to decreased cardiac output (23) or elevated plasma levels of vasopressin (38,39). Renal function was compared in swine receiving continuous positive pressure ventilation (CPPV) with 10 torr PEEP to that in others breathing spontaneously with 10 torr CPAP (31). Animals receiving CPPV responded with increased plasma vasopressin and decreased cardiac output, urine flow, glomerular filtration rate, and sodium excretion. Animals that received CPAP had decreased urine flow and glomerular filtration, but cardiac output, plasma vasopressin, and excretion of sodium did not differ from control values. Since urine flow and glomerular filtration were similarly affected by CPPV and CPAP, these alterations could not have been secondary to changes in cardiac output or vasopressin alone, but may be related to elevated venous pressures. The preservation of pulsatile venous blood flow during spontaneous inspiration may account for the differences. Such flow would be decreased during mechanical inspiration because increased intrapleural pressure would further increase inferior vena cava and renal vein pressures. Thus, a decrease in inspiratory intrapleural pressure during spontaneous breathing minimizes some detrimental renal effects of positive pressure breathing.

In summary, spontaneous ventilation maintains lower airway and intrapleural pressures. This augments venous blood return and does not affect pulmonary vascular resistance adversely. Therefore, cardiac output, and pulmonary blood flow and distribution are better maintained. Presence of spontaneous ventilation is even more important after the application of positive airway pressure. If mechanical ventilation is required, it should be titrated to the level necessary to normalize alveolar ventilation, thereby minimizing deleterious effects.

VENTILATION-PERFUSION RELATIONSHIPS

As previously discussed, spontaneous inspiration directs the majority of ventilation toward dependent regions of the lung (10,40). Gravitational effects insure a similar distribution of blood flow. Thus, the alveolar ventilation-to-perfusion ratio ($\dot{V}_A/\dot{Q}$) normally approaches unity in all lung regions. Significant ventilation-perfusion mismatching usually necessitates therapeutic intervention. Unfortunately, therapy to correct one extreme $\dot{V}A/\dot{Q}$ abnormality frequently induces the other. An increased $\dot{V}A/\dot{Q}$ may require mechanical ventilation, if spontaneous breathing cannot provide adequate alveolar ventilation for carbon dioxide elimination. During mechanical ventilation, the majority of ventilation is directed toward superior lung regions. Blood flow, however, is still greatest in dependent lung regions. As a result, mechanical ventilation increases $\dot{V}A/\dot{Q}$ in the superior lung regions, causing an increase in dead-space. Because dead-space volume increases during mechanical ventilation, an increased ventilator rate may result in a paradoxical increase in P_aCO_2.

A decrease in $\dot{V}A/\dot{Q}$ results in impaired arterial oxygenation. Since the majority of gas exchange occurs during exhalation, improvement in overall $\dot{V}A/\dot{Q}$ must occur primarily during exhalation. Mechanical ventilation usually is not effective in improving such problems since the ratio will increase only during the inspiratory phase of the respiratory cycle. Additionally, Zarins and associates observed a lower PaO_2 in baboons receiving controlled mechanical ventilation than in those receiving IMV with the same level of PEEP (41). This suggests that mechanical ventilation promoted decreased $\dot{V}A/\dot{Q}$ and increased venous admixture. Positive airway pressure applied during exhalation can improve low $\dot{V}A/\dot{Q}$. However, PEEP may increase physiological dead-space and decrease effective alveolar ventilation, especially when applied with mechanical ventilation. Therefore, when ventilatory support is instituted, the goal must be to minimize ventilation-perfusion mismatching in all lung regions. This is best accomplished when spontaneous ventilation is allowed to persist and when mechanical ventilation is used just to prevent acidemia.

Acute respiratory failure often is characterized by a decrease in FRC and an increase in pulmonary venous admixture. Therapy should include PEEP to increase FRC, improve pulmonary gas exchange, increase arterial oxygen tension and decrease pulmonary vascular resistance. It has been recommended that the appropriate (optimal) level of PEEP be determined by titrating PEEP to minimize venous admixture (33,35).

Minimizing venous admixture appears to be least efficient when PEEP is applied during mechanical ventilation. Venous admixture of patients with severe, acute respiratory failure was found to be reduced from 50 to 32% by controlled ventilation with an average of 10 torr PEEP (33). When PEEP was raised above this level, venous admixture increased and PaO_2 decreased. Venous admixture was reduced on an average of 14% by IMV and mean value of 22 torr PEEP in a similar group of patients (35). This difference may be explained by the increased mean airway and intrapleural pressure in patients receiving mechanical ventilation with PEEP. The greater mean airway pressure may overdistend compliant alveoli, increasing pulmonary vascular resistance and redirecting blood flow to less well ventilated areas, thus increasing venous admixture. In contrast, spontaneous breathing during IMV maintains lower mean airway and intrapleural pressure, and allows higher PEEP levels to increase FRC with fewer deleterious effects (35)

During evaluation of pulmonary gas exchange, the effects of inspired oxygen concentration on ventilation and perfusion should be considered. In a normal lung, $\dot{V}A/\dot{Q}$ changes very little from inspiration to expiration. However, this is not true in respiratory failure. The expiratory $\dot{V}A/\dot{Q}$ is less than the inspiratory $\dot{V}A/\dot{Q}$ and will be decreased further by oxygen breathing because more alveolar oxygen is absorbed. Eventually the rate of gas flow from an alveolus into the blood will balance exactly the rate of delivery of gas to the alveolus during inspiration. Such an alveolus will be unstable and any subsequent decrease in inspiratory $\dot{V}A/\dot{Q}$, or increase in oxygen concentration will result in a net flow of gas from the alveolus to the blood, further loss of volume, and collapse. It has been suggested that lung units with an inspiratory $\dot{V}A/\dot{Q}$ of less than 0.08 would be stable only when breathing ambient air (42-45). They have found when oxygen was breathed, blood flow that had been distributed to areas with low $\dot{V}A/\dot{Q}$ during ambient air breathing, subsequently perfused areas with zero ventilation. Thus, oxygen breathing induced atelectasis and shunting.

Other investigators also have found that oxygen breathing increases shunting. When patients with respiratory failure breathe an increased concentration of inspired oxygen, a uniform response occurs (46-48). As the inspired oxygen is increased to 40%, venous admixture decreases and remains unchanged until the inspired oxygen reaches 60%. Venous admixture then increases as inspired oxygen approaches 100%. Increasing inspired oxygen to 40% will minimize oxygen diffusion abnormalities and mask the hypoxemia producing effect of lung areas with low, but finite, $\dot{V}A/\dot{Q}$, thereby accounting for the observed decrease in venous admixture. The observed increase in venous admixture caused by breathing high concentrations of oxygen may result from atelectasis. However, altered pulmonary perfusion may also contribute to this effect (47). In areas of the lung with low $\dot{V}A/\dot{Q}$, hypoxic pulmonary vasoconstriction is thought to limit perfusion by shunting blood to areas with better ventilation. When the inspired oxygen concentration is increased, alveolar PO_2 rises, precapillary pulmonary vasoconstriction decreases, and perfusion to areas with decreased $\dot{V}A/\dot{Q}$ increases. Another possible explanation is that oxygen inhalation increases extra-alveolar shunting of venous blood (49-51). Such right-to-left intrapulmonary shunting of blood can increase venous admixture. We have observed a detrimental effect of short term exposure to 50% inspired O_2 in postoperative patients (52). Thus, detrimental consequences of oxygen breathing should be considered when evaluating lung function and when providing therapy.

In summary, although mechanical ventilation may be necessary for adequate carbon dioxide elimination, spontaneous ventilation insures better matching of ventilation and perfusion. Oxygen administration may be required to prevent hypoxemia, but minimal amounts are best to assure the least detriment to pulmonary function and provide for more precise evaluation of pulmonary dysfunction and therapy. It is apparent that respiratory therapy, based upon measurement of venous admixture during breathing of oxygen-enriched air, may not be directed at the patient's pathophysiology. Acute lung dysfunction often results in lung areas with low $\dot{V}A/\dot{Q}$. Therapy should be directed to correct the dysfunction and improve $\dot{V}A/\dot{Q}$. Therefore, it is preferable for the inspired oxygen concentration to be at a level that will not mask the effects produced by areas of low $\dot{V}A/\dot{Q}$. Such an inspired oxygen concentration will better allow evaluation of low $\dot{V}A/\dot{Q}$ and the effects of therapy.

Work of Breathing

If patients with respiratory failure are to have effective spontaneous breathing, the work of breathing must be maximally efficient. Few clinical studies have attempted to quantify the work of breathing in patients with

222

respiratory failure, perhaps because quantification of work requires techniques which are not readily available (53). For our discussion, only a graphical representation of the elastic work of inspiration will be considered. Any alteration in the volume/pressure relationship of the lung can alter the work of breathing. A normal volume/pressure curve for the lung-thorax system is shown in Figure 1. As a result of a small pressure change, normal tidal breathing from FRC occurs along the volume/pressure curve as indicated by the arrow. The elastic work of inspiration can be estimated by the stippled areas under the curve.

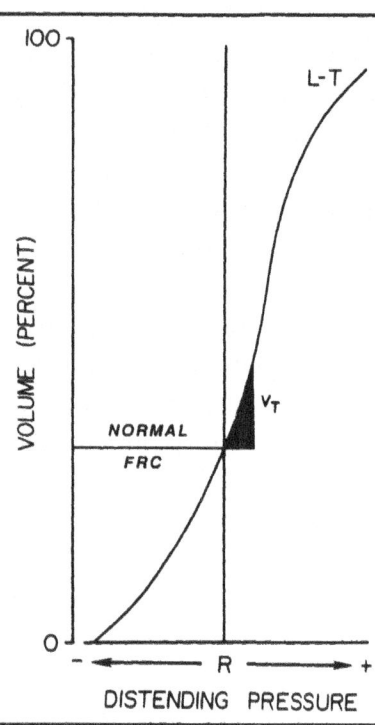

Figure 1. Normal volume/pressure curve of the lung-thorax (L-T). Volume as a percent of total lung capacity, is plotted as a function of distending pressure. Pressure R corresponds to ambient airway pressure. During inspiration, distending pressure is increased and lung volume (VT) increases from normal functional residual capacity (FRC).

In Figure 2, the volume/pressure curves for normal lung, thorax, and lung-thorax are plotted. When the distending pressure of the lung-thorax is zero, which occurs when airway pressure is ambient, the lung volume at this point is the FRC. At FRC, the distending pressure of the lung is equal but opposite to that of the thorax. Any alteration in the volume/pressure relationships for the lung and/or thorax will alter the lung-thorax curve and affect FRC.

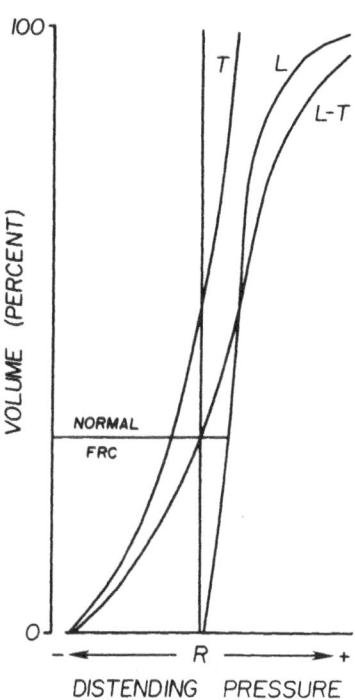

Figure 2. Normal volume/pressure curve of the thorax (T), lung (L), and lung-thorax (L-T). Volume, as a percent of total lung capacity, is plotted as a function of distending pressure. Distending pressure R occurs when airway pressure is ambient. When the distending pressure of the lung-thorax is zero, the distending pressure of the lung is equal, but opposite, to that of the thorax. These equal counter-forces are responsible for determining and maintaining FRC.

The effects of a change in the lung volume/pressure curve, which are likely to occur in patients with acute lung injury, are shown in Figure 3. Because the volume/pressure relationships of the lung and thorax can be altered in an infinite number of ways during respiratory failure, a family of right-shifted lung-thorax curves can result. Each will have a new, but decrementally changed FRC (Fig. 4).

A shift in the volume/pressure curve not only decreases FRC, but can increase the work of breathing. When FRC is decreased, the required pressure change may be increased for the same tidal volume (Fig. 5). When the required pressure change is increased, the area under the curve representing work, also is increased. If this occurs, the patient will decrease tidal volume and increase respiratory rate in an effort to minimize work. Because of these changes, clinicians often have assumed the work of breathing for the patient by instituting mechanical ventilation. However, an increase in FRC and compliance also may decrease the patient's work of breathing.

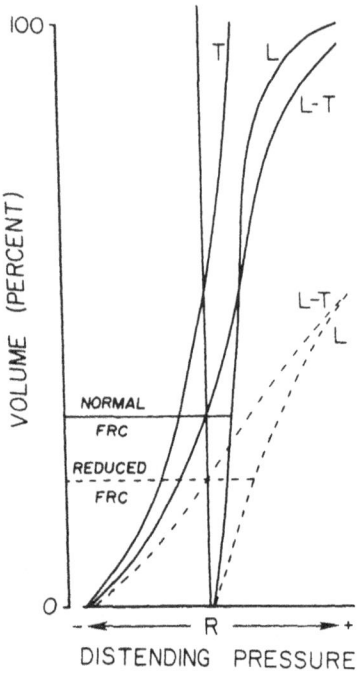

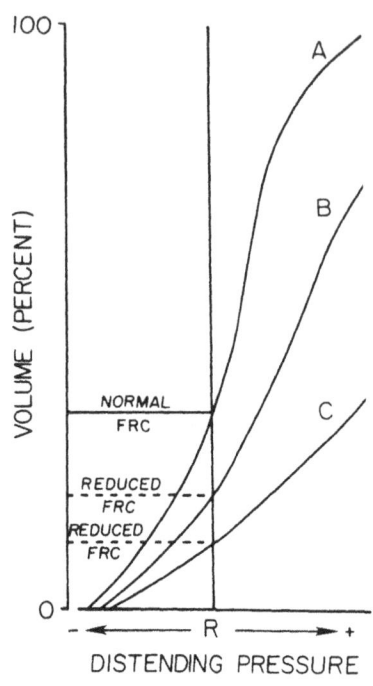

Figure 3. Normal volume/pressure curve of the thorax (T), lung (L), and lung-thorax (L-T) (solid lines). Abnormal volume/pressure curves of the lung (L) and lung-thorax (L-T) (dotted lines). Distending pressure R occurs when airway pressure is ambient. The abnormally right-shifted volume/pressure curve of the lung results in a new volume/pressure curve for the lung-thorax, and a reduction in functional residual capacity (FRC).

Figure 4. Volume/pressure curves of the lung-thorax. Volume, as a percent of total lung capacity, is plotted as a function of distending pressure. Distending pressure R occurs when airway pressure is ambient. Curve A represents a normal volume/pressure relationship for the lung-thorax. Curves B and C are shifted to the right. It should be noted that each curve results in a reduced functional residual capacity (FRC).

Restoration of FRC can be accomplished by applying PEEP to increase distending pressure (Fig. 6). Each volume/pressure curve will require a different level of PEEP to restore FRC and minimize the work of breathing. Therefore, PEEP must be individualized, titrated for each patient, and reassessed frequently. If PEEP is applied to meet these goals, FRC will be increased and often will lie on a favorable portion of the volume/pressure curve, where the required change in pressure to produce a tidal volume will be less. Thus, compliance will be improved and work of breathing reduced.

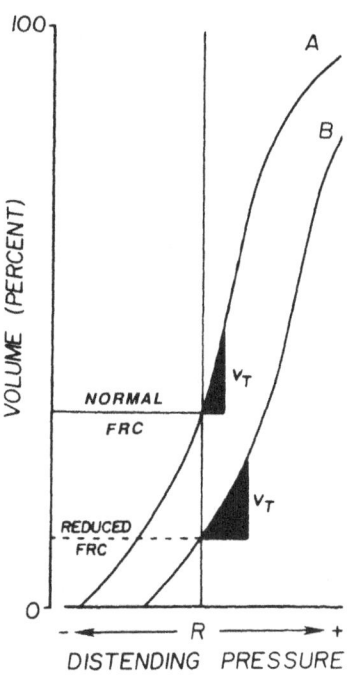

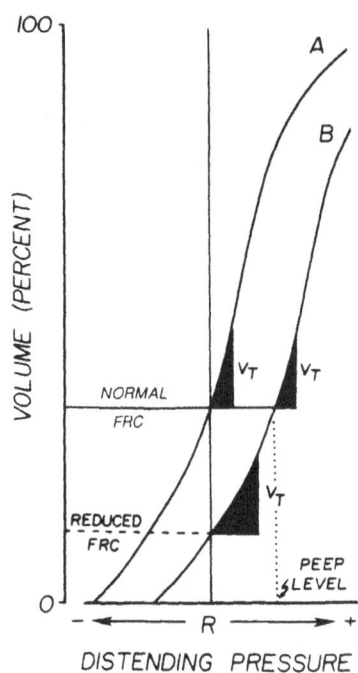

Figure 5. Volume/pressure curves of the lung-thorax. Volume, as a percent of total lung capacity, is plotted as a function of distending pressure. Distending pressure R occurs when airway pressure is ambient. Curve A represents a normal volume/pressure relationship and B represents a right-shifted curve.

Figure 6. Volume/pressure curves of the lung-thorax. These curves are equivalent to those illustrated in Fig 5. When distending pressure is increased by application of positive airway pressure (PEEP), FRC can be normalized. When FRC is increased, the expenditure of work for tidal breathing may be reduced to a value which is nearly normal.

Following application of PEEP to restore FRC, a reduction in the work of breathing will occur only if inspiratory drop in airway pressure is small (54). Again, the spontaneous inspiratory airway pressure change is of clinical significance (28). During CPAP, gas must flow at a rate equalling or exceeding the inspiratory flow rate of the patient. Therefore, airway pressure changes little throughout the respiratory cycle. During spontaneous ventilation with PEEP, gas flow occurs only when inspiratory airway pressure is below ambient pressure. The terms expiratory positive airway pressure (EPAP) and inspiratory pressure (IPAP) have been suggested to help define these respiratory patterns more precisely (55). During CPAP, the expiratory and inspiratory pressures (EPAP and IPAP) are nearly equal. When airway pressure is elevated only during exhalation (EPAP), airway pressure change is greater than with CPAP. Intrapleural pressure change also is greater with EPAP, causing an increase in the work of breathing. As lung compliance decreases, intrapleural pressure change is greater because the stiff lung requires a greater intrapleural pressure change to accomplish tidal breathing, and a further increase in the work of breathing results. Since our goal must be to minimize the patient's work of breathing, CPAP (EPAP and IPAP) should be applied to restore FRC.

In summary, the appropriate ventilatory pattern depends upon intravascular volume, cardiac output, lung volume, compliance and the patient's ability to breathe. Careful evaluation of airway and intrapleural pressure patterns becomes important in providing optimal therapy. Using the principles described, we can define optimal CPAP as the airway pressure that minimizes physiologic intrapulmonary shunting of blood and reduces the work of spontaneous breathing, without causing detrimental cardiovascular effects.

RESPIRATORY CARE

Oxygen Therapy

Patients often have arterial hypoxemia secondary to areas of lung with low, but finite, ventilation-to-perfusion ratio. Arterial hypoxemia produced by such areas is worsened by a low inspired oxygen concentration and usually can be alleviated when oxygen is added to the inspired gas. Another source of arterial hypoxemia is the impairment of oxygen diffusion from alveoli to pulmonary capillary blood. A "diffusion defect" rarely is the only cause of arterial hypoxemia, but may contribute when the inspired concentration is low. Right-to-left intrapulmonary shunting of blood, a third source of hypoxemia, will be unaffected, even during pure-oxygen breathing. Thus, oxygen therapy may improve arterial hypoxemia when it is secondary to two of three abnormalities.

When evaluating and treating arterial hypoxemia, variables which may contribute to the hypoxemia should be considered. Increased oxygen consumption resulting from an increased metabolic rate, or a decrease in cardiac output, will cause lower mixed venous blood lower oxygen tension. A low hemoglobin concentration also will result in a lower mixed venous blood oxygen tension. When mixed venous oxygen tension is reduced, a lower arterial oxygen tension often results. Such factors should be evaluated in patients with arterial hypoxemia. This may require the measurement of mixed venous oxygen saturation and calculation of arterial-mixed venous oxygen content difference and venous admixture (56). Such efforts may prevent inappropriate therapy. Evaluation of hypoxemia is further complicated by the effects of inspired oxygen concentration on pulmonary gas exchange. Breathing an increased oxygen concentration may lead to absorption atelectasis in areas of lung with low, but finite, $\dot{V}_A/\dot{Q}$, as discussed previously. Only if the inspired nitrogen concentration is increased can absorption atelectasis and increased right-to-left intrapulmonary shunting of blood be prevented. Even the application of PEEP will not prevent absorption atelectasis (47). Therefore, administration of high inspired oxygen concentrations, even if limited to 24 hours, is undesirable. Also, prolonged administration of 50% oxygen to patients can no longer be considered therapeutic, rational, or safe (52). Rather, rapid reduction of inspired oxygen is the preferred practice.

In spite of the frequency with which oxygen is used to treat hypoxemia, discontinuation of such therapy has received little attention. Evaluating pulmonary gas exchange in patients with areas of lung with low $\dot{V}_A/\dot{Q}$ when breathing increased concentrations of oxygen might lead to incorrect conclusions, because administration of as little as 30% oxygen may mask the hypoxemic producing effect of areas with low $\dot{V}_A/\dot{Q}$ This should be considered when oxygen therapy is discontinued. For example, a patient breathing 40% oxygen with a PaO_2 of 70 torr might be thought to have adequate pulmonary gas exchange. The clinician might then decide to wean the patient from mechanical ventilation and PEEP. However, ventilation and perfusion could be mismatched to such a degree that breathing only 30% oxygen might decrease P_aO_2 to 50 torr. Were the clinician aware of this abnormality, it is likely that PEEP would be increased rather than decreased. Such evaluations of pulmonary gas exchange and the rational application of PEEP are possible only when the inspired oxygen concentration is low. Often evaluation of pulmonary gas exchange is best when patients breathe room air.

In summary, it is best to use the lowest possible inspired oxygen concentration to maintain an acceptable P_aO_2. This practice maximizes alveolar nitrogen concentration, minimizes absorption atelectasis, minimizes right-to-left intrapulmonary shunting and may decrease the need for PEEP. Since the low, but finite, $\dot{V}A/\dot{Q}$ is more apparent when the inspired oxygen concentration is low, the clinician is better able to evaluate the resolution of lung dysfunction as therapy is applied and time progresses. Oxygen should be viewed as any other drug and should be given only when clinically indicated, only in the amount required, and reduced and removed as soon as feasible. During this period, the sources of hypoxemia should be clarified and specific therapy instituted.

CPAP Therapy

Spontaneous respiration with elevated airway pressure was recognized four decades ago to decrease pulmonary edema in patients with congestive heart failure (57). A motor-driven blower provided an inspiratory gas source and airway pressure was elevated with a face mask and an expiratory valve for constant positive-pressure breathing (CPPB). Shortly thereafter, CPPB was used to treat pulmonary edema secondary to traumatic lung injury (58) and pulmonary contusion in patients with flail chest injuries (59). Thus, there is ample historical precedent for applying elevated airway pressures to spontaneously breathing patients. Much later, mechanical ventilation was emphasized for the treatment of lung injuries and spontaneous breathing with CPPB was abandoned (60). Because of the early emphasis on mechanical ventilation, discontinuation of mechanical ventilatory support often is attempted only after the need for PEEP has been alleviated. This may not be the most rational approach.

Lung compliance and arterial oxygenation are decreased, and work of breathing is increased in patients with acute lung injury. In fact, it is often the increased work of breathing that leads many clinicians to institute mechanical ventilation. By application of CPAP, FRC and compliance can be increased. The increase in FRC will improve $\dot{V}A/\dot{Q}$ and arterial oxygenation. Increased compliance will decrease the work of breathing. Thus, CPAP may reduce the requirement for mechanical ventilation and inspired oxygen supplementation. Since application of CPAP also may alleviate many problems associated with the mechanical ventilator and oxygen, we prefer to wean patients from mechanical ventilation and oxygen before removing CPAP.

Application of CPAP, like oxygen therapy, has been widely discussed for more than four decades. However, little attention has been directed toward the mechanics of weaning patients from CPAP. The clinician would like to insure that a reduction in CPAP will not reduce FRC below normal. Such a decrease in FRC may cause two aspects of pulmonary function to deteriorate. In some regions of the lung $\dot{V}A/\dot{Q}$ may decrease, causing arterial hypoxemia. In addition, lung compliance may decrease. Each of these FRC dependent effects should be evaluated separately as CPAP is reduced. Because a small reduction in CPAP can cause a large fall in FRC, CPAP should be withdrawn in decrements of 2 cm H_2O (61).

To evaluate $\dot{V}A/\dot{Q}$, arterial blood oxygenation must be examined. Alterations in FRC and oxygenation are nearly complete within one minute following a change in CPAP. Therefore, the effect of CPAP on oxygenation should be evaluated within minutes of the addition or removal of CPAP (61). This often requires measurement, not only of P_aO_2, but also of the oxygen tension in mixed venous blood and calculation of venous admixture. If a reduction in CPAP causes a deterioration of these values, CPAP should be increased immediately.

To assess change in lung compliance, respiratory mechanics must be evaluated. A shift to the right of the volume/pressure curve of the respiratory system may decrease both FRC and compliance, causing a greater intrapleural pressure change for tidal breathing and increased work of breathing. The greater negativity of intrapleural pressure may cause subcostal, suprasternal, or intercostal retractions that can be observed clinically. To minimize the work of breathing, the patient will inhale with a smaller tidal volume and increase the respiratory rate in an effort to maintain adequate alveolar ventilation. Thus, after a change in CPAP, the respiratory rate, tidal volume, and physical appearance of the patient should be observed closely. Because change in $\dot{V}A/\dot{Q}$ and compliance may occur independently, it is important that gas exchange and mechanics be evaluated separately. Deterioration in either should be considered a contraindication to further reduction of CPAP and an indication for its return to a higher level. Three additional considerations deserve mention. First, blood gas exchange must be evaluated when the inspired oxygen concentration is low and constant, because venous admixture varies at different concentrations of inspired oxygen (47). For example, a patient breathing 30% oxygen with a calculated venous admixture of 25% may have only a 15% venous admixture breathing 40% oxygen. Were CPAP reduced with the patient breathing 30% oxygen, venous admixture could increase to 30%, indicating a deterioration in pulmonary function. However, if CPAP were decreased and the inspired oxygen simultaneously increased to 40%, venous admixture could be 20%. The clinician erroneously might conclude that the reduction of CPAP is well tolerated when, in fact, the patient's pulmonary status has deteriorated greatly. Thus, it is important to evaluate gas exchange while the concentration of inspired oxygen is constant.

Circuit resistance is the second consideration. In order to evaluate respiratory mechanics accurately, the clinician must be sure that external or mechanical resistance to respiration is minimal and that effective spontaneous respiration exists. Mechanical resistance is best minimized by assuring a continuous flow of gas, or by use of a sufficiently sensitive demand valve in the inspiratory circuit, by use of large-bore tubing and low-resistance valves, and avoidance of acute angles in the system. Such care will prevent inspiratory airway and intrapleural pressures from decreasing to levels which might erroneously suggest a deterioration in pulmonary function.

Currently, there are no commercially available demand valve systems with acceptable sensitivity and flow characteristics. Pressure-assist has greatly improved patient acceptance of such systems, but their complexity and expense seems unwarranted. Therefore, we still prefer continuous flow systems for IMV and CPAP. Care must be taken to insure low inspiratory circuit resistance for reasons mentioned above. In addition, exhalation valve resistance may create excessive inspiratory work of breathing. Where the high flow of gas exits such a valve an increase in airway pressure will result. When the patient inhales, the decrease in flow past the exhalation valve will decrease airway pressure and increase work of breathing. Therefore, low-flow resistance, threshold resistor type exhalation/CPAP valves should be used.

Adequacy of spontaneous respiration is the third consideration. To insure that spontaneous respiration is effective, weaning from CPAP should begin only when the mechanical ventilator rate is low and spontaneous respiration provides the majority of alveolar ventilation. In most instances, weaning from CPAP should not be attempted until the patient is breathing spontaneously and fewer than two mechanical breaths per minute are being provided.

In summary, by applying CPAP, the requirement for oxygen and mechanical ventilatory support may be reduced. IMV and CPAP may allow the patient to be weaned expediently from oxygen and mechanical ventilation.

Mechanical Ventilation

During the last few decades, there has been a trend toward using mechanical ventilation for patients with inadequate arterial oxygenation and increased work of breathing (60). Infrequently, these patients have difficulty eliminating carbon dioxide while breathing spontaneously. Since mechanical ventilation alone usually does not reverse the factors responsible for hypoxemia, a need often exists for an increased concentration of inspired oxygen. Classic criteria for initiating mechanical ventilation based on respiratory strength and drive often are not applicable to such patients. Without specific guidelines for patients with acute respiratory failure, the decision to initiate and terminate mechanical ventilatory support often is subjective. Such difficulty can be avoided if mechanical ventilation is reserved only for patients unable to sustain adequate spontaneous ventilation.

When IMV is used, mechanical ventilation can be applied to prevent acidemia and CPAP can be optimally applied, thereby reducing the need for an increased inspired O_2 concentration and mechanical ventilation. Weaning may be accomplished by lowering the IMV rate in decrements. When mechanical ventilation has been completely discontinued and spontaneous respiration is adequate to prevent acidemia, the patient is considered weaned from mechanical ventilation. It is important to emphasize the difference between acidemia and respiratory acidosis.

Compensatory respiratory acidosis has been thought to occur only rarely in conscious patients. However, use of IMV has led us to observe some patients who decrease ventilation to maintain a normal arterial pH even though P_aCO_2 may exceed 60 torr. If the patient has no history of lung disease or chronic carbon dioxide elevation, therapy aimed at correction of the coexisting metabolic alkalosis will result in prompt reduction of P_aCO_2. Therefore, P_aCO_2 may not be the best index of adequacy of spontaneous respiration, nor should it be a criterion for IMV rate reduction in many patients. Rather, arterial pH should be used as a guide and the rate of IMV should be reduced as long as arterial pH remains greater than 7.35. In this way, patients can be weaned rapidly and safely from mechanical ventilatory support, even when metabolic alkalosis is present.

By promoting spontaneous respiration and rapid termination of mechanical ventilation, IMV may avoid several problems observed during conventional therapy. Occasionally, during prolonged mechanical ventilatory support, patients develop a psychological dependence upon the ventilator that may cause weaning problems. It appears that those allowed to breathe spontaneously throughout the period of ventilatory support do not develop such dependence (62). In addition, for reasons that are not clear, a pronounced neuromuscular discoordination of the respiratory muscles may occur in patients who have prolonged mechanical ventilatory support. Some reports have indicated that almost all patients requiring ventilatory support for more than 24 hours develop discoordination of abdominal and accessory muscles of respiration (63). Such discoordination may be sufficient to prevent adequate spontaneous respiration and may prolong ventilator dependence. This discoordination does not occur in patients who maintain spontaneous breathing. Recently, Andersen and associates confirmed the absence of respiratory muscle discoordination in patients who received IMV (64).

Initially, IMV was used on adult patients only as a weaning technique. Currently, we employ IMV as a ventilatory support mode to allow greater flexibility in oxygen therapy, CPAP, and mechanical ventilation. Each is applied and weaned separately to meet established goals. Controversy still exists whether IMV can speed the weaning process more than conventional techniques. A prospective investigation compared the efficacy of IMV criteria with traditional criteria for weaning patients from mechanical ventilatory support. The study concluded that IMV results in faster and safer weaning for a majority of patients (22).

In summary, the advantages of IMV depend on the ability to apply therapy in a goal-oriented manner, rather than rapidity of weaning from mechanical ventilation. Only IMV allows oxygen therapy and mechanical ventilation to be reduced early in the therapy of patients with respiratory failure, through the use of optimal CPAP.

Current Practice

Ventilatory care of patients with acute respiratory failure often proceeds in the following fashion. Initially, oxygen is added to the inhaled gas to alleviate arterial hypoxemia. If a satisfactory arterial oxygen tension is not achieved, or maintained, the trachea is intubated and mechanical ventilation instituted. If an adequate P_aO_2 still cannot be obtained with inspired oxygen concentration less than 60%, an arbitrary amount of PEEP is added. Weaning from ventilatory support proceeds in re-verse fashion. PEEP is decreased in decrements, as long as P_aO_2 remains satisfactory and inspired oxygen is "nontoxic". After successful removal of PEEP, mechanical ventilation is withdrawn and the patient breathes spontaneously from a T-piece for increasingly longer periods. Once totally spontaneous respiration is deemed to be satisfactory, patients are extubated and an elevated inspired oxygen concentration administered to prevent arterial hypoxemia. By using IMV we have developed a practice that proceeds in a more objective and efficient fashion.

Patients suffering acute respiratory failure often require oxygen therapy, mechanical ventilatory support, and CPAP. In general, patients are orotracheally intubated. Initially, mechanical ventilatory support is supplied to normalize alveolar minute ventilation. To treat arterial hypoxemia, an elevated inspired oxygen concentration is administered. Pulmonary mechanics and gas exchange are evaluated and CPAP titrated to minimize abnormalities. Once optimal CPAP is obtained, mechanical ventilation is reduced, as long as arterial pH remains greater than 7.35. Simultaneously, the inspired oxygen concentration is reduced decrementally to a level that will not mask the hypoxemic-producing effect of areas of lung with low $\dot{V}A/\dot{Q}$, yet, that will maintain P_aO_2 at an acceptable level. Often this may be accomplished with 30% oxygen, or less. Pulmonary gas exchange and mechanics are evaluated frequently and when considered adequate, CPAP is reduced without allowing detrimental change to occur. Finally, the patient is extubated. It is important to note that patients are weaned from mechanical ventilation and oxygen first and from CPAP last. This order is the reverse of the standard mode of therapy. Because this general approach may not apply to all patients, specific therapy for those who have had a major operation, acute respiratory failure, chest trauma or acute exacerbation of chronic obstructive lung disease may vary. Most patients who have undergone major operations have little or no underlying lung disease. They may require mechanical ventilation and oxygen therapy for a short time because of the effects of anesthesia and operation. Initially, we provide these patients with 100 ml•kg^{-1}•min^{-1} of total minute ventilation using a mechanical tidal volume of 12-15 ml/kg and a rate of 7.5 breaths/min (16). Because they usually have no problem with arterial oxygenation, the initial inspired oxygen is 30%. A PEEP of 5 cm H_2O is added to the expiratory limb of the ventilator circuit. Within 10 minutes of the time mechanical support is instituted, an arterial blood sample is analyzed and gas exchange is evaluated. The rate of mechanical ventilation is adjusted to the point that it just prevents acidemia. As the patient recovers from the sedatives, narcotics, and/or muscle relaxants used for anesthesia, the ventilator rate is reduced rapidly. When arterial oxygenation is adequate with 30% inspired oxygen and 5 cm H_2O PEEP, and arterial pH is greater than 7.35 without ventilatory assistance, the patient is extubated. As mentioned previously, the use of IMV for managing such patients has decreased the period of mechanical ventilatory support slightly and has made weaning safer. It is likely that pulse oximetry will become more popular, will decrease the requirement for frequent arterial blood analysis and will further speed the weaning process (22).

Ventilatory management of patients with acute respiratory failure with decreased FRC and lung compliance is more difficult. Occasionally, lung compliance may deteriorate so that patients cannot support adequate respiration and must have mechanical ventilatory support. Even though mechanical support may be necessary at first, CPAP often lessens this need by increasing both FRC and lung compliance, thereby reducing the work of breathing. Thus, only a very short period of mechanical ventilatory support may be required (65). Thereafter, spontaneous respiration with CPAP and a slightly increased inspired oxygen concentration are usually the only required therapeutic adjuncts.

This approach is beneficial in several respects. Weaning from mechanical ventilatory support may occur within minutes or hours of the initiation of therapy (67). Patients who require controlled mechanical ventilation with PEEP often need intravenous infusions of large amounts of fluids to stabilize cardiovascular function (23). Such intravascular fluid loading may increase pulmonary capillary hydrostatic pressure and cause deterioration in pulmonary function secondary to increased lung water, when weaning from mechanical support is attempted. If spontaneous breathing is allowed to persist in the early phase of therapy and mechanical ventilatory support is discontinued as soon as possible, intravascular volume expansion often is unnecessary and CPAP and oxygen may be withdrawn more rapidly. Barotrauma probably is caused by increased airway pressure during mechanical inspiration. If patients are weaned rapidly from mechanical ventilation, exposure to elevated airway pressure and barotrauma may be reduced. Available evidence suggests that barotrauma is lessened when IMV is used (65).

Controlled mechanical ventilation has long been the standard form of therapy for patients with lung contusion and flail chest (66). However, the efficacy of such therapy has been questioned (67). The treatment of patients with severe chest trauma should be similar to that just described. Patients with lung injury and flail chest often cannot breathe spontaneously with ambient airway pressure because of the reduction in lung compliance. Elevation of airway pressure with CPAP may increase FRC and lung compliance, so that mechanical ventilatory support is unnecessary (68). In such cases, stabilization of the chest wall occurs without mechanical ventilation. However, if the chest wall is very unstable, mechanical ventilatory support should not be discontinued. Thus, the appropriate function of mechanical ventilation in the treatment of chest trauma should be to allow immobilization of the chest wall, but only until lung compliance improves enough that spontaneous respiration can occur without disruption of unstable segments. In many instances, mechanical ventilatory support can be discontinued within a matter of hours. Only in the rarest cases, when totally unstable chest wall segments make spontaneous respiration ineffectual, is mechanical ventilatory support necessary for more than a week (68). These patients should be weaned from mechanical ventilation, oxygen and CPAP according to evaluation of gas exchange an pulmonary mechanics, as outlined previously.

Ventilatory support of patients with acute exacerbation of chronic obstructive lung disease is difficult. These patients have a high rate of mortality, and their clinical course often is marked by extreme fluctuation in blood pressure, barotrauma, electrolyte imbalance, and other undesirable side effects of mechanical ventilatory support (69). Weaning them from mechanical support often is hampered by respiratory and metabolic alkalosis, malnutrition, and sedation. Although currently popular, allowing patients to "rest" with mechanical ventilation may not be therapeutic. The longer mechanical ventilation is maintained, the smaller is the chance of survival. Within 24 to 48 hours, the cause of the acute respiratory failure usually is resolving, so that such a rest is unnecessary. Furthermore, controlling the patient's respiration and administering sedatives often leads to problems with weaning. Using IMV we have developed the following clinical approach. A patient with chronic obstructive lung disease often has a hypoxemic drive to breathe. Therefore, the initial inspired oxygen concentration usually does not exceed 30%. Spontaneous respiration is encouraged. If mechanical ventilation is required, the initial ventilator rate is low, in most cases no more than 2 or 3 breaths per minute, with a tidal volume of 10 ml/kg. This amount of support usually results in a slow, but consistent fall in P_aCO_2 and an increase in arterial pH. In this manner, rapid reduction in P_aCO_2 and alkalosis may be avoided (70). Such patients usually have increased FRC and lung compliance. Therefore, PEEP may not improve $\dot{V}A/\dot{Q}$. Once ventilatory support has been instituted, a vigorous regimen of bronchodilation and tracheo-bronchial toilet is initiated. As the patient improves, mechanical ventilation can be withdrawn rapidly. When IMV has been reduced to zero, the patient should be extubated without a prolonged trial of spontaneous respiration.

SUMMARY

Respiratory therapy should be directed at underlying pathology, not symptomatology. Mechanical ventilation, oxygen, and CPAP therapy should be administered to patients in independently prescribed amounts. Removal should follow suit. The method of determining optimal mechanical ventilation, oxygen, and CPAP is not unlike that recommended for many other therapeutic modalities. Each should be applied to achieve a predetermined goal, each should be continually re-evaluated, and each should be withdrawn when no longer required. Optimal CPAP should be applied to improve matching of ventilation and perfusion and to assist lung mechanics so that the requirement of oxygen and mechanical ventilation is reduced. Reduced inspired oxygen may promote resistance to atelectasis and allow more rapid discontinuation of mechanical ventilation and CPAP. Minimal mechanical ventilatory support will eliminate iatrogenic respiratory alkalosis, and improve distribution of ventilation. This approach minimizes the detrimental effects of mechanical ventilation on acid-base balance and cardiovascular function, as well as decreasing the possibility of barotrauma. Sixteen years of prospective evaluation have demonstrated numerous clinical advantages of IMV. This approach has simplified the clinical management of patients with compromised respiratory function and has decreased morbidity and mortality.

GENERAL REFERENCES

1. Campbell EJM, Agostoni E, Davis JN: The Respiratory Muscles: Mechanical and Neural Control. 2nd ed., Philadelphia, WB Saunders, 1970.
2. Fenn WO, Rahn H (eds.): Handbook of Physiology, Section Respiration, Vol. I. Washington, D.C., American Physiological Soc, 1959
3. Nunn JF: Applied Respiratory Physiology. 2nd ed., London, Boston, Butterworth, 1977
4. Shapiro BA: Airway pressure therapy for acute restrictive pulmonary pathology. In: Critical Care: State of the Art, Vol. II. Shoemaker WC, Thompson WL (eds.) Fullerton, California. The Society of Critical Care Medicine, 198, p. II(C):1-53.

SPECIFIC REFERENCES

5. Nunn JF: Applied Respiratory Physiology. 2nd ed., London, Boston, Butterworth, 1977,p. 112-43
6. Nunn JF: Applied Respiratory Physiology. 2nd ed., London, Boston, Butterworth, 1977, p. 45-73
7. Chapin JC, Downs JB, Douglas ME, Murphy EJ, Ruiz BC: Lung expansion, airway pressure transmission, and positive end-expiratory pressure. Arch Surg 114:1193-97, 1979
8. Nunn JF: Applied Respiratory Physiology. 2nd ed., London, Boston, Butterworth, 1977, p. 74-111
9. Bynum LJ, Wilson JE III, Pierce AK: Comparison of spontaneous and positive-pressure breathing in supine normal subjects. J Appl Physiol 41:341-347, 1976
10. Rehder K, Sessler AD, Rodarte JR: Regional intrapulmonary gas distribution in awake and anesthetized-paralyzed man. J Appl Physiol 42:391-402, 1977
11. Rehder K, Knopp TJ, Brusasco V, Didier EP: Inspiratory flow and intrapulmonary gas distribution. Am Rev Respir Dis 124:392-6, 1981
12. Froese AB, Bryan AC: Effects of anesthesia and paralysis on diaphragmatic mechanics in man. Anesthesiology 41:242-55, 1974
13. Nunn JF: Applied Respiratory Physiology. 2nd Ed., London, Boston, Butterworth, 1977, p. 177-208
14. Downs JB, Mitchell LA: Pulmonary effects of ventilatory pattern following cardiopulmonary bypass. Crit Care Med 4:295-300, 1976
15. Downs JB, Douglas ME: Intermittent mandatory ventilation and weaning. In: Intermittent Mandatory Ventilation. Kirby RR, Graybar GB (eds.). Int Anesthesiol Clin 18(2):81-95, 1980
16. Downs JB, Marston AW: A new transport ventilator: An evaluation. Crit Care Med 5:112-14, 1977
17. Llewellyn MA, Swyer PR: Assisted and controlled ventilation in the newborn period: Effect of oxygenation. Br J Anaesth 43:926-31, 1971
18. Downs JB, Douglas ME, Ruiz BC, Miller NL: Comparison of assisted and controlled mechanical ventilation in anesthetized swine. Crit Care Med 7:5-8, 1979
19. Downs JB, Perkins HM, Modell JL: Intermittent mandatory ventilation. An evaluation. Arch Surg 109:519-23, 1974
20. Campbell EJM, Agostoni E, Davis JN: The Respiratory Muscles: Mechanics and Neural Control. 2nd Ed., Philadelphia, WB Saunders, 1970, p. 115-142
21. Nunn JF: Applied Respiratory Physiology. 2nd Ed., London, Boston, Butterworth, 1977, p. 144-176
22. Millbern SM, Downs JB, Jumper LC, Modell JH: Evaluation of criteria for discontinuing mechanical ventilatory support. Arch Surg 113:1441-43, 1978

23. Qvist J, Pontoppidan H, Wilson RS, Lowenstein E, Laver MB: Hemodynamic responses to mechanical ventilation with PEEP: The effect of hypervolemia. Anesthesiology 42:45-55, 1975

24. Downs JB, Douglas ME, Sanfellippo PM, Stanford W, Hodges MR: Ventilatory pattern intrapleural pressure and cardiac output. Anesth Analg 56:88-96, 1977

25. Downs JB: A technique for direct measurement of intrapleural pressure. Crit Care Med 4:207-10, 1976

26. Mead J, Gaensler EA: Esophageal and pleural pressures in man, upright and supine. J Appl Physiol 14:81-3, 1959

27. Milic-Emili J, Mead J, Turner JM, Galuser EM: Improved technique for estimating pleural pressure from esophageal balloons. J Appl Physiol 19:207-11, 1964

28. Sturgeon CL Jr, Douglas ME, Downs JB, Dannemiller FJ: PEEP and CPAP: Cardiopulmonary effects during spontaneous ventilation. Anesth Analg 56:633-41

29. Weinstein ME, Rice CL, Peters RM, Virgilio RW: Hemodynamic and respiratory response to varying gradients between end-expiratory pressure and end-inspiratory pressure in patients breathing on continuous positive airway pressure. J Trauma 18:231-35, 1978

30. Kirby RR, Perry JC, Calderwood HW, Ruiz BC, Lederman DS: Cardiorespiratory effects of high positive end-expiratory pressure. Anesthesiology 43:533-39, 1975

31. Marquez JM, Douglas ME, Downs JB, Wu WH, Mantini EL, Kuck EJ, Calderwood HW: Renal function and cardiovascular responses during positive airway pressure. Anesthesiology 50:393-98, 1979

32. Nunn JF: Applied Respiratory Physiology. 2nd Ed., London, Boston, Butterworth, 1977 p. 209-31

33. Downs JB, Klein EF Jr, Modell JH: The effect of incremental PEEP on PaO2 in patients with respiratory failure. Anesth Analg 52:210-15, 1973

34. Suter PM, Fairley HB, Isenberg MD: Optimum end-expiratory airway pressure in patients with acute airway pressure in patients with acute pulmonary failure. N Engl J Med 292:284-89, 1975

35. Kirby RR, Downs JB, Civetta JM, Modell JH, Dannemiller FJ, Klein EF Jr, Hodges M: High level positive end expiratory pressure (PEEP) in acute respiratory insufficiency. Chest 67:156-63, 1975

36. Shapiro BA, Harrison RA, Walton JR, Davison R: Intermittent demand ventilation (IDV): A new technique for supporting ventilation in critically ill patients. Respir Care 21:521-25, 1976

37. Heenan TJ, Downs JB, Douglas ME, Ruiz BC, et al: Intermittent mandatory ventilation—is synchronization important? Chest 77:598-602, 1978

38. Baratz RA, Philbin DM, Patterson RW: Plasma antidiuretic hormone and urinary output during continuous positive-pressure breathing in dogs. Anesthesiology 34:510-13, 1971

39. Kumar A, Pontoppidan H, Baratz RA, Laver MB: Inappropriate response to increased plasma ADH during mechanical ventilation in acute respiratory failure. Anesthesiology 40:215-21, 1974

40. Landmark SJ, Knopp TJ, Rehder K, Sessler AD: Regional pulmonary perfusion and V/Q in awake and anesthetized-paralyzed man. J Appl Physiol 43:993-1000, 1977

41. Zarins CK, Bayne CG, Rice Cl, et al: Does spontaneous ventilation with IMV protect from PEEP induced cardiac output depression? J Surg Res 22 (3):299-304, 1977

42. Briscoe WA, Cree EM, Filler J, Houssax HEJ, Cournand A: Lung volume, alveolar ventilation and perfusion interrelationships in chronic pulmonary emphysema. J Appl Physiol 15:785-95, 1960

43. Wagner PD: Recent advances in pulmonary gas exchange. In: Anesthesia and Respiratory Function. Kafer ER (ed.) Int Anesthesiol Clin 15(2):81-111, 1977

44. West JB: Blood flow to the lung and gas exchange. Anesthesiology 41:124-38, 1974

45. West JB: New advances in pulmonary gas exchange. Anesth Analg 54:409-18, 1975

46. Suter PM, Fairley HB, Schlobohm RM: Shunt, lung volume and perfusion during short periods of ventilation with oxygen. Anesthesiology 43:617-27, 1975

47. Douglas ME, Downs JB, Dannemiller FJ, Hodges MR, Munson ES: Change in pulmonary venous admixture with varying inspired oxygen. Anesth Analg 55:688-95, 1976

48. Barany JS, Saltzman AR, Locke RA: Oxygen-related intrapulmonary shunting in obstructive pulmonary disease. Chest 74-34-38, 1978

49. Strauss HW, Hurley PJ, Rhodes BA, Wagner HN Jr: Quantification of right-to-left transpulmonary shunts in man. J Lab Clin Med 74:597-607, 1969

50. Tobin CE: Arteriovenous shunts in the peripheral pulmonary circulation in the human lung. Thorax 21:197-204, 1966.

51. Balchum OJ, Jung RC, Turner AF, et al: Pulmonary artery to vein shunts. Current research in chronic airway obstruction. In: Proceedings of the Ninth Annual Aspen Emphysema Conference, Aspen, Colorado, 223-38, 1968

52. Register SD, Downs JB, Stock, MC, Kirby RR: Is 50% Oxygen harmful? Crit Care Med 15:598-601, 1987

53. Gherini S, Peters RM, Virgilio RW: Mechanical work on the lungs and work of breathing with positive end-expiratory pressure and continuous positive airway pressure. Chest 76:251-6, 1979

54. Douglas ME, Downs JB: Cardiopulmonary effects of PEEP and CPAP, Special correspondence. Anesth Analg 57:347-50, 1978

55. Greenbaum DM, Miller JE, Eross B, Snyder JV, Grenvik A, Safar P: Continuous positive airway pressure without trachael intubation in spontaneously breathing patients. Chest 69:615-20, 1976

56. Mitchell LA, Downs JB, Dannemiller FJ: Extrapulmonary influences on A-aDO2 following cardiopulmonary bypass. Anesthesiology 43:583-6, 1975

57. Barach AL, Martin J, Eckman M: Positive pressure respiration and its applications to the treatment of acute pulmonary edema. Ann Intern Med 12:754-95, 1988

58. Burford TH, Burbank B: Traumatic wet lung. Observations on certain physiologic fundamentals of thoracic trauma. J Thorac Surg 14:415-24, 1945

59. Jensen NK: Recovery of pulmonary function after crushing injuries of the chest. Dis Chest 22:319-46, 1952

60. Ashbaugh DG, Petty TL, Bigelow DG, et al: Continuous positive-pressure breathing (CPPB) in adult respiratory distress syndrome. J Thorac Cardiovasc Surg 57:31-41, 1969

61. Rose DM, Downs JB, Hennan TJ: Temporal responses of functional residual capacity and oxygen tension to changes in positive end-expiratory pressure. Crit Care Med (9): 79-82, 1981

62. Downs JB, Klein EF Jr., Desautels D, Modell JH, Kirby RR: Intermittent mandatory ventilation: A new approach to weaning patients from mechanical ventilators. Chest 64:331-5, 1973

63. Chiang H, Pontoppidan H, Wilson RS, et al: Respiratory muscle discoordination following prolonged mechanical ventilation. In: Abstracts of the 1973 Annual Meeting of the American Society of Anesthesiologists. San Francisco, California, p. 211-12, 1973

64. Andersen JB, Kann T, Rasmussen JP, et al: Respiratory thoracoabdominal coordination and muscle fatigue in acute respiratory failure. Am Rev Respir Dis Annual Meeting Supplement. (Abstract) 117(4): 89-90, 1978

65. Douglas ME, Downs JB: Pulmonary function following severe acute respiratory failure and high levels of positive end-expiratory pressure. Chest 71:18-23, 1977

66. Avery EE, Morch ET, Benson DW: Critically crushed chests: A new method of treatment with continuous mechanical hyperventilation to produce alkalotic apnea and internal pneumatic stabilization. J Thorac Surg 32:291-309, 1956

67. Trinkle JK, Richardson JD, Franz JL, Grover FL, Aron KV, Holmstrom FMG: Management of flail chest without mechanical ventilation. Ann Thorac Surg 19:355-63, 1975

68. Downs JB (commentor), Parham AM, Yarbrough DR III, Redding JS: Flail chest syndrome and pulmonary contusion. Editorial comment. Arch Surg 113:903, 1978

69. Kilburn KH: Shock, seizures and coma with alkalosis during mechanical ventilation. Ann Intern Med 65:977-84, 1966

70. Downs JB, Block AJ, Vennum KB: Intermittent mandatory ventilation in the treatment of patients with chronic obstructive pulmonary disease. Anesth Analg 53:437-41, 1974

PULMONARY EMBOLIC DISEASE: DIAGNOSIS AND TREATMENT

R. C. Bone

One of the most difficult diagnoses to make in medicine today is that of pulmonary embolic disease. In a study done in the early 1970s (1), evidence of pulmonary embolism at autopsy correlated poorly with an antemortem diagnosis of pulmonary embolic disease; in only one-third of the cases were emboli correctly identified. A batting average of .333 may be terrific for a professional baseball player, but for a physician attempting to make a diagnosis of a potential lethal disease, such a statistic is unsatisfactory (2).

Although more than 500,000 pulmonary emboli are estimated to occur annually, the vast majority are not clinically evident. This estimate is derived from the known number of deaths per year that result from pulmonary emboli, 50,000 to 100,000. More than one-third of these deaths occur within the first hour after the embolic event, many occurring as terminal events in hospitalized patients. Occasionally, the diagnosis is difficult or delayed because of the clinical similarity to other acute medical events or because of superimposed embolic phenomena in patients with pre-existing pulmonary or cardiovascular disease. Most emboli of small to medium arteries do not require intensive care monitoring unless they occur in sufficient numbers or in patients with decreased pulmonary reserve. However, emboli that occlude 40 to 50% of the pulmonary vasculature (massive emboli) are often associated with shock and usually cause sufficient respiratory embarrassment to require intensive care monitoring and therapy.

Prophylaxis for pulmonary emboli is briefly reviewed. Clinical presentation, diagnosis, and medical and surgical intervention in patients with "massive emboli" (those who require intensive care) are discussed.

T. H. Stanley and R. J. Sperry (eds.), Anesthesia and the Lung 1992, 243–251.
© 1992 Kluwer Academic Publishers.

Pulmonary emboli remain a cause of considerable morbidity and mortality in hospitalized and institutionalized patients. In the intensive care setting, pulmonary emboli are serious, and often fatal. In these critically ill patients, measures to decrease the incidence of deep vein thrombosis, and thereby prevent pulmonary emboli, are warranted.

Physical findings in patients with massive pulmonary emboli are those associated with cardiovascular compromise and right ventricular overload. Tachypnea, tachycardia, hypotension, and cyanosis are often found. Jugular distention, hepatojugular reflux, parasternal heave, right ventricular gallop, murmur of tricuspid insufficiency, and an increased pulmonic component of the second heart sound indicate significant right heart strain. Pulmonary hypertension usually does not occur until 50% of the pulmonary vasculature is occluded. Pulmonary artery pressures of greater than 40 mmHg do not occur in acute embolism—even massive embolism—unless chronic recurrent embolization or other non-embolic causes of pulmonary hypertension exist. The differential diagnosis of patients with massive pulmonary emboli includes conditions associated with hypotension and central chest pain, such as acute myocardial infarction, acute aortic dissection, and ruptured esophagus.

DIAGNOSTIC AIDS

Laboratory findings that are most helpful include arterial blood gas levels, chest radiograph, electrocardiogram, lung scan, and pulmonary angiograms. Biochemical tests such as bilirubin, lactic dehydrogenase, and serum glutamic oxalic transaminase are rarely helpful. Leukocytosis or elevated fibrin split products are also nonspecific and of little use. Blood gases reveal hypoxemia, as related to the widened alveolar/arterial gradient. Although blood gases may be normal with smaller emboli, hypoxemia associated with massive embolization is striking.

Chest radiographs may be normal, even with massive emboli. Pleural effusion, infiltrates, areas of consolidation, Hampton's hump, plate-like atelectasis, elevated hemidiaphragm, and Westermark's sign may be associated with pulmonary emboli. In patients with massive emboli and acute or chronic pulmonary emboli, enlarged pulmonary arteries or cardiomegaly (representing right ventricular enlargement) may be present.

Electrocardiograms of patients with massive pulmonary emboli are most likely to be abnormal (80%). Transient changes, indicating right heart compromise, such as right axis deviation (S_1, Q_3, T_3) and p-pulmonale may be seen with smaller emboli, but persistent changes indicate more massive emboli (50% or more vascular occlusion). Many arrhythmias are associated with pulmonary emboli, and unexplained arrhythmias should bring pulmonary embolism to mind. However, complete right bundle branch block tends to occur only in patients with massive embolism. Although history, physical findings, blood gases, chest radiographs, and electrocardiograms can be helpful in indicating the possibility of pulmonary embolism, definitive diagnosis is only possible with a lung scan and pulmonary angiogram.

Many methods have been proposed and studied for prophylaxis of deep vein thrombosis. These include full anticoagulation therapy with heparin or Coumadin, low-dose heparin, platelet inhibitors, dextrans, and devices that enhance blood flow from the lower extremities, such as pneumatic compression boots. With the use of I-fibrinogen scanning, many studies have been conducted to compare various prophylactic regimens.

Much has been written, since the early 1970s, about prophylaxis of thromboembolic disease with low-dose heparin. Heparin, in small amounts, increases the rate of combination of antithrombin III with activated factor X (Xa), as well as with thrombin. This enhances the body's mechanism for antithrombotic processes. Low-dose heparin is given as 5000 units subcutaneously every 12 hours. Studies evaluating the efficacy of giving heparin every 8 hours revealed a slightly greater decrease in overall frequency of thrombosis but not in the frequency of fatal emboli. More frequent heparin dosage is associated with greater numbers of hemorrhagic complications, and is therefore not recommended. With the evidence on hand, coupled with the low incidence of complications of therapy, routine use of prophylactic low-dose heparin in critically ill patients is warranted unless specific contraindications exist.

ACUTE MASSIVE PULMONARY EMBOLISM

Patients in whom pleuritic chest pain, pleural rub, hemoptysis, and mild hypoxemia develop pose very few diagnostic or therapeutic problems. However, thromboembolic events in patients with other acute cardiopulmonary diseases are difficult to diagnose. Once a diagnosis is made, the majority of such patients pose no special problems for therapeutic maneuvers. However, there exists a subset of patients for whom the entire gamut of diagnostic and therapeutic interventions must, at least, be considered.

CLINICAL PRESENTATION

Massive pulmonary embolism is most likely to present as an acute cardiovascular event. Symptoms such as sudden syncope or collapse (80%), dyspnea (72%), and central chest pain (34%) often present initially. Cardiac arrest may occur in 20 to 30% of these patients.

LUNG SCAN

To diagnose pulmonary embolism, a microembolism technique, employing an isotope (usually technetium-99), is commonly used to generate perfusion lung scans. Images in four to six views are obtained for interpretation. A persistent absence of flow on several views is interpreted as a positive defect. The false-negative rate is extremely low; a normal or negative perfusion scan correlates more than 99% of the time with normal pulmonary angiograms. The false-positive rate, however, can range as high as 50 to 60%. In some studies, positive angiograms correlate with perfusion scans exhibiting segmental or larger defects as much as 89% of the time. Ventilation lung scans using inhaled xenon document mismatched areas, that is, regions where there is no perfusion but ventilation continues. It is well-documented that pulmonary vascular occlusion is associated with areas of decreased ventilation secondary to bronchoconstriction and atelectasis. These events are more likely to occur with smaller defects. In patients suspected of having massive embolism, lung scans are most likely to be positive, with a high degree of confidence.

However, before using thrombolytic agents or surgical interventions (e.g., inferior vena cava interruption, embolectomy), further studies (e.g., angiography) are indicated.

In the PIOPED study (3), an investigation of major importance, giving us information on the sensitivity and specificity of ventilation-perfusion scans in pulmonary embolism, is published. Nearly all patients with acute pulmonary embolism had abnormal scans (high, intermediate, or low probability), but so did most patients without emboli (sensitivity 98%, specificity 10%). This study of more than 900 patients shows that the sensitivity of this technique is 41% for high probability scans, 82% for intermediate or high probability scans, and 98% for low, intermediate, or high probability scans. Specificities were 97%, 52%, and 10%, respectively.

This study was a multi-center investigation that was extremely well done. One very surprising result is that 4% of patients with normal or near-normal perfusion lung scans were found to have pulmonary emboli. The popular "clinical pearl" that patients having normal or near-normal perfusion scans are free of pulmonary embolic disease is, therefore, incorrect 4% of the time.

Ventilation-perfusion lung scans were criticized in the 1970s because of their non-specificity. Robin humorously referred to the situation as being akin to the Emperor who had no clothes (3). After that time, several studies documented that carefully performed lung scans do have reasonable sensitivity and specificity. The major conclusions for the PIOPED study is that both the dismal and optimistic projections do not tell the full story. There are significant problems in using only ventilation-perfusion scans for definitive diagnosis of pulmonary embolic disease (3, 5). The relatively low sensitivity of high-probability scans (41%) means that scans, alone, are inadequate to ascertain the presence of pulmonary embolism. On the other hand, only 3% of patients in the PIOPED study who did not show thromboemboli on angiography had high-probability ventilation-perfusion scans (97% specificity). When combined with the clinical picture, therefore, the sensitivity and specificity of ventilation-perfusion lung scans makes them an important adjunct to diagnosis. Among PIOPED patients for whom clinical impressions and ventilation-perfusion scans were both high probability, 96% had pulmonary emboli.

In my opinion, the greatest recent advance has occurred in the non-invasive diagnosis of deep venous thrombi (which are the usual antecedents to pulmonary emboli) using either impedance studies or duplex ultrasound of the legs (6-8). In diagnosing pulmonary embolic disease today, the clinical history, used in conjunction with evaluation of arterial blood gases, ventilation-perfusion scans, and non-invasive studies of the deep veins of the legs should markedly improve the physician's batting average. If the post-mortem studies of the 1970s were repeated today, using this recent information, the batting averages should be much better. My suggestions for diagnostic evaluation are included in an algorithm that utilizes information published on the diagnostic accuracy of non-invasive studies for deep venous thrombosis (see figure) (3,6-8).

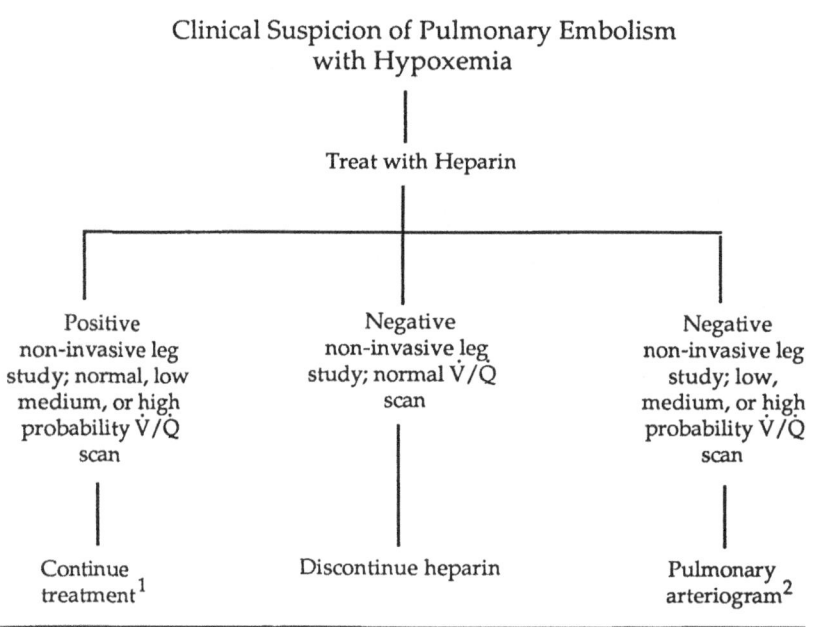

Clinical Suspicion of Pulmonary Embolism
with Hypoxemia

Treat with Heparin

| Positive non-invasive leg study; normal, low medium, or high probability V̇/Q̇ scan | Negative non-invasive leg study; normal V̇/Q̇ scan | Negative non-invasive leg study; low, medium, or high probability V̇/Q̇ scan |

| Continue treatment[1] | Discontinue heparin | Pulmonary arteriogram[2] |

1. If high quality non-invasive leg study is able to be performed. If doubt about quality of non-invasive study, a venogram should be done.

2. In selected cases with a very high suspicion of pulmonary embolism (i.e., previous documented pulmonary embolism), a high probability V̇/Q̇ scan might be accepted as proof of pulmonary embolism without an angiogram.

The ventilation-perfusion lung scan, taken in isolation is neither "the Emperor has no clothes," nor "the Emperor is fully clothed." Indeed, the Emperor may have some clothes on, but unfortunately he is, as yet, incompletely attired. In the majority of cases of suspected pulmonary embolism, the emperor has a "well-clothed" appearance. When there is significant doubt, a pulmonary angiogram should be done.

PULMONARY ANGIOGRAPHY

At present, definitive diagnosis of pulmonary embolus is made on the basis of pulmonary angiograms. Limitations to this procedure appear to be related to the experience of the angiographer and the interpreter. The mortality rate is 0.2%, and deaths are usually associated with severe pulmonary hypertension. The most important indication of embolism is a filling defect. Vasculature cut-off with and without regional delay in arterial flow is also significant. A flow-directed catheter with selected pulmonary angiograms in abnormal segments (demonstrated by lung scan) is a technique used to decrease the use of contrast dye and avoid exacerbating already high pulmonary artery pressures in selected patients. Digital angiography, using lower volumes of contrast in central venous lines, is promising. This technique also avoids the previously mentioned problems, and dye can be introduced through already existing central venous lines.

Overall, angiography is of low morbidity and mortality and is indicated when patients may be subjected to high-risk or high-morbidity therapies (e.g., thrombolytic agents, inferior vena cava interruption, embolectomy). Clinicians who prefer to use long-term anticoagulation for patients with pulmonary emboli are more likely to desire angiographic evidence.

MEDICAL INTERVENTION

Medical therapy for pulmonary emboli consists of anticoagulant and thrombolytic agents. The majority of patients with pulmonary emboli, that is, those without significant respiratory or cardiovascular deterioration, are treated with anticoagulants. Heparin infusions are used during the acute phase, followed by warfarin compounds for as long as 4 to 6 months. Although accepted practice, laboratory monitoring of such therapy varies from area to area, and complication rates may be as high as 25%. For situations in which major complications of therapy or significant respiratory and cardiovascular embarrassment exist, other modes of therapy (e.g., thrombolytic agents or surgery) must be considered.

REFERENCES

1. Modan B, Sharon E, Jelin N: Factors contributing to the incorrect diagnosis of pulmonary embolic disease. Chest 62:388-93, 1972
2. Bone RC. Ventilation/perfusion scan in pulmonary embolism: The emperor is incompletely attired (editorial). JAMA 263:2794-95, 1990
3. Terrin ML, and the PIOPED Investigators: Value of the ventilation/perfusion scan in acute pulmonary embolism: Results of the prospective investigation of pulmonary embolism diagnosis (PIOPED). JAMA 263:2753-59, 1990
4. Robin ED: Overdiagnosis and overtreatment of pulmonary embolism: The Emperor may have no clothes. Ann Intern Med 87:775-581, 1977
5. Hull RD, Hirsh J, Carter CJ, et al: Diagnostic value of ventilation-perfusion lung scanning in patients with suspected pulmonary embolism. Chest 88:819-28, 1985
6. Hull RD, Hirsh J, Carter CJ, et al: Diagnostic efficacy of impedance plethysmography for clinically suspected deep-vein thrombosis. Ann Intern Med 102:21-28, 1985
7. Polak JF, Culter SS, O'Leary DH: Deep veins of the calf: Assessment with Doppler flow imaging. Radiol 171:481-485, 1989
8. White RH, McGahan JP, Daschbach MM, Hartling RP: Diagnosis of deep-vein thrombosis using duplex ultrasound. Ann Intern Med 111:297-304, 1989

SUGGESTED READING

Bedard CK, Bone RC: Westermark's sign in the diagnosis of pulmonary emboli in patients with the adult respiratory distress syndrome. Crit Care Med 5:137-40, 1977

Collins R, Scrimgeour A, Yusuf S, Peto R: Reduction in fatal pulmonary embolism and venous thrombosis by perioperative administration of subcutaneous heparin. Overview of results of randomized trials in general, orthopedic, and urologic surgery. N Engl J Med 318(18): 1162-73, 1988

Glenny RW: Pulmonary embolism: Complications of therapy. South Med J 80(10):1266-76, 1987

Hayes S, Bone RC: Pulmonary emboli with respiratory failure. Med Clin North Am 67(6):1179-91, 1983

Kessler CM, Druy E, Goldhaber SZ. Acute pulmonary embolism treated with thrombolytic agents: Current status of tPA and future implications for emergency medicine. Ann Emerg Med 17(11):1216-20, 1988

Marder VJ, Sherry S: Thrombolytic therapy: Current status. N Engl J Med 318(24):1585-95, 1988

McCann RL, Sabiston DC: Current management of venous thrombolytic disease. Br J Surg 76(2):113-4, 1989

Mohr DN, Ryu JH, Litin SC, Rosenow EC: Recent advances in the management of venous thromboembolism. Mayo Clin Proc 63(3):281-90, 1988

Pingleton SK, Bone RC, Ruth WE, Pingleton WW: Low-dose heparin for pulmonary emboli in an intensive care unit. Chest 79:647-50, 1981

Schmidt GA, Hall JB: Acute on chronic respiratory failure: Assessment and management of patients with COPD in the emergent setting. JAMA 261(23)3444-53, 1989

Valenzuela TD: Pulmonary embolism. Ann Emerg Med 17(3):209-13, 1988

ADULT RESPIRATORY DISTRESS SYNDROME

R. C. Bone

The Adult Respiratory Distress Syndrome (ARDS) is often the first manifestation of Multiple System Organ Failure (MSOF). The MSOF syndrome is defined as the presence of two or more organ systems with impaired function. The syndrome of multi-organ failure is characterized by a hyperdynamic, hypermetabolic state identical to that seen in the septic syndrome. The mortality rate associated with multi-organ failure exceeds 60%, and the emergence of MSOF and the septic syndrome as important clinical entities is related to improvements in the technology of life-support systems.

TREATMENT OF ACUTE RESPIRATORY FAILURE

Treatment of acute respiratory failure of any cause includes provision of adequate tissue oxygenation by respiratory and circulatory support. Since the clinical problems are similar no matter what inciting agent leads to ARDS, the therapeutic goal is to support patients until alveolocapillary membrane integrity is re-established. Critical factors in ARDS treatment include: 1) optimal distention of alveoli to increase functional residual capacity, 2) maintenance of tissue perfusion, and 3) control of the primary problem.

Because alveolar collapse leads to a basic pathophysiologic defect, major efforts are directed toward obtaining optimal distention of alveoli. PEEP is used to increase functional residual capacity (FRC) and to correct the tendency toward progressive atelectasis. Ventilatory assistance is frequently required. Indications for supplemental oxygen include arterial oxygen tension lower than 60 mmHg (room air; patient with previously normal lungs). If arterial oxygen tension does not increase satisfactorily

253

T. H. Stanley and R. J. Sperry (eds.), Anesthesia and the Lung 1992, 253–267.
© 1992 Kluwer Academic Publishers.

with high concentrations of oxygen, ventilatory assistance may be necessary.

PEEP is indicated if an F_IO_2 above 50% is required to maintain satisfactory arterial oxygen tension in a mechanically ventilated patient. Continuous positive airway pressure (CPAP) is a technique whereby PEEP can be given to a patient by mask. This method of PEEP administration is to be condemned in obtunded or stuporous patients, but may be useful in alert patients. The P_aO_2/F_IO_2 ratio and its response to therapy can be used as an index of survival (Fig. 1).

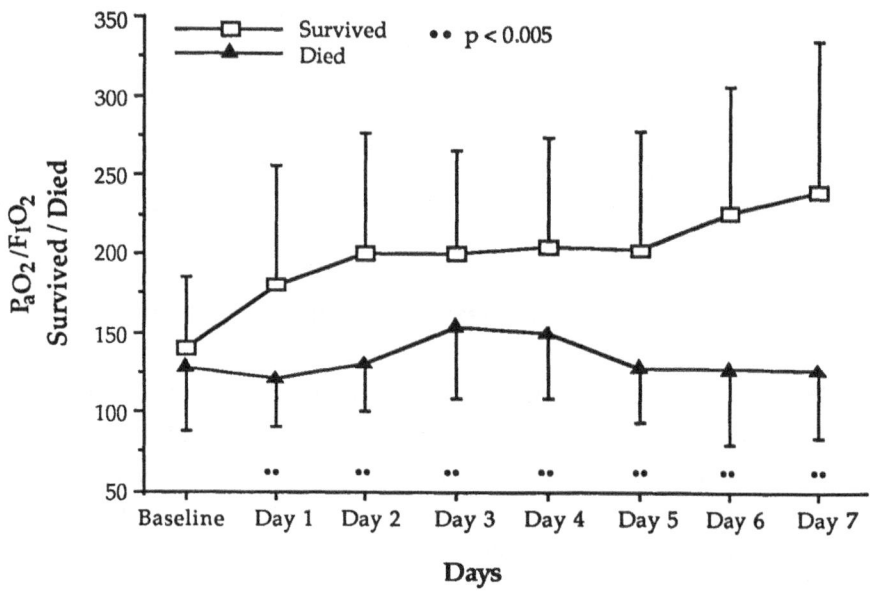

Figure 1. P_aO_2/F_IO_2 ratios and survival in acute respiratory failure.

Further treatment includes: 1) correction of factors that led to decreased red blood cell oxygen transport, 2) provision of appropriate nutritional support, and 3) avoidance of complications.

POSITIVE END EXPIRATORY PRESSURE

Since its introduction for use in the management of adult patients with diffuse lung injury more than 20 years ago, PEEP has become an integral component in the treatment of ARDS. PEEP is still a mainstay in the treatment of diffuse lung processes, since it supports the P_aO_2 and allows reduction in inspired oxygen concentrations (F_IO_2). PEEP produces increases in the alveolar and airway pressures at the end of expiration—to levels greater than atmospheric pressure. A continuous positive distending pressure is therefore produced across alveolar and airway walls, regenerating (through the process of recruitment) patency in many closed or atelectatic gas exchange units. Areas of shunt and ventilation/perfusion mismatch may be corrected, which would improve oxygenation. Fluid-filled alveoli may be stabilized by allowing fluid to occupy relatively flat layers on alveolar walls; this would also improve gas exchange. It is important to recognize, however, that PEEP does not decrease absolute amounts of extravascular lung water; in fact, lung water may actually increase at high lung volumes.

The beneficial effects of PEEP therapy include its ability to increase FRC; increase pulmonary compliance; decrease shunt fractions ($\dot{Q}s/\dot{Q}T$); increase P_aO_2 for given F_IO_2 levels; and possibly, conserve alveolar surfactant, thereby reducing alveolar surface tension. These attributes have made PEEP a standard in the treatment of respiratory failure secondary to diffuse parenchymal lung disease. Intrapulmonary shunting may also decrease in association with the decreased cardiac output produced by high levels of PEEP.

Although PEEP helps to improve several of the physiologic alterations associated with diffuse lung injury, there is no evidence to substantiate that PEEP therapy is anything more than supportive. Further, despite aggressive supportive therapy, there has been no appreciable change in survival of ARDS patients over the past two decades. The use of PEEP has been advocated in the treatment of flail chest and mechanical dysfunction of the chest, in infant respiratory distress syndrome, in postoperative patients (to improve oxygenation), and in the treatment of obstructive sleep apnea. Several reports have even suggested that early use of PEEP might protect susceptible patients from developing ARDS, but investigations of possible benefit of prophylactic PEEP in patients at high risk for the development of ARDS have proven inconclusive. This has been a controversial topic, and the issue will prove difficult to resolve because of the heterogeneity of the adult respiratory distress syndrome.

Another controversial issue in PEEP therapy has been appropriate levels of PEEP to administer. Most would agree that PEEP should be increased or decreased in small increments and that each patients's cardiac output and tissue oxygen delivery need to be carefully monitored. If cardiac output decreases, it must be supported with volume infusions and inotropic agents. The literature contains numerous attempts to specify "optimal" or "best" levels of PEEP. The common theme among these efforts appears to define some "ideal" level of PEEP as that level that allows inspired oxygen concentrations to be reduced to less toxic ranges while maintaining adequate tissue oxygen delivery.

Unfortunately, PEEP therapy has some undesirable effects—intra-alveolar pressures may exceed intracapillary pressures (leading to increased dead space ventilation $[V_D/V_T]$) and cardiac output and organ perfusion may decrease. While the use of PEEP is usually associated with increases in P_aO_2, this parameter may actually decline as a result of decreased cardiac output, alveolar over-distention, or increased pulmonary arterial resistance and decreased pulmonary capillary size. With administration of PEEP, blood may be diverted from well-preserved and ventilated lung units to more poorly ventilated ones, exacerbating pulmonary shunting. PEEP may even elevate cerebral venous and intracranial pressures, potentiating cerebral dysfunction.

It is important to reiterate that PEEP does not decrease extravascular lung water, but can significantly decrease intravascular pulmonary fluid volume as a consequence of reduced cardiac output. This PEEP-related decrease in cardiac output is primarily based on diminished venous return caused by elevated intrathoracic pressure. In addition, PEEP is capable of increasing pulmonary vascular resistance, decreasing left ventricular after-load, decreasing myocardial blood flow, and altering the geometry and compliance of the right and left ventricles. PEEP-induced decreases in cardiac output leads to declining hepatic, adrenal, bronchial, fundal mucosal, renal, coronary, and subendocardial arterial blood flow. These changes appear to return to baseline levels when PEEP is discontinued. PEEP may also predispose patients to pulmonary barotrauma, especially when large tidal volumes are used. Physicians need to be aware of this potential complication and realize that tension pneumothorax may develop rapidly in patients ventilated with PEEP.

Despite its potential detrimental effects, PEEP therapy has a beneficial role in the management of respiratory failure secondary to diffuse parenchymal lung disease. When using PEEP, however, attention must be directed toward maintaining organ perfusion and function. At present, there is no evidence that PEEP decreases extravascular lung water or prevents the development of ARDS in susceptible patients. The primary goal of PEEP therapy, therefore, is to obtain adequate arterial oxygen saturation (on non- toxic F_IO_2 levels) while maintaining cardiac output and tissue oxygen delivery.

SEPSIS

While many advances have occurred recently in our understanding of the pathogenetic mechanisms and treatment of septic shock, our ability to rescue a patient from it has unfortunately lagged behind. Its definition is simply the deranged metabolic state that arises from systemic sepsis in a hypotensive patient unresponsive to fluid management. Septic shock may be precipitated by a variety of organisms. Invasion into the bloodstream by bacteria or their toxic metabolites triggers various pathophysiologic sequelae that eventually lead to hypotension and multi-organ failure.

Gram-negative sepsis is now a major concern in immunosuppressed patients. Each year in the United States there are an estimated 300,000 to 500,000 cases of gram-negative sepsis, with mortality rates ranging from 20 to 75%. Given that sepsis is more often considered a complication of disease rather than the lethal end-point of a serious underlying disease, these mortality figures may be underestimates. The literature on gram-negative sepsis is limited to case reports from the pre-antibiotic era. Today, gram-negative sepsis accounts for 1% of all university hospital admissions.

Septic shock should not be viewed as a single entity, since a vast array of organisms presenting in a variety of fashions may culminate in moribund patients (Table 1). Vasomotor collapse can result from decreased intravascular volume (as in patients with cholera). Organisms (e.g., meningococcemia, Rocky Mountain spotted fever, viral myocarditis) may invade the myocardium and lead to hypotension. The myriad of organisms that cause endocarditis may cause shock from progressive destruction of endovalvular structures. Probably the most intensely studied form of shock—and one of increasing importance—is that of gram-negative sepsis. Shock with this form of sepsis is linked to activation of several inherent metabolic pathways, which will be discussed later.

Table 1. Mechanisms of shock in sepsis.

Decreased intravascular volume (e.g., cholera, toxic shock syndrome, dengue)

Myocardial depression

Myocardial cell invasion or pump failure (e.g., meningococcemia, viral myocarditis, diphtheria)

endovalvular destruction (e.g., endocarditis)

Decreased venous return to heart (e.g., gram-negative sepsis)

Perhaps the single most important determinant of outcome in patients with septic shock is severity of underlying disease. Patients with malignancies or cirrhosis, asplenics, and those of advanced age or with multiple diseases (diabetes, renal failure, heart disease, etc.), or patients treated with immunosuppressive agents are at greatest risk of dying from septic shock. The source of infection and virulence of the organism have significant effects on patient outcome. Nosocomial infections and sepsis due to gram-negative bacilli are associated with higher mortality rates than community-acquired infections and gram-positive infections.

CLINICAL ASPECTS

The Septic Syndrome can be defined as hypothermia (T < 96°F rectal) or hyperthermia (T > 101°F rectal), tachycardia (> 90 bpm), tachypnea (>20 bpm), a presumed site of infection, and evidence of inadequate perfusion (as evidenced by either poor or altered cerebral function), arterial hypoxia (P_aO_2 < 75 mmHg), and elevated plasma lactate level or urine output less than 0.5 ml/kg body weight/hour.

The clinical presentation of a patient in septic shock may evolve over days or may take an explosive course (as in meningococcemia), killing the patient in a matter of hours. One of the keys to successful therapy, therefore, is to recognize septic shock as quickly as possible. The earliest changes may occur in the patient's vital signs or mental status. The presence of fever or hypothermia, hyperventilation, tachycardia, or a change in mental status (none of which are specific for septic shock) should prompt acquisition of several blood cultures and possible initiation of therapy. Early in its course, blood pressure may be normal or slightly reduced, and perfusion to the extremities is usually adequate; as septic shock progresses, hypotension results, and as perfusion to the extremities drops, the skin becomes mottled, cyanotic, and cold. The skin in occasional patients may show classic changes as the ecthyma gangrenosum lesion of bacteremia with *Pseudomonas aeruginosa*, and sometimes, *Aeromonas hydrophila*. Bullae and desquamation of the palms and soles may suggest toxic shock syndrome in menstruating women or post-surgical patients. Petechiae occur with several types of bacteremia; however, with gram-negative bacilli they are less common. They may accompany pneumococcal sepsis in asplenic patients. Meningococcemia may present rather dramatically, with diffuse petechial, purpuric, and ecchymotic lesions. Petechiae should also alert clinicians to the possibility of disseminated intravascular coagulation (DIC). If the coagulation cascade is activated (as with gram-negative bacteremia), DIC may result. DIC is characterized by thrombocytopenia, coagulation factor consumption, fibrin split products, decreased fibrinogen levels, and often, significant hemorrhaging (most frequently in the gastrointestinal tract, lungs, and skin). DIC is viewed by many to be an incidental pre-terminal event. Janeway lesions, Osler nodes, splinter hemorrhages, palatal and conjunctival petechiae would, of course, suggest endocarditis, but these are seen in only a minority of cases.

With the wide availability of Swan-Ganz monitoring, the cardiovascular changes of septic shock have been well-documented. Traditionally, these changes have been characterized by a spectrum, beginning with decreased systemic vascular resistance and increased cardiac output (warm shock), then progressing to decreased cardiac output and increased systemic vascular resistance (cold shock). Even though patients are best managed with hemodynamic monitoring, a reasonable assessment of tissue perfusion can be made quickly by feeling the temperature of the extremities and looking for mottling, cyanosis, etc. Lactic acid levels have been followed in septic patients. High levels are associated with hypoperfusion and ineffective aerobic glycolysis; decreasing levels correlate with improvement of the septic state.

Pulmonary manifestations of septic shock may include dyspnea, tachypnea, and diffuse rales. Early on, arterial blood gases usually show respiratory alkalosis, with or without hypoxemia. This proceeds to respiratory and metabolic acidosis as the patient further decompensates. Shunt physiology is present when 100% F_IO_2 fails to correct the hypoxemia. Chest x-rays may show diffuse pulmonary infiltrates. A diagnosis of adult respiratory distress syndrome (ARDS)—or non-cardiogenic pulmonary edema—can be made if these factors are present in conjunction with a normal wedge pressure. Some series document ARDS in 20% of patients in septic shock.

Acute tubular necrosis and oliguric renal failure may develop in patients with septic shock. Optimal fluid management to simultaneously maintain renal perfusion and avoid congestive heart failure further argues for invasive hemodynamic monitoring. The liver may acutely show striking elevations in transaminase levels if significant hypotension is present. SGOT and SGPT usually fall as quickly as they rose if blood pressure is restored and the patient survives. Elevated bilirubin levels should alert physicians to bacteremia with Bacteroides species or hemolysis as occurs with Clostridial infections or DIC (Table 2).

Table 2. Clinical manifestations of septic shock.

---

1. Vital signs—hypotension, tachycardia, tachypnea, hypo- or hyperthermia, chills

2. Skin—petechia, ecthyma gangrenosa, bullae, ecchymoses, purpura, mottling, cyanosis

3. Coagulation abnormalities—bleeding, DIC

4. Hematologic—granulocytosis with left shift, thrombocytopenia, leukopenia

5. Multi-organ failure—lung, liver, kidney, heart

THERAPY

One way of organizing a treatment strategy is to divide various modalities into the following groups: 1) Essential—including antibiotics, fluids, oxygen, and cardiotropic agents; 2) Controversial—including steroids, heparin, naloxone, and cyclo-oxygenase inhibitors; and 3) Future—monoclonal antibodies and passive immunizations for bacterial antigens and toxins may, some day, come into clinical usage (Table 3).

Table 3. Therapies for septic shock.

1. Essential—antibiotics, fluids, oxygen, cardiotropics

2. Controversial—steroids, morphine antagonists, prostaglandin inhibitors

3. Future—monoclonal antibodies, passive immunization

Essential

Therapy for patients with septic shock should be started immediately. Several studies have shown the mortality rate of bacteremia can be reduced with appropriate use of antibiotics. They should be begun empirically and in maximum doses *before* culture results are available. Antibiotic coverage should include gram-positive and gram-negative organisms, as well as those suggested by the clinical situation. These might include anaerobes if a pelvic or gastrointestinal source of infection is suspected. Metronidazole and clindamycin are drugs that would be added to cover for anaerobic bacteria. *Pseudomonas aeruginosa* in cancer patients or those with ecthyma gangrenosa skin lesions, *Streptococcus pneumoniae* in asplenics, or *Staphylococcus aureus* pneumonia complicating influenza epidemics, for example, would necessitate utilization of antibiotics to cover these organisms. Combination therapy with a third-generation cephalosporin or anti-pseudomonal beta lactam and an aminoglycoside has theoretical advantages of increased spectrum, more rapid killing, prevention of resistance, and synergy. These concepts, however, have not been proven in clinical studies, and except for *Pseudomonas* infections in immunocompromised hosts, have not been universally accepted. Newer antibiotics with broad spectra of activity (including against *Pseudomonas aeruginosa*) are ceftazadime and imipenim-cilastatin. If blood cultures become positive, therapy can be adjusted to include antibiotics with lower toxicity and narrower spectra.

Narrowing the spectrum of coverage is important, since prolonged use of broad-spectrum agents is more often associated with superinfections, bleeding, pseudomembranous colitis, etc. In immunosuppressed patients, vancomycin is sometimes used empirically, to cover coagulase-negative staphylococci and Corynebacterium JK bacilli; both of these skin organisms may become invasive in the presence of intravenous lines and Hickman catheters.

The hypotension of sepsis should first be corrected with volume.[a] The proper amount of IV cystalloid to administer is best judged with the clinical response or with Swan-Ganz monitoring. In patients with underlying heart disease, right heart filling pressures should be kept at levels that maximize cardiac output. Pulmonary capillary wedge pressures should be kept below 18 mmHg (in the absence of obvious heart disease). Studies are underway to evaluate the efficacy of hypertonic albuminated fluids.

As septic shock progresses, volume administration becomes inadequate to maintain normal blood pressure, and cardiotropic agents are needed. Dopamine is probably the drug of choice, since at low infusion rates (2-3 $\mu g \bullet kg^{-1} \bullet min^{-1}$), it increases renal, mesenteric, cerebral, and coronary flow. At higher levels (20-50 $\mu g \bullet kg^{-1} \bullet min^{-1}$), greater alpha-adrenergic vasoconstrictive action is seen. Dobutamine enhances cardiac output, decreases systemic vascular resistance (with little change in heart rate), and may be used synergistically with dopamine in some cases. Alpha-adrenergic agents (such as phenylephrine and methoxamine) are not usually dependable in septic shock, since tissue perfusion is not elevated (especially in acidosis) and tissues are unresponsive to these sympathomimetic amines.

Vasodilators like nitroprusside may be indicated in the setting of congestive heart failure and high systemic vascular resistance. Digitalis has not proven useful in septic shock, with the possible exception of meningococcemia sepsis. In some refractory cases, intra-aortic balloon pump counterpulsations may be necessary until other measures control the septic state.

---

[a] We prefer crystalloid (0.9 normal saline or Ringers lactate) to colloid because crystalloids are (1) less expensive, (2) do not activate the killikrenin-kinin system, and (3) do not cause bleeding.

The last two therapies in the essential group include oxygen in hypoxemic patients and bicarbonate in acidotic patients. Arterial blood gas levels should be obtained serially and hypoxemia corrected, with increasing concentrations of inspired oxygen (F_iO_2) and positive end-expiratory pressure (PEEP), if necessary. Caution with both of these modalities must be taken; prolonged use of O_2 at high concentrations (>50% over several days) can lead to irreversible pulmonary fibrosis, and PEEP can decrease cardiac output. With increasing PEEP (>20 cm H_2O), the risk of pneumothorax increases.

Controversial

Controversial therapies of septic shock include the use of steroids, heparin, opiate antagonists, and cyclo-oxygenase inhibitors. In order to discuss each of these properly, a knowledge of drug actions on the underlying pathophysiologic mechanisms and metabolic pathways activated in septic shock is necessary. Most of the studies to-date have dealt with shock associated with experimental gram-negative rod bacteremia for several reasons. The incidence of shock in patients with gram-negative bacteremia is much greater than with gram-positive organisms. Shock seems to be a more integral part of gram-negative sepsis, not only because of its frequency, but its timing as well—occurring much earlier (within 4-10 hours). Experimental infusion of minute amounts of endotoxin released from gram-negative bacteria have reproduced the clinical manifestations and metabolic changes of septic shock. There are many problems correlating these studies with clinical septic shock, but the mechanism of their deleterious effect in animals provides hope for future therapies in controlled human trials.

Endotoxin (lipopolysaccharide) is thought to be an initiating factor in gram-negative septic shock. After entry into the bloodstream, endotoxin activates several proposed mediators, which are, in turn, responsible for the pathophysiologic changes observed (see Table 4). Both endotoxin and intact gram-negative bacilli are capable of activating the complement system, through both the classical and alternate (properdin) pathways. The latter pathway is thought to be a first-line of defense and doesn't require antibody to initiate the complement cascade. This may account for some of the early clinical differences between gram-positive and gram-

Table 4. Proposed mediators in septic shock.

1. Complement components C_{3a}, C_{5a}
2. Coagulation factors
3. Kinins
4. Endorphins
5. Histamine
6. Prostaglandins
7. Lysosomal enzymes
8. Macrophage products (interleukins, monokines)
9. Catecholamines, acetylcholine
10. Glucocorticoids

negative sepsis. Two vasodilatory anaphylotoxins C_{3a} and C_{5a} are released after activation of the complement cascade. C_{3a} induces histamine release (mast cell degranulation); resulting vasodilation constitutes the first wave of inflammation. C_{5a} and the terminal (C_3-C_9) complex activate polymorphonuclear cells (PMNs). Arachidonic acid products, lysosomal enzymes, and oxygen radicals released from these PMNs create a capillary leak syndrome, and thus, comprise the second wave of inflammation.

Endotoxin also initiates the coagulation system through its affects on Hageman factor. If the compensatory fibrinolytic mechanisms fail, a state of DIC—with coagulation factor consumption, bleeding, and ischemia—may ensue. The kallikrein-kinin system is also activated by Hageman factor, causing production of the very potent vasodilator, bradykinin. One of the major inhibitors of Hageman factor is antithrombin III, whose activity is enhanced by heparin.

Lastly, the vasodilatory properties of endotoxin may be due to activation of phagocytic cells that produce various compounds (e.g., leukocyte endogenous mediator, endogenous pyrogen, lymphocyte activating factor). These substances, in turn, induce endorphin release from the pituitary gland, reset the hypothalamic thermostat, suppress granulopoiesis and neutrophil release, and set in motion a variety of metabolic activities in the liver, pancreas, and muscle.

The controversial therapeutic modalities used in septic shock are known to act on the above-mentioned pathways. It was hoped that heparin could be used to inhibit coagulation factor consumption and activation of the kallikrein-kinin system, but the efficacy of heparin in accomplishing these effects has never been proven. There is a definite risk of bleeding with heparin use, so we very rarely advocate its use for septic shock—other than to use it in low-doses to prevent pulmonary emboli.

Naloxone, an opiate antagonist, has been used in septic shock because animal models suggest that the hypotension of endotoxin shock is at least partly mediated by endogenous opiates (endorphins). Naloxone increases mean systolic blood pressure in laboratory animals in shock, but has no effect on normal controls. Several prospective, randomized, double-blinded studies in humans, however, have failed to demonstrate any significant effect on blood pressure or clinical outcome. However, in these studies, no dose-response curve was generated to define an efficacious dose. Thyroid-releasing hormone has similar actions on hypotensive laboratory animals as naloxone, but it does not reverse analgesia—which has some theoretical advantages in the treatment of patients. Steroids may also block endorphin release because of their inhibition of ACTH (a relative of β–lipotropin).

A spin-off of complement activation is C_5A, which is chemotactic for polymorphonuclear cells. PMNs, in the presence of C_5A, become more adhesive. Aggregation and degranulation then occur. Release of toxic metabolites (oxygen radicals, neutral proteases, and arachidonic acid metabolites) leads to tissue injury and greater influx of PMNs. Prostaglandins produced in endothelial cells may also account for some of the tissue damage. It seems that the host must pay the price of a small amount of tissue damage from normal inflammatory processes in order to control microbial invasion. Steroids have been used in septic shock in attempts to control the host response to the inciting stimulus. In high concentrations steroids are believed to: 1) block binding of chemotactic substances to PMNs; 2) blunt the effects of activated complement on PMNs; 3) inhibit lysosomal degranulation; and 4) block phospholipase A_2.

High-dosage steroids have been shown to reduce mortality from lethal doses of endotoxin in some experimental animal models. In other animals, however, the LD_{50} of infused organisms is lowered by steroid administration. The results of several human studies are equally contradictory. The results of two recent multi-center, prospective, randomized trials did not show decreased mortality rate in "steroid" groups.

Leukotriene infusion produces a shock-like scenario when given to experimental animals. Antiprostaglandin therapy has had success in reducing the mortality of experimental septic shock in various animal models. Aspirin and nonsteroidal agents improve survival in dogs given otherwise lethal doses of endotoxin or gram-negative bacteria. Many studies suggest that thromboxane A_2 is responsible for the pulmonary hypertension, capillary leakage, and leukocyte activation seen in the lungs of humans with ARDS. Prostacyclin (PGI_2), a membrane stabilizer and inhibitor of platelet aggregation, appears to counteract the activities of thromboxane products. The balance between PGI_2 and thromboxane A_2 may therefore be important in determining the degree of lung injury in septic shock. Infusion of PGI_2 30 minutes after endotoxin administration increases survival in experimental animals. Thromboxane synthetase and cyclo-oxygenase inhibitors (non-steroidal anti-inflammatory drugs) have the same effect. Studies are now underway to evaluate various prostaglandin inhibitors and their ability to halt the metabolic pathways triggered by sepsis in experimental animals.

Future

Future therapies for septic shock will most likely include forms of passive immunization (e.g., human antisera, monoclonal antibodies to common bacterial antigens). Several researchers are studying antisera to endotoxin. In general, bacterial lipopolysaccharides are composed of oligosaccharide side chains, core polysaccharide, and lipid A. Development of antiserum to the side chains would be difficult because of variation from strain to strain. The core polysaccharide-lipid A complex, however, is much more uniform amongst species of *Enterobacteriaceae*.

Antiserum to a mutant strain of *E. coli* (the core moiety is exposed for greater immunogeneity) has been shown to reduce mortality in a randomized, controlled study of more than 200 gram-negative bacteremic patients. This approach is appealing, in that the effects of endotoxin are neutralized quickly and the harmful inflammatory reactions are avoided. Monoclonal antibody therapy may, one day, prove to be a cost-effective and efficacious manner of treating septic shock. Therapies currently under investigation are illustrated in Figure 2.

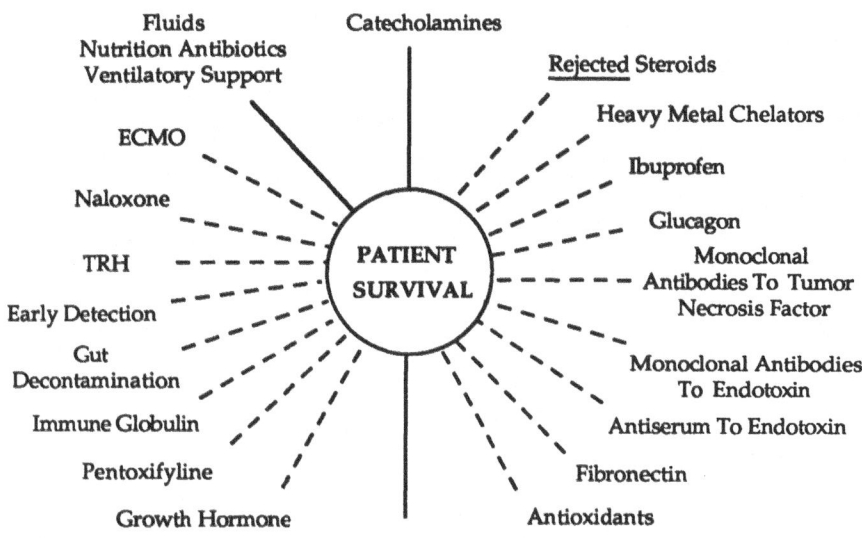

Figure 2. Conventional and proposed treatment of septic shock and multi-organ failure. Conventional therapies are represented by solid lines. Dashed lines indicate agents currently subjected to animal studies or clinical trials.

REFERENCES

Bone RC, Fisher CJ Jr, Clemmer TP, et al: A controlled clinical trial of high-dose methylprednisolone in the treatment of severe sepsis and septic shock. N Engl JMed 317:653-8, 1987

Goris RJ, Nuytinck HK, Redl H: Scoring systems and predictors of ARDS and MOF. Prog Clin Biol Res 236B:3-15, 1987

Jacobs ER, Bone RC: Sepsis. In Pulmonary Disease Reviews, Volume IV. (Bone RC, ed). New York, Wiley Publications, 1983, pp 99-117

Jacobs ER, Bone RC: Clinical indicators in sepsis and septic adult respiratory distress syndrome. Med Clin North Am 70(4):921-32, 1986

Schuster HP: Multisystem organ failure. Prog Clin Biol Res 236A:459-62, 1987

Schwartz DB, Bone RC, Balk RA, Szidon JP: Hepatic dysfunction in the adult respiratory distress syndrome. Chest 95(4):871-75, 1989

Tracey KJ, Lowry SM, Cerami A: Cachetin/TNF-alpha in septic shock and septic adult respiratory distress syndrome. Am Rev Resp Dis 138(6): 1377-79, 1988

HEMODYNAMICS AND THERAPY IN ARDS

W. M. Zapol

DIAGNOSIS

ARDS patients suffer from diffuse injury of the pulmonary microvasculature with increased permeability to plasma proteins. A definitive diagnosis of ARDS requires evidence of the following:

a) increased venous admixture (e.g., $\dot{Q}s/\dot{Q}T > 30\%$ or $P_aO_2 / F_IO_2 < 250$);

b) acute bilateral diffuse radiographic infiltrates;

c) an appropriate cause (see Table 1, not pulmonary embolism, atelectasis or congestive heart failure). Many clinicians lump diffuse pneumonia (bacterial, viral etc.) in the ARDS group. Sepsis syndrome and post-traumatic ARDS account for over half the ARDS patients in our ICU;

d) a pulmonary capillary wedge pressure of less than 18 mmHg. Thus a Swan-Ganz catheter is necessary to make a definitive diagnosis (unless an LA line is present). Congestive heart failure and ARDS may be coincident. The precise causes for the development of ARDS in man are poorly understood and despite advanced supportive treatment with mechanical ventilation, diuretics and other pharmacological therapies to improve organ function, more than half of all ARDS patients will die (1).

PATHOPHYSIOLOGY:

The pulmonary artery pressure (PAP) and vascular resistance (PVR) are elevated in moderate and severe ARDS of diverse etiology (2,3). This occurs despite a normal P_aO_2 and can occur within a few hours after acute lung injury. We remain uncertain as to the precise cause of the increased

269

T. H. Stanley and R. J. Sperry (eds.), Anesthesia and the Lung 1992, 269–276.
© 1992 Kluwer Academic Publishers.

Table 1. Some injuries causing ARDS.

Severe trauma (thoracic or extra-thoracic)	Fat embolization
Bacteremia	Aspiration of gastrointestinal contents
Smoke or toxic gas inhalation (including O_2)	Surface burns
Hydrocarbon ingestion	Toxic drugs (heroin, paraquat)
Neurogenic pulmonary edema	Viral, mycoplasma, bacterial pneumonia
Legionnaire's disease, Pittsburgh agent	Acute vasculitis
Goodpasture's syndrome	Anaphylactic reaction to drugs and blood
Radiation of thorax	Immunosuppression and infection (pneumocystis)
Thrombus, amniotic fluid, or tumor embolism to the lung	

PVR but its effect, pulmonary hypertension, places a severe load on the lung which exchanges fluid in the face of both an increased microvascular permeability and an increased hydrostatic pressure. Late in ARDS the PVR cannot be reduced by infusing vasodilators (nitroprusside, phentolamine, ibuprofen). However, early in ARDS, infusing nitroprusside reduced the PAP and pulmonary capillary wedge pressure (PCWP), while increasing cardiac output, thus vasodilation or vascular recruitment occurred (3,4). Prostacyclin (PGI_2) infusion also has been given to reduce the pulmonary vascular resistance (5). All the intravenous vasodilators dilate vessels to both ventilated and unventilated alveoli, thus the shunt fraction $\dot{Q}s/\dot{Q}T$ or the level of pulmonary oxygenation inefficiency increases. Recently, Frostell et al. reported that inhaling NO, an endothelium derived relaxing factor, caused marked and selective pulmonary vasodilation without any decrease of the systemic vascular resistance (6). Falke et al. gave 18 ppm NO to a patient with severe ARDS and caused marked pulmonary vasodilation without systemic vasodilation. That patient's $\dot{Q}s/\dot{Q}T$ level decreased, probably because inhaled NO selectively dilates ventilated alveoli (7).

What is the structural basis of the elevated PVR in ARDS? Two techniques have provided information on pulmonary vascular alterations in ARDS. Balloon occlusion pulmonary arteriography was employed by

Greene et al. to study the pulmonary vasculature in over 220 patients with ARDS. He learned that 80 of the patients had multiple PA filling defects (PAFD). These filling defects were associated with DIC, an elevated PVR, increasing severity of ARDS, and death of the patients (approximately 85% died). On the other hand, ARDS patients without PAFD often survived their illness (8).

These angiographic studies were correlated with morphologic examinations of post-mortem and lung biopsy specimens. K. Kobayashi et al. used silicone rubber perfusions to demonstrate widespread arterial occlusions of ARDS lungs. Greene et al. reported that most patients with PAFD had pulmonary artery thromboembolism at autopsy. We were surprised by the large number of PA vascular occlusions in ARDS lungs. Jones et al. (9) and Tomashefski et al. (10) subsequently reported that 21 of 22 ARDS lungs cast with gelatin barium at autopsy had thromboemboli. In addition, Tomashefski et al. described major remodeling of the pulmonary arteries with marked medial muscular thickening and growth of smooth muscle into distal regions of the pulmonary artery where muscle is not normally present. Muscle may encroach upon the lumen and increase the PVR in later stages of ARDS.

The right ventricle faces an increased afterload in ARDS. As the PAP increases this thin-walled muscular cavity must eject blood into the pulmonary artery at higher pressures. There is a general finding that in ARDS as PAP increases the right ventricular ejection fraction (RVEF) decreases. This has been confirmed by gated and first pass (11,12,13) radionuclide studies as well as thermodilution measurements of RVEF. In late stage ARDS with the PAP greater than 40 mmHg the patient can exhibit a low cardiac output, high PCWP and RVEDP and an enlarged poorly contracting right ventricle with a small, hyperdynamic left ventricle. Strategies to improve survival require increasing RV contractility (e.g., inotropic agent infusion) and possibly efforts to reduce the elevated PVR (e.g., thrombolytic therapy with streptokinase infusions in selected patients). Falke et al. reported a reduction of PVR and increased RVEF with inhalation of NO in a patient with ARDS (7). Greene et al. have reported a pilot trial of streptokinase infusions in ARDS patients (14). Such supportive maneuvers may be required to buy time to allow pulmonary healing.

MEDIATORS IN ARDS

A large number of possible mediators have been proposed to cause the diffuse lung injury due to increased capillary permeability that is diagnosed the adult respiratory distress syndrome (ARDS) (15). Perhaps the most common cause of ARDS is sepsis, whether the primary focus is within the lung or elsewhere. Therefore, release of a number of mediators of lung injury are directly and indirectly stimulated by exposure to gram negative bacterial lipopolysaccharide (LPS) (16). LPS given intravenously to sheep causes leukopenia, fever and an increased transpulmonary flux of protein rich edema fluid. LPS causes the release of a host of secondary mediators of injury including thromboxane and the endoperoxide metabolites of arachidonic acid (17). Thromboxane is a profound pulmonary vasoconstrictor, since endothelial injury in the presence of hypertension causes much greater rates of edema formation, the release of vasoconstrictor compounds by LPS is especially dangerous. Many additional mediators (serotonin, histamine, platelet activating factor, leukotrienes, complement anaphylatoxins, etc.) are also possible mediators of ARDS that will be mentioned but will not be discussed.

TNFα

Tumor necrosis factor alpha, also known as cachectin, is a macrophage and monocyte produced polypeptide hormone with a subunit of approximately 17 kilodaltons. Recent studies increasingly implicate TNFα as a key agonist producing shock and death following endotoxemia (18). Animal research shows TNFα appears in the circulation within minutes after endotoxin is injected and peaks at blood levels near 0.3M. Of singular significance is the finding that mice passively immunized against this hormone are protected against the lethal effects of endotoxin injection. Researchers are hoping to determine whether this effect can be exploited to man's benefit, a task made possible largely because rapid advances in molecular biologic engineering have yielded ample amounts of highly purified recombinant human TNFα(rh-TNFα). Researchers are now able to examine *in vivo* the effects of infusing this hormone.

It has been determined that TNFα, infused intravenously into rats and dogs in quantities similar to those produced endogenously after endotoxin injection, causes hypotension, metabolic acidosis, hemoconcentration and death within a few hours (18,19). Autopsy reveals diffuse pulmonary inflammation and hemorrhage. The similarity of these effects of cachectin to the acute lung injury which occurs when ARDS arises in the context of bacterial sepsis gives added importance to the study of this hormone. Focusing on its pulmonary and systemic effects in larger animals, we have found that infusing human recombinant TNFα (25-150 µg/kg) into sheep with a lung lymph fistula produces immediate neutropenia and progressive hypotension with hemoconcentration. A major fluid infusion is required to replace the intravascular fluid lost. Progressive increase of lung lymph flow rate occurs at an unchanged L/P ratio. This suggests that rh-TNFα may increase pulmonary microvascular permeability (20). One study suggests passive immunization to TNFα in monkeys 1 to 2 hours before I.V. gram negative bacterial challenge protects against septic hypotension and death (21). Whether treatment of humans with antibodies to TNFα can prevent septic shock or ARDS is unknown but of great interest.

ENDOTOXIN NEUTRALIZATION BY ANTIBODIES

Gram negative endotoxin releases mediators which cause acute lung injury, pulmonary hypertension and increase lung microvascular permeability. In order to fortify cells against such an attack, we begin with the known fact that immunity to specific bacterial types protects many animals against challenge by the homologous bacterial species.

Ziegler et al. (22) have found that transfusion of polyclonal anti E. coli J5 human sera reversed clinical gram negative endotoxin shock. Teng et al. (23) recently produced a human monoclonal antibody (MAb) to J5 strain E. coli. This monoclonal antibody protects rabbits from the lethal effects of many gram negative endotoxins and shields mice from gram negative bacterial infections.

A recent report by Feeley et al. (20) has shown that pretreating rats with 0.6 mg/kg of this human anti-endotoxin MAb 15 minutes before infusing I.V. 3 mg/kg endotoxin prevented increased [99mTc] DTPA clearance from lung into blood at 24 hours as well as the increase of serum lipid peroxidation products but did not prevent neutrophil accumulation in the lung. Recently, 30 centers assessed this human monoclonal antibody raised against J5 in a double-blind, prospective and randomized multicenter study of patients with a known source of sepsis, fever and evidence of the early onset of single organ failure. Of 543 patients with sepsis who were treated, 200 (375) had gram negative bacteremia proven by blood culture. For these 200 patients followed to death or study day 28, there were 45 deaths among 92 patients receiving placebo (49%) and 32 deaths among 105 recipients of MAb (30%, p < 0.014). MAb therapy given early during a gram negative infection may prevent the subsequent release of noxious mediators or even possibly prevent ARDS (or other organ failure).

This study was sponsored by Centocor (Malvern, PA) and we analyzed the effects of this MAb on the incidence and progression of ARDS (26). Another prospective randomized study of a murine MAb against E. coli J5 was sponsored by Xoma Corp (Berleley, CA). It is possible that neutralizing gram negative endotoxins with antibodies can prevent or increase survival of patients with ARDS due to sepsis syndrome.

REFERENCES

1. Montgomery BA, Stager MA, Carrico CJ, Hudson LD: Causes of mortality in patients with the adult respiratory distress syndrome. Am Rev Resp Dis 132:485-9, 1985
2. Zapol WM, and Snider MT: Pulmonary hypertension in severe acute respiratory failure. N Engl J Med 296:476-80, 1977
3. Zapol WM, Snider MT, Rie M, Frikker M, and Quinn D: Pulmonary circulation during ARDS. In Acute Respiratory Failure, Zapol WM, Falke K (eds.). In the series, Lung Biology in Health and Disease. New York, Marcel Dekker, 1985, pp 241-73
4. Radermacher P, Huet Y, Lemaire F: Comparison of Ketanserin and sodium nitroprusside in patients with severe ARDS. Anesthesiology 68:152-7, 1988
5. Radermacher P, Borislav S, Wüst HJ, Tarnow J, Falke KJ: Prostacyclin for the treatment of pulmonary hypertension in the adult respiratory distress syndrome: Effects on pulmonary capillary pressure and ventilation-perfusion distributions. Anesthesiology 72:238-44, 1990

6. Frostell C, Fratacci M-D, Wain JC, Jones R, Zapol WM: Inhaled nitric oxide: A selective pulmonary vasodilator reversing hypoxic pulmonary vasoconstriction. Circulation (in press)

7. Falke K, et al: Am Rev Resp Dis 133 (Suppl May), 1991

8. Greene R, Boggis CRM, Jantsch HS: Radiography and angiography of the pulmonary circulation in ARDS. In Acute Respiratory Failure, Zapol WM, Falke K (eds.). In the series, Lung Biology in Health and Disease. New York, Marcel Dekker, 1985, pp 275-302

9. Jones R, Reid LM, Zapol WM, et al: Pulmonary vascular pathology: human and experimental studies. In Acute Respiratory Failure, Zapol WM, Falke K (eds.). In the series, Lung Biology in Health and Disease. New York, Marcel Dekker, 1985, pp 23-160

10. Tomashefski JF, Zapol WM and Reid LM: The pulmonary vascular lesions of the adult respiratory distress syndrome. Am J Pathol 112:112-26, 1983

11. Laver MB, Strauss WA, and Pohost GM: Right and left ventricular geometry: adjustments during acute respiratory failure. Crit Care Med 7:509-19, 1979

12. Rajagopalan B, Lowenstein E, Zapol WM: Cardiac function in the adult respiratory distress syndrome. In Acute Respiratory Failure, Zapol WM, Falke K (eds.). In the series, Lung Biology in Health and Disease. New York, Marcel Dekker, 1985, pp 555-76

13. Sibbald WJ, Driedger AA, Cunningham DG, Cheung H: Right and left ventricular performance in acute hypoxemic respiratory failure. Crit Care Med 1986; 14:852

14. Greene R, Lind S, Jantsch H, et al: Pulmonary vascular obstruction in severe ARDS: angiographic alterations after i.v. fibrinolytic therapy. Am J Roentgenol 148:501-8, 1987

15. Simon RH: Predictors of the adult respiratory distress syndrome. J Crit Care 2:81-5, 1987

16. Meyrick BO: Endotoxin mediated pulmonary endothelial cell injury. Fed Proc 45:19, 1986

17. Huttemeier PC, Watkins WD, Peterson MB, Zapol WM: Acute pulmonary hypertension and lung thromboxane release following endotoxin infusion in normal and leukopenic sheep. Circ Res 50:688-94, 1982

18. Beutler B, Cerami A: Cachectin: More than a tumor necrosis factor. N Engl J Med 316:319, 1987

19. Tracy K, Lowry SF, Fahey III, TJ, et al: Cachectin/tumor necrosis factor induces lethal shock and stress hormone response in the dog. S Gyn Obst 164:415-22, 1987

20. Kreil EA, Greene E, Fitzgibbon C, et al: Effects of recombinant human tumor necrosis factor alpha, lymphotoxin, and escherichia coli lipopolysaccharide on hemodynamics, lung microvascular permeability, and eicosanoid synthesis in anesthetized sheep. Circ Res 65:502-14, 1989

21. Tracey KJ, Fong Y, Hesse DG, et al: Anticachectin/TNF monoclonal antibodies prevent septic shock during lethal bacteraemia. Nature 330:662-4, 1987

22. Ziegler EJ, McCuthchan A, Fierer J, et al: Treatment of gram-negative bacteremia and shock with a human antiserum to a mutant Escherichia coli. N Engl J Med 307:1225-30, 1982

23. Teng NN, Kaplan HS, Hebert JM, et al: Protection against gram-negative bacteremia and endotoxemia with human monoclonal IgM antibodies. Proc Natl Acad Sci 82:1790-94, 1985

24. Feeley TW, Minty BD, Scudder CM, et al: The effect of human antiendotoxin monoclonal antibodies on endotoxin induced lung injury in the rat. Am Rev Respir Dis 135:665-70, 1987

25. Ziegler EJ, Fisher, Jr., CJ, Sprung CL, et al: Treatment of gram-negative bacteremia and septic shock with HA-1A human monoclonal antibody against endotoxin. N Eng J Med 1991;324:429-36

26. Bigatello LM, Greene RE, Sprung CL, et al: A randomized trial of a human monoclonal antibody against endotoxin in sepsis: Effects on the adult respiratory distress syndrome. (Submitted)

RESPIRATORY MECHANICS IN ARDS PATIENTS

N. T. Eissa and J. Milic-Emili

DEFINITION AND HISTORICAL BACKGROUND

Although the current definition of adult respiratory distress syndrome (ARDS) was made by Ashbaugh et al. (1), the syndrome was actually described much earlier. A progressive form of pulmonary collapse was known to physicians treating battlefield casualties during World War I (2). As noted by Matthay (3), Osler's textbook of medicine (4) provides an excellent description of the early phase of the syndrome. In 1927, Osler wrote "uncontrolled septicemia leads to frothy pulmonary edema that resembles serum, not the sanguineous transudative edema fluid seen in dropsy or congestive heart failure." There were no mechanical ventilators or intensive care units in Osler's time, so he could not tell us more about ARDS because the development of this type of exudative pulmonary edema was usually a terminal complication. Lung injury following trauma was later described in causalities of World War II as "traumatic wet lung" (5). In this report the authors provided clinical and physiological features of the syndrome and asserted, "It cannot be overemphasized that the lung reacts to trauma just as uniquely as the brain or any highly specialized organ." In 1950 a pathological state called "congestive atelectasis" was described by Jenkins et al. (6). They accurately described airless, congested, heavy lungs with alveolar debris and hyaline membrane formation in autopsy cases. ARDS became a recognized clinical entity, however, only in 1967 when it was described by Ashbaugh et al. (1), who defined the syndrome as a sudden onset of permeability pulmonary edema as a result of a triggering event e.g trauma, aspiration, etc. Later, it became apparent that the syndrome is more complicated than that. For instance, this definition would also fit non-cardiogenic pulmonary edema

277

T. H. Stanley and R. J. Sperry (eds.), Anesthesia and the Lung 1992, 277–296.
© 1992 *Kluwer Academic Publishers.*

due to exertion at high altitudes or due to drug reactions. These states resolve rapidly and often do not require mechanical ventilation. Clinicians have recognized ARDS as a syndrome characterized by severe dyspnea, hypoxemia refractory to supplemental oxygen, reduced lung compliance and roentgenographic evidence of diffuse bilateral pulmonary infiltrates which occur 6 to 48 hours after a catastrophic event, e.g., sepsis, trauma (7). These criteria, however, should not be applied in a strict fashion. For instance, roentogenographic findings could manifest late in the course of the disease or could be unilateral. Recently, Murray et al. (8) proposed a more refined definition of the syndrome with a unified scoring system that takes into account the degree of lung injury, the underlying disorder and any associated non-pulmonary organ dysfunction. This was done to facilitate collecting and comparing epidemiologic and experimental data.

GENERAL CONSIDERATIONS

Although altered respiratory mechanics has helped to define ARDS and mechanical ventilation remains the keystone for supportive therapy, quantitive determination of respiratory mechanics in patients with this syndrome is not routinely performed. This probably reflects the preconception that measurements of respiratory mechanics in these patients are difficult to perform. In fact, in mechanically ventilated patients, a detailed analysis of respiratory mechanics can be performed readily with simple and commonly available equipment, namely a pneumotachograph to measure flow, an integrator to obtain volume changes from the flow signal, and a pressure transducer to measure the pressure at the airway opening or, preferably, in the trachea some distance beyond the distal end of the endotracheal tube (9). Several commercial ventilators allow direct measurements of these variables (e.g., Siemens 900C, Siemens-Elema AB, Solna, Sweden; and Puritan-Bennett 7200, Puritan-Bennet Corp., Kansas City, Mo). With this equipment it is possible to determine, non-invasively, the static and dynamic compliance of the respiratory system; the flow resistance of the respiratory system, airways and thoracic tissues; and intrinsic PEEP (PEEPi) (9,10,11). The ability and use of these measurements would be expected to aid in clinical decision making in the management of such critically ill patients. The quantitative changes in respiratory system mechanics and the influence of these on the ability to discontinue ventilatory support or ultimate patient outcome are largely unknown. Serial evaluation of respiratory system mechanics may aid in the investigation of these and other important clinical issues in the management of ARDS patients receiving mechanical ventilation.

Since the earliest reports of the syndrome (1,5,6), it has been recognized that ARDS patients exhibit a reduction in lung volume and in respiratory compliance. Recently increased airway, pulmonary, and thoracic tissues flow resistance and presence of PEEPi have been described in these patients (9,10,12). In this review we will discuss the mechanical disturbances associated with the syndrome; pertinent information about methodology and therapeutic interventions will be provided as well.

LUNG VOLUME

Reduction in lung volume is known to occur in ARDS. Indeed, in 1945 Burford et al. (5), in their description of "traumatic wet lung," predicted that this "wet" phase of the lung could be the precipitating event for the "silent" massive collapse in post-operative patients described in 1908 by Pasteur (13). Later, functional residual capacity (FRC) was found to be reduced in ARDS patients (14,15). In these studies, FRC was measured by gas dilution techniques. These techniques do not measure the total thoracic gas volume, but rather the gas contained in airspaces with open airways. Changes in total thoracic volume (including gases, liquids, and solids) can be estimated by non-invasive methods such as radiography, computed tomography, strain gauges, magnetometers, bellows pneumographs, and inductive plethysmographs. The latter technique (16) allows for partitioning of the respiratory movements into the motion of the rib cage and of the abdomen-diaphragm.

COMPLIANCE

Static Compliance of the Respiratory System (Cst,rs)

Cst,rs in mechanically ventilated patients is conventionally measured by dividing V_T by end-inspiratory static elastic recoil pressure of the respiratory system (Pst,rs) obtained by end-inspiratory airway occlusion until a plateau is reached (usually several seconds). In this case the adequacy of respiratory muscle relaxation is indirectly assessed by the presence of a plateau in airway pressure during the occlusion. This approach assumes that the end-expiratory lung volume during mechanical ventilation corresponds to the relaxation volume of the respiratory system (Vr) and hence end-expiratory airway pressure equals zero. This assumption, however, is often not valid due to the presence of PEEPi (17). This problem can be easily dealt with by performing airway occlusions at end-expiration in addition to end-inspiration. Cst,rs is then computed as VT divided by the difference in airway pressure between end-inspiratory and end-expiratory occlusions (17). Failure to recognize and measure PEEPi will lead to underestimation of Cst,rs measurements.

The above measurements require patients to be relaxed otherwise the use of an esophageal balloon to estimate pleural pressure is needed. The esophageal balloon technique has been validated in critically ill patients (18). Cst,rs varies considerably with changes in tidal volume (9,11). Therefore, its measurement becomes mainly useful to follow the progress of a given patient at a given ventilation setting. Increase in Cst,rs in this case can be taken as a sign of improvement and vice versa.

Static Volume-Pressure (V-P) Relationship of the Respiratory System

The elastic properties of the respiratory system may be best assessed by constructing the static V-P relationship of the respiratory system obtained under conditions in which airflow is absent and respiratory muscle relaxation is complete. This measurement can be readily performed in relaxed mechanically ventilated patients using the rapid airway occlusion technique (19). In this procedure V_T is changed for one breath (test breath) and end-inspiratory airway occlusion is maintained until a plateau pressure is reached (usually 2-3 seconds). This plateau pressure corresponds to the end-inspiratory Pst,rs (Fig. 1). If a series of end-inspiratory airway occlusions is performed at different V_T's, the static V-P relationship can be constructed by plotting Pst,rs against the corresponding inflation volume. Relaxation of the respiratory muscles can be achieved by administration of muscle relaxants and/or sedatives. The use of mechanical hyperventilation to relax patients by reducing their P_aCO_2 and hence their respiratory drive is problematic since hypocapnia will lead to increased airway resistance (20).

The airway occlusion technique mentioned above is an appealing approach compared to the earlier method ("super-syringe technique") used to construct static V-P curves in mechanically ventilated patients (21,22) for it is simple, does not require disconnecting the patient from the ventilator, and minimizes the artifacts due to continued gas exchange during the procedure (19).

Reduced Cst,rs (increased stiffness) is generally considered as a hallmark of ARDS (1,15). Reduced lung compliance in ARDS has been attributed to pulmonary edema (23), loss of ventilated lung units (24), and increased lung surface tension (25). Katz et al. (26) reported reduced compliance of the chest wall in patients with acute respiratory failure of different etiologies, including ARDS. This was attributed to the presence of

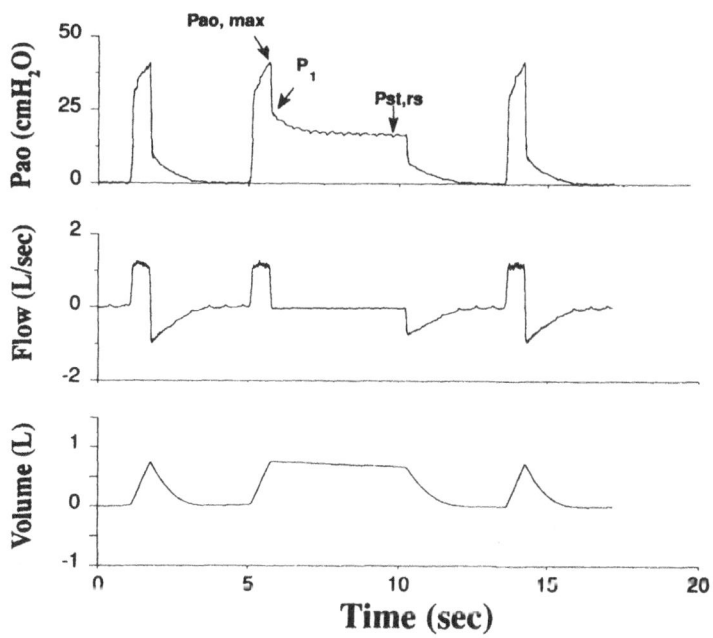

Figure 1. Records of pressure at the airway opening (Pao), flow, and changes in lung volume from a sedated-paralyzed ARDS patient which illustrate the technique of rapid airway occlusion. After end-inspiratory airway occlusion there is an immediate drop in pressure from Pao,max to P_1, followed by a slow decay to a plateau value that represents static elastic recoil pressure of the respiratory system (Pst,rs). The decrease in pressure from Pmax to P_1 includes the resistive pressure due to the endotracheal tube. For further explanations see text. From ref. #32.

abdominal distension, chest wall edema, pleural effusion and restrictive bandages.

Slutsky et al. (24) noted that, after inducing pulmonary edema with oleic acid in dogs, the V-P curves of the lungs were shifted downward and to the right. However, when volume was determined in terms of rib cage expansion (anteroposterior diameter) using a magnetometer, the pre- and post-oleic acid curves were virtually superimposed. Since the changes in rib cage magnetometer signal reflect the changes in total volume of the thorax (gas, liquid, and solid), these findings are consistent with the notion that the presence of pulmonary edema does not alter the intrinsic compliance of the lung tissue, but rather that the excess edematous fluid simply competes with gas for space. In fact, recent work by Gattinoni et al. (22) using computed tomography has demonstrated that the lungs in ARDS patients are not homogeneously affected and that V-P curves performed on theses patients investigate only healthy or recruitable zones which have essentially normal intrinsic properties. Thus in ARDS, the clinician might be effectively dealing with a functionally small lung ("baby lung"), rather than with a stiff lung of normal dimensions.

The above findings have important clinical implications. Large tidal volumes (10-15 ml/kg) and high levels of PEEP (10-15 cmH_2O) are recommended in the management of ARDS patients to improve arterial oxygenation (27). Several mechanisms have been postulated to account for this effect: recruitment of previously collapsed alveolar units (23), reduction of cardiac output (28), improvement in ventilation-perfusion mismatch (29), and redistribution of lung water (30). In the absence of significant alveolar recruitment application of PEEP will result in hyperinflation of the functional lung units and increased risk of pulmonary barotrauma (11,15,31). Application of high levels of PEEP and/or large tidal volumes in patients whose lungs are severely affected (i.e. with "baby lungs") will be expected to result in dangerous alveolar overdistension. In eight ARDS patients studied on zero end-expiratory airway pressure (ZEEP) and with variable V_T's, six patients showed evidence of alveolar overdistension (i.e., reduced compliance) when they were ventilated with V_T's within the conventionally recommended range (10-15 ml/kg) (31). The stiffer the patient's respiratory system was, the less V_T was needed to reach alveolar overdistension.

Figure 2 illustrates the static V-P curves in two ARDS patients obtained both on ZEEP and on PEEP of 10 cmH$_2$O. Lung volume is expressed relative to end-expiratory lung volume on ZEEP. Changes in FRC due to PEEP were determined using the procedure previously described (11, 32). In the patient of panel A the static V-P curve on ZEEP exhibited a convexity towards the x-axis indicating progressive alveolar recruitment with increasing inflation pressure. Application of 10 cmH$_2$O of PEEP in this patient resulted in an upward shift of the static V-P curve which should mostly reflect recruitment of new lung units (11,33). By contrast, in the patient of panel B the static V-P curve on ZEEP reflected a curvilinear relationship with concavity towards the x-axis indicating that this patient was already operating on the flat portion of the V-P curve. With application of PEEP the data points moved along a fixed V-P relationship indicating no alveolar recruitment but rather overdistention of lung units, with increased risk of pulmonary barotrauma. The above results imply that measurement of the static V-P curve can provide useful information in terms of alveolar recruitment with PEEP and risk of pulmonary barotrauma (11,15).

Apart from pulmonary barotrauma, severe alveolar overdistension has been shown to cause acute lung injury characterized by pulmonary edema through epithelial and endothelial damage (34). Surfactant deficiency was also produced in normal dogs' lungs by ventilation with large V_T's (35). Since the same end-inspiratory lung volume can be reached by various combinations of PEEP and V_T's, further studies are needed to elucidate the optimal combination of PEEP and V_T.

Dynamic Compliance of the Respiratory System (Cdyn,rs)

"Effective" Cdyn,rs is commonly determined in by dividing V_T by the difference between peak airway pressure (Pao,max) and end-expiratory airway pressure (36). This variable does not represent the true Cdyn,rs, as Pao,max includes a resistive pressure component (9,37,38). Furthermore, this measurement does not take into account PEEPi. It is a useful index, however, of the effective "inspiratory impedance" of the respiratory system. The true Cdyn,rs is obtained by dividing V_T by the difference in pressure between the end-inspiratory and end-expiratory points of zero flow

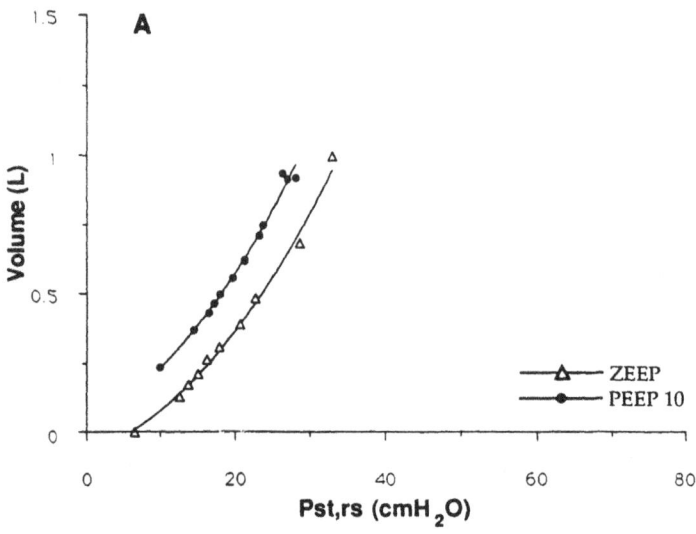

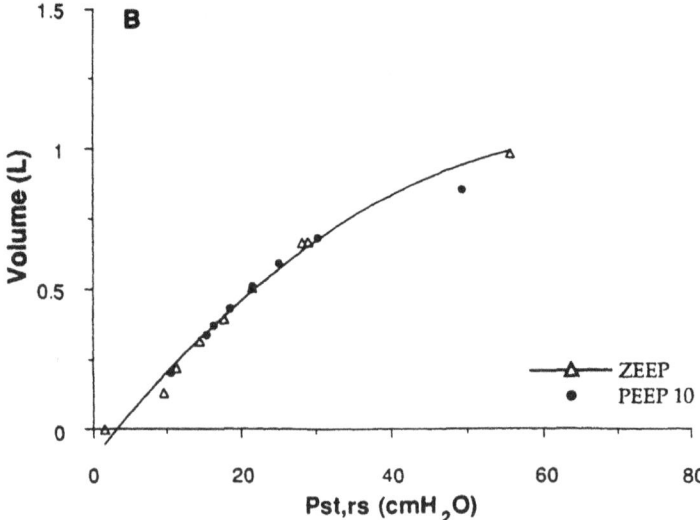

Figure 2. Static volume-pressure relationships obtained in two ARDS patients on ZEEP and on PEEP of 10 cmH$_2$O. Volume is expressed relative to end-expiratory lung volume on ZEEP. Pst,rs: static elastic recoil pressure of the respiratory system. For further explanations see text.

(37). The end-inspiratory point of zero flow corresponds to the airway pressure immediately following end-inspiratory occlusion (P_1) (Fig. 1), (9,38) while the end-expiratory point of zero flow corresponds to dynamic PEEPi (see below). P_1 can be readily measured breath-by-breath by applying a brief end-inspiratory pause (e.g., 0.1 sec) available on most ventilators. In both normal subjects (38) and ARDS patients (9) Cdyn,rs is markedly flow, volume and inspiratory time dependent.

FLOW RESISTANCE

There are four approaches available for measuring flow resistance: (a) the elastic subtraction method (39), (b) the interrupter method (39), (c) the forced oscillation method (40); and (d) the plethysmographic method (41). For obvious reasons, the last of these cannot be applied in mechanically ventilated patients. In the past, the forced oscillation technique could not be applied in these patients because of technical problems caused by the tracheal tube; however, a possible solution has been proposed recently (42). The technique of rapid airway occlusion during constant flow inflation, previously described in detail (9,10,38) is essentially a combination of two of the basic approaches for measuring flow resistance described in 1927 by von Neergaard and Wirz: the interrupter and the elastic subtraction methods (39). This technique was originally proposed by Rattenborg in 1956 (43). A virtue of the technique is that flow resistance can be measured at a fixed inspiratory flow but different tidal volumes, or at fixed tidal volumes but different inflation flows. Furthermore, with this approach the measurements can be carried out with any preselected previous lung volume history. This technique is appealing both for its simplicity and because it provides a comprehensive on-line assessment of respiratory mechanics. It can not only be applied in patients with relaxed respiratory muscles, but also in patients who trigger the ventilator provided that most of the inspiration is passive (relaxed). Furthermore, if pleural pressure is measured by the use of an esophageal balloon, flow resistance can be partitioned into its lung and chest wall components.

This technique allows for measurements of the interrupter resistance which in humans is thought to reflect airway resistance (10,44) and the effective additional resistance due to viscoelastic properties of the respiratory system and time constant inequalities. The latter which is also called tissue resistance (37), is flow, volume and inspiratory time dependent (9,38).

Measurement done with this technique in ARDS patients showed an increase of both airway and tissue flow resistance (9,10,12). Factors leading to increased airway resistance in ARDS include airway flooding, reduced lung volume, vagal reflexes, and bronchial hyperreactivity (9,10,12). In 1958, Briscoe et al. (45) showed that in normal subjects airway resistance decreases with increasing lung volume according to a hyperbolic function, reflecting the concomitant increase in airway diameters (46). A similar behavior of airway resistance as measured by the interrupter technique (interrupter resistance, Rint,rs) has been recently found in normal anesthetized paralyzed subjects (38). By contrast, in ARDS patients, on average, Rint,rs showed an initial decrease and a distinct terminal rise with increasing lung volume (Fig. 3). With application of
PEEP the distinct terminal rise becomes more pronounced (10). This paradoxical behavior may be explained as follows. In normal seated subjects, Vincent et al. (47) studied lower pulmonary flow resistance, by intratracheal catheter and esophageal balloon, using the oscillation technique at frequency of 4 Hz. At this frequency pulmonary tissue resistance should be negligible (48) and hence their measurements should essentially reflect lower airway resistance. In line with Briscoe et al. (45), they found that at lung volumes lower than about 80% of the vital capacity, lower airway resistance decreased with increasing lung volume while at lung volumes approaching the total lung capacity it exhibited a distinct increase. The explanation for that is not readily available, but it is possible that at high lung volumes the longitudinal stretching of large airways produces a decrease in calibre such that lower airway resistance increases (49). This easily testable possibility has not been explored to date.

Patients with ARDS, respond differently to application of PEEP. Figure 4 depicts the relationships between Rint,rs and overall inflation volume (i.e. relative to end-expiratory lung volume on ZEEP) in two representative ARDS patients studied on ZEEP and on PEEP of 10 cmH_2O. Patient 5 (Figs. 2A and 4A) was not close to maximal inflation, as indicated by the fact that on both ZEEP and PEEP the slope of the V-P (Fig. 2A) curves actually increased with increasing inflation volume. In this patient, Rint,rs decreased progressively with increasing lung volume (Fig. 4A), in line with the previous observations of Briscoe et al. (45). By contrast, patient 6 (Figs. 2B and 4B) was operating at a relatively high lung volume, as reflected by the fact that the V-P curve was flat (Fig. 2B). In this patient, Rint,rs increased progressively over virtually the entire range of lung volume studied (Fig. 4B).

These results have important clinical implications. In critically ill patients PEEP is generally assumed to reduce airway resistance by inducing bronchodilatation either directly (50) or as a result of increasing lung volume (45). These results show that this is not the case in most ARDS patients. In fact, the effect of PEEP on Rint,rs depends on the degree of prevailing lung distension. In ARDS patients, the number of aerated lung units is markedly reduced (22), and as a result the magnitude of inflation volumes required to reach the flat portion of their static V-P curve is narrower. If ARDS patients are mechanically ventilated with high PEEP and large tidal volumes they should exhibit a paradoxical rise of Rint,rs during the prevailing lung inflation.

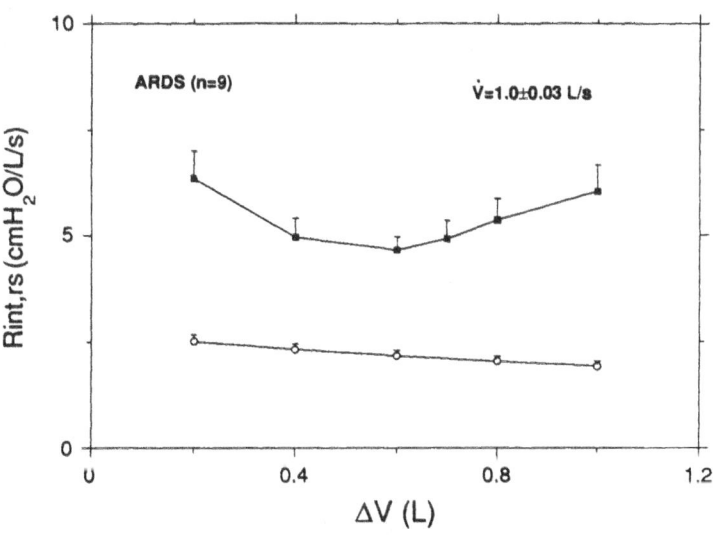

Figure 3. Average relationships between Rint,rs and inflation volume (ΔV) obtained during constant flow inflation ($\dot{V}$ of 1.0 ± 0.03 L/s in 9 ARDS patients and in 16 normal anesthetized paralyzed subjects (38). Bars, SEM. From ref. #32.

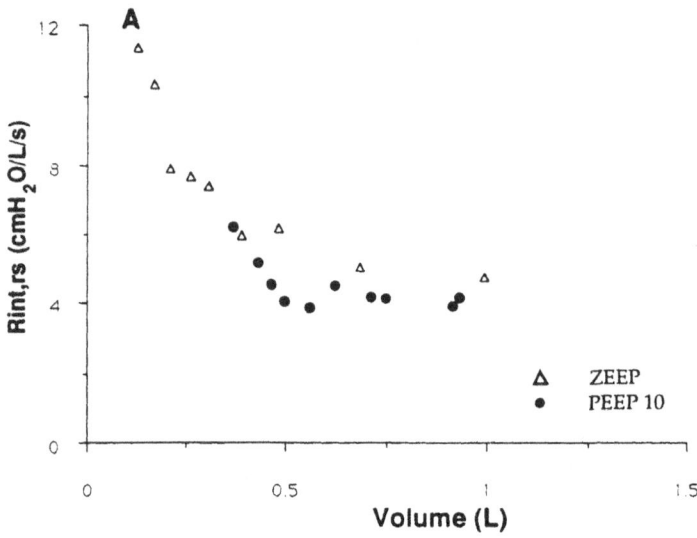

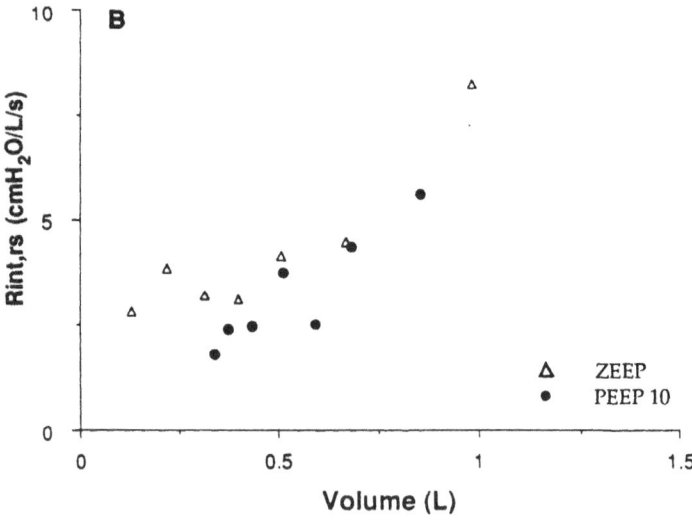

Figure 4. Relationships between interrupter resistance (Rint,rs) and inflation volume, expressed relative to end-expiratory lung volume on ZEEP obtained in two ARDS patients on ZEEP and on PEEP of 10 cmH$_2$O. For further explanations see text. Modified from ref. #10.

Tissue resistance is markedly flow, volume and time dependent (9). It is high at low respiratory frequencies (<15 breaths/min) where it accounts for most of the total resistance of the respiratory system (9). At high frequencies (>30 breaths/min), it becomes negligible (9).

Endotracheal Tube Resistance

It should be stressed that in mechanically ventilated patients the endotracheal tube contributes markedly to total flow resistance (51). The flow resistance offered by the endotracheal tubes increases markedly with increasing flow and varies with the size of the tube (51).

INTRINSIC PEEP

In 1972 Bergman (52) described a state of dynamic hyperinflation in patients who were mechanically ventilated at rapid frequencies. Under such conditions, incomplete exhalation due to insufficient available time will lead to an increase in end-expiratory lung volume above Vr. Bergman (52) also predicted that the alveolar pressure at end expiration will be positive and he postulated that in some patients this might be desirable. Bergman, however, did not measure that pressure. In 1975 Jonson et al. (53) measured the end-expiratory pressure in mechanically ventilated patients by maintaining end expiratory airway occlusion using the end-expiratory hold button on the Servo 900C ventilator and found that pressure to be elevated in patients with chronic obstructive pulmonary disease (COPD) and pointed out that this pressure has to be taken in account for correct measurement of static compliance. The incidence and ramifications of this pressure, later called intrinsic PEEP, occult PEEP, and auto-PEEP, were fully addressed by Pepe et al. (54) and Rossi et al. (17). PEEPi can have adverse effects on the venous return and cardiac output (54). For correct measurement of static respiratory compliance allowance has to be made for PEEPi (17). Furthermore, since PEEPi imposes a threshold pressure that the respiratory muscles must overcome before the onset of inspiratory flow, PEEPi can be regarded as an inspiratory threshold load (55).

In mechanically ventilated patients PEEPi is not detected by the ventilator manometer (54). During exhalation, the exhalation valve is open and only resistive pressure due to applied PEEP will register on the ventilator manometer. If the expiratory port is occluded at end expiration, alveolar pressure and circuit pressure equilibrate, and PEEPi is then seen on the ventilator manometer. External valves are needed to perform end expiratory occlusions in patients ventilated with ventilators which are not equipped with end-expiratory hold buttons.

In spontaneously breathing patients PEEPi can be determined as the negative deflection in esophageal pressure from the start of inspiratory effort to the onset of inspiratory flow (55,56). This pressure has been termed dynamic PEEPi (55,56). Values of dynamic PEEPi are usually lower than those obtained by the end-expiratory occlusion technique (static PEEPi). Static measurement of PEEPi necessarily reflect alveolar pressure after readjustment of dynamic regional volume and pressure differences due to time constant inequalities within the lung (pendelluft). In other words, in this case PEEPi reflects the equilibrium or static increase in end-expiratory Pst,rs caused by dynamic hyperinflation. In the presence of pendelluft (and hence regional difference in PEEPi) it is axiomatic that static PEEPi should exceed the lowest regional alveolar pressure present at the end of an unoccluded expiration. By contrast, the dynamic PEEPi should reflect the lowest regional end-expiratory alveolar pressure (or regional PEEPi) within the lung. Indeed, as soon as esophageal pressure during inspiration balances the lowest regional PEEPi, air begins to flow into the lung. In the case of a mechanically uniform lung, static and dynamic PEEPi should be identical but in the presence of time constant inhomogeneities within the lung, static and dynamic PEEPi differ, the latter reflecting the lowest regional PEEPi. In a recent study on patients with severe COPD, Petrof et al. (55) found that dynamic PEEPi represented, on average, 57% of static PEEPi.

Implications of PEEPi during Mechanical Ventilation

The putative role of mechanical ventilation is to reduce the activity of the inspiratory muscles to tolerable levels during patient-triggered mechanical ventilation (e.g., assisted mechanical ventilation, pressure support). This end is not achieved in patients who exhibit high PEEPi since the inspiratory effort required from the patient to trigger the ventilator may be excessive (57). By contrast, during controlled mechanical ventilation all of the work of breathing is done by the ventilator. Nevertheless, as pointed out above, PEEPi must be taken into account for correct measurement of respiratory compliance (17), and more importantly in terms of adverse effects on venous return and cardiac output (54). Patients with high PEEPi are implicitly difficult to wean from mechanical ventilation and they become ventilator-dependent (58).

PEEPi IN ARDS PATIENTS

Moderate values of PEEPi (up to 6.5 cmH_2O) have been reported in mechanically ventilated patients with no history of COPD, including patients with ARDS (11,59). While in COPD patients PEEPi is caused primarily by expiratory flow limitations (55,56), the nature of PEEPi in ARDS patients is not clearly understood. In the absence of respiratory muscle activity, the rate of lung deflation is determined by the elastic recoil pressure stored during the preceding lung inflation and the opposing total flow resistance offered by the respiratory system (including endotracheal tube, ventilator tubing and additional equipment, if any). Accordingly, the stiffer the respiratory system (i.e., decreased compliance) the faster will be the rate of lung emptying. Conversely, increased flow resistance will impede the rate of lung deflation. From the above, it appears that PEEPi in ARDS should reflect a disproportionate increase of expiratory flow resistance.

PEAK AIRWAY PRESSURE (Pao,max)

Pao,max is the sum of (a) the end-inspiratory Pst,rs, (b) the pressure losses due to viscoelastic mechanisms and/or time constant inequalities within the respiratory system, and (c) the resistive pressure dissipations due to the resistance of the airways, endotracheal tube and tubing connecting the patients to the ventilator. Figure 5 illustrates the relationship between Pao,max and several of its components with flow in an ARDS patient during constant-flow inflations with a fixed V_T of 0.683 L delivered

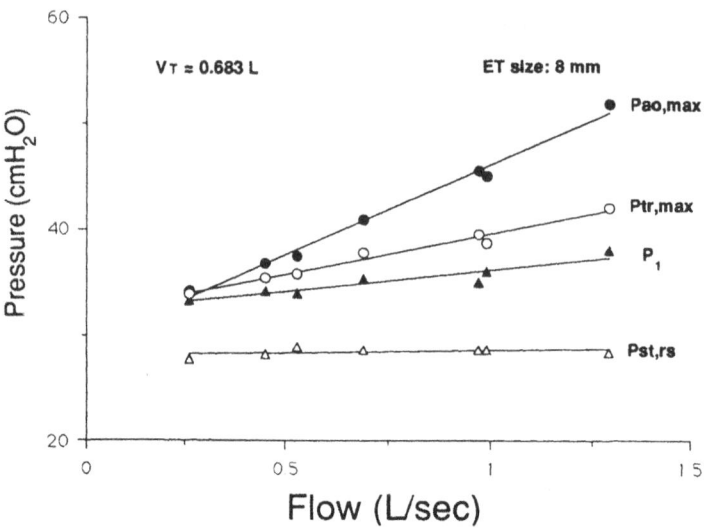

Figure 5. Relationship of peak airway pressure (Pao, max) and its components with flow in a sedated-paralyzed ARDS patient during constant-flow inflations with a fixed tidal volume (VT) of 0.683 L delivered at the same end-expiratory lung volume but at different inspiratory flows. Ptr, max: peak tracheal pressure; P_1: airway pressure immediately following end-inspiratory airway occlusion; Pst,rs: static elastic recoil pressure of the respiratory system. From ref. #32.

at the same end expiratory lung volume but at different inspiratory flows. Ptr,max is tracheal pressure measured 3 cm past the carinal end of the endotracheal tube. The end-inspiratory lung volume was fixed, as evidenced by the constancy of the end-inspiratory Pst,rs. By contrast, Pao,max increased markedly with increasing flow, reflecting in part the increase the resistive pressure due to the endotracheal tube (represented by the difference between Pao,max and Ptr,max). P_1 is the airway pressure immediately following end-inspiratory airway occlusion. The difference between Ptr,max and P_1 is the resistive pressure offered by the airways. The difference between P_1 and Pst,rs reflects the pressure losses due to viscoelastic mechanisms and/or time constant inequalities within the respiratory system (9,38). From the above, it appears that under changing conditions of inspiratory flow Pao,max will be a poor parameter for monitoring respiratory mechanics and risk of pulmonary barotrauma. For instance, an increase in Pao, max in a patient could be due to change in one or more of its components: (a) reduced compliance with a concomitant increase in Pst,rs; (b) increased PEEPi; (c) increased pressure dissipations due to viscoelastic behavior and/or time constant inequalities within the respiratory system which lead to an increase in the difference between P_1 and Pst,rs; (d) increased airway resistance with an increase in the difference between Ptr,max and P_1; (e) increased endotracheal tube resistance due to accumulations of bronchial secretions or tube kinking as reflected by an increase in the difference between Pao,max and Ptr,max. Therefore, making a correct assessment, requires determining each component of Pao,max. This can readily be obtained using the technique of rapid airway occlusion (Fig. 1). Nevertheless, in any given patient the Pao, max is useful to follow his/her progress if ventilator settings remain unchanged.

REFERENCES

1. Ashbaug DG, Bigelow DB, Petty TL, Levine BE: Acute respiratory distress in adults. Lancet 2:319-23, 1967
2. Elliot TR, Dingley LA: Lancet 1:1305, 1914
3. Matthay MA: The adult respiratory distress syndrome—New insights into diagnosis, pathophysiology, and treatment . West J Med 150:187-94, 1989
4. Osler W: The Principles and Practise of Medicine (10th ed.). New York, D. Appleton, 1927
5. Burford TH, Burbank B: Traumatic wet lung. J Thoracic Sug 14:415-24, 1945
6. Jenkins MT, Jones RF, Wislon B, Moyer CA: Congestive atelectasis a complication of intravenous infusion of fluid. Ann Surg 132:327-47, 1950
7. Petty TL: Acute Respiratory Distress Syndrome (ARDS), Disease-a-month. Edited by Bone R. Vol 36. Chicago, Year Book Medical Publ, 1990, pp. 1-58
8. Murray JF, Matthay MA, Luce JM, Flick MR: An expanded definition of the adult respiratory distress syndrome. Am Rev Respir Dis 138: 720-23, 1988
9. Eissa NT, Ranieri VM, Corbeil C, et al: Analysis of behavior of respiratory system in ARDS patients: effects of flow, volume and time. J Appl Physiol 70: 2719-29, 1991
10. Eissa NT, Ranieri MV, Corbeil C, et al: Effects of positive end-expiratory pressure, lung volume and inspiratory flow on interrupter resistance in ARDS patients. Am Rev Respir Dis (in press)
11. Ranieri MV, Eissa NT, Corbeil C, et al: The effect of PEEP on alveolar recruitment and gas exchange in ARDS patients. Am Rev Respir Dis (in press).
12. Wright PE, Bernard GR: The role of airflow resistance in patients with the adult respiratory distress syndrome. Am Rev Respir Dis 139: 1169-74, 1989

294

13. Pasteur W: Massive collapse of the lung. Lancet 7:1352-55, 1908
14. Ramachandran PR, Fairly HB: Changes in functional residual capacity during respiratory failure. Can Anaesth Soc J 17:359-69, 1970
15. Falke KJ, Pontoppidan H, Kumar A, et al: Ventilation with end-expiratory pressure in acute lung disease. J Clin Invest 51:2315-23, 1972
16. Sackner MA, Krieger BP: Noninvasive respiratory monitoring. Heart-lung Interactions in Health and Disease. Edited by Scharf SM, Cassidy SS. New York, Marcel Dekker, 1989, pp 663-805
17. Rossi A, Gottfried SB, Zocchi L, et al: Measurement of static compliance of the total respirator system in patients with acute respiratory failure during mechanical ventilation. Am Rev Respir Dis 131:672-7, 1985
18. Fleury B, Murciano D, Talamo C, et al: Work of breathing in patients with chronic obstructive pulmonary disease in acute respiratory failure. Am Rev Respir Dis 131:822-7, 1985
19. Levy P, Similowski T, Corbeil C, et al: A method for studying the static volume-pressure curves of the respiratory system during mechanical ventilation. J Crit Care 4:8389, 1989
20. Don HF, Robson JG: The mechanics of the respiratory system during anesthesia: The effect of atropine and carbon dioxide. Anesthesiology 26:168-78, 1965
21. Metamis D, Lemaire F, Harf A, et al: Total respiratory pressure volume curves in the adult respiratory distress syndrome. Chest 86:54-7, 1984
22. Gattinoni L, Pesenti A, Avalli L, et al: Pressure-volume curve of total respiratory system in acute respiratory failure. Am Rev Respir Dis 136:730-6, 1987
23. Malo J, Ali J, Wood LDH: How does positive end-expiratory pressure reduce intrapulmonary shunt in canine pulmonary edema? J Appl Physiol 57:1002-10, 1984
24. Slutsky AS, Scharf SM, Brown R, Ingram RH: The effect of oleic acid-induced pulmonary edema on pulmonary and chest wall mechanics in dogs. Am Rev Respir Dis 121:91-6, 1980
25. Petty TL, Silvers GW, Stanford RE: Abnormalities in lung elastic properties and surfactant function in adult respiratory distress syndrome. Chest 75:571-4, 1979
26. Katz JA, Zinn SE, Ozanne GM, Fairley HB: Pulmonary chest wall, and lung-thorax elastance in acute respiratory failure. Chest 80:304-11, 1981
27. Downs JB, Douglas ME: Physiologic effects of respiratory therapy, Textbook of Critical Care (2nd ed.). Edited by Shoemaker WC, Ayres S, Grenvik A, Holbrook PR, Thompson WL. Philadelphia, WB Saunders, 1989, pp. 599-606
28. Dantzker DR, Lynch JP, Weg JG: Depression of cardiac output is a mechanism of shunt reduction in the therapy of acute respiratory failure. Chest 77:636-42, 1980

29. Dantzker DR, Brook CJ, Dehart P, et al: Ventilation-perfusion distribution in the adult respiratory distress syndrome. Am Rev Respir Dis 120:1039-52, 1979
30. Paré PD, Warriner B, Baile EM, Hogg JG: Redistribution of pulmonary extravascular water with positive end-expiratory pressure in canine pulmonary edema. Am Rev Respir Dis 127:590-3, 1983
31. Eissa N, Ranieri M, Corbeil C, et al: The effects of inflation volume on the elastic properties of the total respiratory system and the risk of pulmonary barotrauma in ARDS patients. Intensive Care Med 16 (S1): S39, 1990
32. Eissa NT, Milic-Emili J: Modern concepts in monitoring and management of respiratory failure: Respiratory mechanics, Anesthesiology Clinics of North America. Vol 9. Edited by Kvetan V. Philadelphia, WB Saunders, 1991, pp. 199-218
33. Katz JA, Ozanne GM, Zinn SE, Fairley HB: Time course and mechanisms of lung-volume increase with PEEP in acute pulmonary failure. Anesthesiology 54:9-16, 1981
34. Dreyfuss D, Soler P, Basset G, Saumon G: High inflation pressure pulmonary edema: Respective effects of high airway pressure, high tidal volume, and positive end-expiratory pressure. Am Rev Respir Dis 137: 1159-64, 1988
35. Greenfield LJ, Ebert PA, Benson DW: Effects of positive pressure ventilation on surface tension properties of lung extracts. Anesthesiology 25:312-6, 1964
36. Fairly HB: Respiratory monitoring, Monitoring in Anesthesia and Critical Care Medicine. Edited by Blitt CD. New York, Churchill Livingstone, 1985, pp 229-264
37. Milic-Emili J, Robatto FM, Bates JHT: Respiratory mechanics in anesthesia. Br J Anaesth 65:4-12, 1990
38. D'Angelo E, Calderini E, Torri G, et al: Respiratory mechanics in anesthetized paralyzed humans: Effects of flow, volume, and time. J Appl Physiol 67:2556-64, 1989
39. Neergaard K von, Wirz K: Die Messung der Strömungswiederstande in der Atemwege des Menschen, insbesondere bei Asthma und Emphysem. Zeitschrift für Klimische Medizin 105:51-82, 1927
40. Dubois AB, Brody AW, Lewis DH, Burgess BF Jr: Oscillation mechanics of lungs and chest in man. J Appl Physiol 8:587-94, 1956
41. Dubois AB, Botelho SY, Comroe JH Jr: A new method for measuring airway resistance in man using a body plethysmograph: Values in normal subjects an in patients with respiratory disease. J Clin Invest 35:322-6, 1956
42. Navajas D, Farré R, Rotger M, Canet J: Recording pressure at the distal end of the endotracheal tube to measure respiratory impedance. Eur Respir J 2:178-84, 1989
43. Rattenborg C: Basic mechanics of artificial ventilation in management of life-threatening poliomyelitis. Edited by Lassen HCA. London, Livingstone, 1956, pp. 23

44. D'Angelo E, Robatto FM, Calderini E, et al: Pulmonary and chest wall mechanics in anesthetized paralyzed humans. J Appl Physiol 70:2602-10, 1991
45. Briscoe WA, Dubois AB: The relationship between airway resistance, airway conductance and lung volume in subjects of different age and body size. J Clin Invest 37:1279-85, 1958
46. Heinbecker P: A method for the demonstration of calibre changes in the bronchi in normal respiration. J Clin Invest 4:459-69, 1927
47. Vincent NJ, Knudson R, Leith DE, et al: Factors influencing pulmonary resistance. J Appl Physiol 29:236-43, 1970
48. Hantos Z, Daróczy B, Suki B, et al: Forced oscillatory impedance of the respiratory system at low frequencies. J Appl Physiol 60:123-32, 1986
49. Ingram RH, Pedley TJ: Pressure-flow relationships in the lungs, Handbook of Physiology. Vol III, sect. 3, The Respiratory System. Edited by Macklem PT, Mead J. Bethesda, MD, Am Physiol Soc, 1986, pp. 277-93
50. Barach AL, Swenson P: Effect of breathing gases under positive pressure on lumens of small and medium-sized bronchi. Arch Intern Med 63:946-48, 1939
51. Gottfried SB, Rossi A, Higgs BD, et al: Noninvasive determination of respiratory system mechanics during mechanical ventilation for acute respiratory failure. Am Rev Respir Dis 131:414-20, 1985
52. Bergman NA: Intrapulmonary gas trapping during mechanical ventilation at rapid frequencies. Anesthesiology 37:626-33, 1972
53. Jonson B, Nordström, Olsson SG, Akerback D: Monitoring of ventilation and lung mechanics during automatic ventilation. A new device. Bull Physiopath Resp 11:729-743, 1975
54. Pepe PE, Marini JJ: Occult positive end-expiratory pressure in mechanically ventilated patients with airflow obstruction. Am Rev Respir Dis 126:166-170, 1982
55. Petrof BJ, Legaré M, Goldberg P, et al: Continuous positive airway pressure reduces work of breathing and dyspnea during weaning from mechanical ventilation in severe obstructive pulmonary disease. Am Rev Respir Dis 141:281-89, 1990
56. Haluszka J, Chartrand DA, Grassino AE, Milic-Emili J: Intrinsic PEEP and arterial PCO_2 in stable patients with chronic obstructive pulmonary disease. Am Rev Respir Dis 141:1194-97, 1990
57. Smith TC, Marini JJ: Impact of PEEP on lung mechanics and work of breathing in severe airflow obstruction. J Appl Physiol 65:1488-99, 1988
58. Kimball WR, Leith DE, Robins AG: Dynamic hyperinflation and ventilator dependence in chronic obstructive pulmonary disease. Am Rev Respir Dis 126:991-5, 1982
59. Broseghini C, Brandolese R, Poggi R, et al: Respiratory mechanics during the first day of mechanical ventilation in patients with pulmonary edema and chronic airway obstruction. Am Rev Respir Dis 138:355-61, 1988

NEW MODES OF VENTILATORY SUPPORT

J. B. Downs

Since the advent of intermittent positive pressure ventilation (IPPV), positive end-expiratory pressure (PEEP), intermittent mandatory ventilation (IMV), continuous positive airway pressure (CPAP), mandatory minute ventilation (MMV), and high frequency ventilation, several ventilatory modalities have been introduced for the treatment of ventilatory insufficiency. Pressure support ventilation (PSV) and airway pressure release ventilation (APRV) are most recent. Although PSV was introduced seven years ago, there is little data concerning its usefulness in patient care. Nevertheless, PSV is a standard feature of several commercially available ventilators. APRV is presently an experimental technique and, therefore, not in general use.

PRESSURE SUPPORT VENTILATION

Pressure support ventilation, also termed inspiratory assist or assisted spontaneous breathing, originally was developed as an adjunct to IMV and MMV to augment spontaneous respiration and to overcome high circuit resistance during spontaneous breathing. During PSV, the patient's spontaneous inspiration triggers the ventilator to provide a variable flow of gas that increases until airway pressure reaches a preselected level. A servo mechanism adjusts the flow to keep inspiratory airway pressure constant. When the patient's inspiratory effort wanes, flow decreases. When patient demand for inspiratory flow is sufficiently reduced, flow is terminated, and airway pressure returns to baseline. Thus, during each attempted spontaneous inhalation, the patient receives assisted ventilation with a mechanism that is pressure limited and flow cycled. The inspiratory work of breathing performed by the ventilator during PSV

T. H. Stanley and R. J. Sperry (eds.), Anesthesia and the Lung 1992, 297–301.
© 1992 *Kluwer Academic Publishers.*

depends on the pressure level and the patient's respiratory mechanics and cannot be determined directly. If the pressure support level is elevated sufficiently, most of the respiratory work is performed by the ventilator, and the ventilatory mode is similar to conventional assisted positive pressure ventilation, but with a pressure limit. The major theoretical advantage of PSV is adjustable breath-to-breath ventilatory assistance, in which each respiratory cycle is similar in configuration and equally assisted by the ventilator. This may facilitate adaptation of the patient to the ventilator and weaning from the ventilatory support. Since the patient controls respiratory rate and the duration of inspiration, the development of respiratory alkalosis, frequently seen during conventional assisted ventilation, should be less likely.

Prakash and Meij compared controlled ventilation and PSV in 26 patients who were recovering from coronary artery bypass surgery. The authors claimed that the use of PSV was associated with shorter time of endotracheal intubation. However, the weaning protocols used for PSV and controlled ventilation were not described, nor were results tested with adequate statistical analysis. MacIntyre compared SIMV and PSV in 15 patients who required mechanical ventilatory support. PSV was administered with a pressure limit (range from 13 to 41 cm H_2O) adjusted to minimize respiratory rate. The author observed that respiratory rate during PSV was lower than total respiratory rate during SIMV with similar minute ventilation. Peak airway pressure was lower and mean airway pressure higher during PSV. Upon interview, all but one patient expressed a subjective preference for PSV. Experiments conducted in a lung model by MacIntyre suggest that PSV may alter the pressure/volume characteristics of the lung and decrease respiratory muscle work with smaller change in pressure and larger change in volume, a type of work better suited for an endurance muscle system. This finding has not been confirmed in experimental animals or in humans.

To appropriately use PSV, one must recognize that it is a method of administering variable positive pressure mechanical ventilatory support and not a form of spontaneous breathing. While it is clear that spontaneous respiratory work can be reduced using PSV, difficulties in determining the level of assistance provided by a given pressure do not allow comparisons between ventilatory modalities on the basis of existing data.

Cardiovascular and pulmonary complications of PSV probably depend on airway and intrathoracic pressure and lung volume as they do during other forms of assisted ventilation. Some ventilators that have unacceptably high flow resistance may require the use of PSV if conventional mechanical breaths are not delivered. In these cases, use of a well designed low resistance CPAP system may be a more efficacious and simple alternative. Available data show that PSV may be used to provide ventilatory support to patients with mild to moderate respiratory failure and that weaning from ventilatory support may be accomplished using decremental PSV. There are no comparative investigations that establish PSV as the method of choice for ventilatory assistance, or for weaning from ventilatory support in any patient group. Theoretically, however, PSV differs sufficiently from other ventilatory modalities, that it warrants further clinical investigation on a large scale to determine its role in modern respiratory therapy.

AIRWAY PRESSURE RELEASE VENTILATION

Airway pressure release ventilation is a new ventilatory support technique introduced by Downs and Stock. APRV is designed to augment alveolar ventilation in patients who require ventilatory assistance despite reduction of respiratory work with CPAP. Currently, the utility of APRV is being evaluated in experimental and clinical investigations. APRV equipment is not yet commercially available, nor can it be reliably produced with any existing ventilator.

During APRV, changes in lung volume that are required for augmentation of alveolar ventilation are produced using intermittent release of CPAP. The APRV system includes a CPAP circuit in which baseline airway pressure is maintained above ambient using a threshold resistor valve and either a high gas flow, a pressurized volume reservoir, or possibly a sensitive demand valve. A release valve is situated in the expiratory limb of the CPAP circuit to allow rapid decrease in airway pressure. The release valve must have extremely low flow resistance to allow adequate emptying of the lungs during pressure release. The release valve is driven by a timing device that allows adjustment of the extent, length, and frequency of pressure release. Use of APRV requires that a level of CPAP has been adjusted to optimize expiratory lung volume and pulmonary gas exchange. When the timer opens the release valve, airway pressure falls rapidly, gas exits the lungs, and lung volume decreases below baseline allowing excretion of carbon dioxide. When the release valve closes, CPAP and lung volume are rapidly re-established. Augmentation of alveolar ventilation depends on release volume and the APRV rate. Release volume of the APRV breath is determined by lung compliance, airway resistance, release time, and the gradient between CPAP and the release pressure level. The patient can breathe freely between, or during, the APRV breaths at all times. If sufficient release volume and rate are used, controlled ventilation will result. Weaning from APRV is accomplished by lowering the frequency of airway pressure release, until the patient is breathing only with CPAP.

APRV is distinguished from any other form of ventilatory support because ventilation is accomplished by decreasing lung volume below baseline. Reverse I:E ratio ventilation with a pressure limit may mimic closely APRV. However, reverse I:E ratio ventilation seldom is combined with spontaneous breathing, and weaning is accomplished by decreasing the time of increased airway pressure, rather than increasing it, as is the case with APRV. The theoretical advantages of APRV, compared to other forms of positive pressure ventilation, are related to low peak and mean airway and intrathoracic pressures. Peak airway pressure during APRV never exceeds the CPAP level, and maximum lung volume corresponds to functional residual capacity. Therefore, the incidence of barotrauma should be minimal. Changes in intrathoracic pressure during APRV are similar to those that occur during spontaneous breathing with CPAP.

Stock et al. compared APRV and IPPV in anesthetized dogs with normal lungs and found no significant differences in gas exchange or cardiovascular function between the two ventilatory modalities. We then induced high permeability pulmonary edema in the animals with intravenous oleic acid, and compared APRV with IPPV+PEEP, maintaining constant mean airway pressure. APRV was associated with significantly lower peak airway pressure and improved oxygenation of arterial blood. No differences in cardiac function were observed, likely because mean intrathoracic pressures were similar. Garner et al. compared conventional controlled ventilation and APRV in 14 patients with mild acute lung injury following cardiac operation. Except for lower peak airway pressure during APRV, both ventilatory modalities produced similar results in cardiopulmonary function. When anesthesia resolved, weaning was easily accomplished using APRV.

Experimental and clinical investigations have shown that APRV can augment alveolar ventilation in dogs with or without lung injury and in postoperative patients with mild pulmonary insufficiency. Results of several ongoing studies in patients with varying degrees of respiratory insufficiency will determine or disprove the usefulness of APRV in clinical practice.

SUMMARY

A considerable disparity presently exists between the marketing of new modalities of positive pressure ventilation and the scientific evaluation of their utility in patient care. A ventilator that would include only features proven effective clinically, likely would be considerably lighter in weight, smaller in size, and less expensive than most currently marketed ventilators. Neither of the ventilatory techniques presented here are supported by sufficient clinical and experimental data so that recommendations can be made for their routine application in patient care. PSV, breath-to-breath adjustable assisted ventilation, may be useful in some clinical situations, but requires further investigation. APRV is an entirely new concept of ventilatory assistance that is undergoing clinical evaluation with encouraging preliminary results.

SUGGESTED READING LIST

Downs JB, Stock MC: Airway pressure release ventilation: a new concept in ventilatory support. Editorial. Crit Care Med 15:459-61, 1987

MacIntyre NR: Respiratory function during pressure support ventilation. Chest 89: 677-83, 1986

Prakash O, Meij S: Cardiopulmonary response to inspiratory pressure support during spontaneous ventilation vs conventional ventilation. Chest 83:103 7, 1985

Räsänen J, Downs JB, Stock MC: Cardiovascular effects of conventional positive pressure ventilation and airway pressure release ventilation. Chest 93:911-15, 1988

Stock MC, Downs JB, Frolicher DA: Airway pressure release ventilation. Crit Care Med 15:462-66, 1987

SEPTIC SHOCK

R.C. Bone

Sepsis can be defined as the systemic response to the presence in the body of microorganisms or their toxic products. Previous clinical studies have required *in vitro* laboratory growth of the organisms to confirm the diagnosis of sepsis. The septic syndrome is defined by specific clinical criteria and has a significant mortality rate in addition to other sequelae commonly associated with sepsis.

The criteria for the sepsis syndrome identify a population of patients at imminent risk for development of septic shock and ARDS. The sepsis syndrome itself carries a clinically significant mortality rate. Identification and definition of this syndrome may allow for earlier detection and treatment of patients with sepsis and could potentially result in improved survival through prevention of shock and multiple system organ failure. Since the septic syndrome has the potential for earlier identification of septic patients, it may allow for earlier therapeutic intervention, aid in the search to uncover pathophysiologic mechanisms, and provide a useful clinical point at which to evaluate new therapeutic modalities.

INTRODUCTION

The high frequency and often devastating consequences of sepsis make it a major cause of death from infection in the United States today (1). Although bacteremia may be asymptomatic, it too often comes to clinical attention as an acute catastrophic event recognized by a characteristic constellation of signs and symptoms. Indeed, the term sepsis implies bacteremia coupled with a host response to the circulating microorganisms.

303

T. H. Stanley and R. J. Sperry (eds.), Anesthesia and the Lung 1992, 303–312.
© 1992 Kluwer Academic Publishers.

Factors that determine the presence or absence of clinical symptoms are largely unknown, though they are of obvious importance in the therapy of bacteremic patients. Conversely, several clinical and laboratory features of bacteremic patients mitigate for or against survival and the development of a particularly devastating manifestation of sepsis, the adult respiratory distress syndrome (ARDS). This review will discuss risk factors, incidence, and prognostic indicators of sepsis and septic ARDS, and conclude with a brief review of two controversial aspects of therapy for septic lung injury: corticosteroids and prophylactic positive end expiratory pressure (PEEP).

CLINICAL MANIFESTATIONS OF SEPSIS

Manifestations of bacteremia are diverse in their range and representation in individual patients (Table 1). Skin lesions such as septic

Table 1. Clinical manifestations of bacteremia.

Fever or hypothermia
Chills
Skin lesions
Altered mental status
Organ dysfunction

    Kidney
    Gastrointestinal
    Lung
    Cardiovascular

bulla, Janeway lesions, Roth spots, and others may be observed (2). Fever and chills, thought to be pathophysiologically dependent upon the production of endogenous pyrogen (interleukin 1), frequently are present. Altered mental status may be observed and may, in fact, be the first manifestation of sepsis in elderly patients. Decreasing urine output, which may be associated with peripheral edema, is a reflection of inadequate perfusion and, more ominously, early renal failure (2). Also, the gastrointestinal, pulmonary, and cardiovascular systems frequently show evidence of dysfunction in the presence of bacteremia (3). Dysfunction of each of these organ systems is prognostically important, since mortality rate is well correlated to the number of organ systems injured (4). Early dysfunction involving the cardiovascular system, however, is the single most reliable predictor of early death in endotoxemia (5) and is the most frequent immediate cause of death in septic patients in the first 24 hours.

Laboratory abnormalities may be helpful in the evaluation of bacteremic patients (Table 2). Arterial blood gases obtained early in the course

---

Table 2. Clinical abnormalities associated with bacteremia.

Arterial blood gases

Respiratory alkalosis → metabolic (lactic) acidosis
Increased alveolar-arterial oxygen gradient

Coagulation abnormalities
Granulocytosis/granulocytopenia
Complement system activation

---

of bacteremia are likely to reflect respiratory alkalosis secondary to stimulation of central respiratory centers. If cardiovascular compensation is inadequate to maintain vital organ perfusion, lactic acidosis will supervene. Hypoxemia may be present, though abnormal arterial-alveolar oxygen ratios or gradients are earlier indicators of pulmonary dysfunction. Coagulation abnormalities, most commonly thrombocytopenia with or without other evidence of disseminated intravascular coagulation, are frequently observed (6). Granulocytosis with predominance of immature forms, or granulocytopenia and falling white blood cell counts are suggestive of bacteremia. Patients with gram-negative bacteremia may have evidence of complement system activation (7).

Many investigators find it helpful to define a subset of bacteremic patients whose clinical features portend poorer prognosis. The term sepsis or septic syndrome implies that a patient has good evidence of a serious infection and a systemic response to that infection (Table 3). Criteria for definition of a serious infection include such factors as hyperthermia or hypothermia, granulocytosis or granulocytopenia, positive blood culture for a recognized pathogen, or gross pus in an enclosed space. Systemic response to infection is implied by the presence of clinical manifestations, such as otherwise unexplained arterial hypotension, low systemic vascular resistance, or metabolic acidosis. While most patients who are bacteremic and febrile but lack other manifestations of sepsis do well, the mortality rate for patients with cardiovascular collapse, even when the site of

Table 3. Definition of sepsis.

Serious infection is evidenced by two or more of the following:

- Core temperature > 39°C or < 35°C
- Neutrophil count > 12,000 μl or < 3000/μl or > 20% immature forms
- One positive blood culture for a commonly accepted pathogen
- A known or suspected source for systemic infection (such as the urinary tract) from which a recognized pathogen has been cultured
- Gross pus in an enclosed space

Systemic response is evidenced by one of the following:

- Unexplained arterial hypotension
- Systemic vascular resistance (SVR) < 800 dynes/sec•cm^{-5}
- Unexplained metabolic acidosis (base deficit > 5 mEq/L)

infection is known and appropriate antibiotics are given, is between 50 and 70% (6,8). Interestingly, treatment in an intensive care unit does not appear to alter the outcome of pneumococcal bacteremia once shock is established (9). Thus, a more specific definition of sepsis may guide us toward the features of sepsis that can be used to predict outcome.

SEPTIC SYNDROME

The sepsis syndrome can be defined in terms of the systemic response to sepsis expressed as tachycardia, fever or hypothermia, tachypnea, and evidence of inadequate organ perfusion or organ dysfunction. More specifically, it can be defined as hypothermia (T < 96°F), fever (T > 101°F), tachycardia (> 90 bpm), tachypnea (> 20 respirations/min), clinical suspicion of infection, and evidence of inadequate organ perfusion or function expressed as poor or altered cerebral function, hypoxemia (P_aO_2 < 75 mmHg), elevated plasma lactate, or oliguria (urine output <30 ml/hr or <0.5 ml/kg body weight per hour) (10). When sepsis syndrome is accompanied by hypotension unresponsive to fluid therapy it is referred to as septic shock. Although the exact incidence is not known, 70,000-300,000 cases of sepsis are estimated to occur in the United States each year (11). Shock develops in approximately 40% of these patients and adversely affects survival (6). A number of recent innovations in medical practice may have actually increased the likelihood of sepsis and septic shock (11). These innovations include: aggressive oncologic chemotherapy, cortico-steroid or immunosuppressive therapy for organ transplantation or inflammatory diseases, increasing survival of patients predisposed to sepsis, and more frequent use of invasive medical procedures (11,12).

Patients with the sepsis syndrome (n = 191) were prospectively evaluated and comprised the placebo group of a multicenter trial of methylprednisolone in sepsis syndrome and septic shock (10). Forty-five percent of the patients were found to be bacteremic; 31% were in septic shock (sepsis syndrome plus systolic blood pressure <90 mmHg or decreased from baseline systolic blood pressure >40 mm Hg) at study entry. An additional 24% of the patients developed shock after admission, with 70% doing so within 24 hours of study entry; shock reversal occurred with a frequency of 73%. Twenty-five percent of the patients developed the Adult Respiratory Distress Syndrome (ARDS). Mortality for patients with sepsis syndrome who did not develop shock was 13%. Mortality for the groups of patients with shock at admission and shock subsequent to admission was 27.5% and 43.2%, respectively. Forty-seven percent of bac-teremic patients developed shock after study admission compared to 29.6% of non-bacteremic patients (p < 0.05). Other than development of shock, there were no significant differences between the bacteremic and non-bacteremic patients. Also, the outcomes for patients with gram-negative and gram-positive bacteremias did not differ significantly.

PROGNOSTIC INDICATORS IN SEPSIS

A large series of bacteremic patients reported by Kreger and McCabe detailed the clinical features and effects of antibiotic therapy in 612 patients with gram-negative bacteremia over a 10-year period (6). For purposes of evaluation, patients were classified according to their underlying illness as being rapidly fatal, ultimately fatal, or nonfatal. Historical features that were associated with increased mortality in patients in any of the underly-ing disease categories are listed in Table 4. Factors that also were examined but did not materially affect the outcome of bacteremia included race, gen-der, and the coexistence of neoplastic diseases. The majority of factors listed in Table 4 impair the immune response of the host, and may be pos-tulated to influence survival by this mechanism.

Table 4. Pre-existing factors that adversely influence the outcome of sepsis.

> Antecedent antibiotics
> Antecedent antimetabolites
> Antecedent corticosteroids
> Azotemia
> Congestive heart failure
> Diabetes mellitus
> Nosocomial infection
>
> Adapted from Kreger et al. (6).

The single best clinical indicator of sepsis and poor outcome was the presence of shock. Shock occurred in 44% of the patients evaluated in this study; fatality in patients with shock was 47%, in contrast to mortality of 7% in patients who did not manifest shock. These data are in close accordance with those of Winslow (8), who noted that 64% of patients with septic shock from gram-positive or gram-negative bacteremia died. Additional clinical factors in Kreger's patients that were associated with the development of shock were age >65 years; antecedent corticosteroid, antimetabolite, or antibiotic therapy; azotemia; and congestive heart failure (6). In a prospective study of serial cardiopulmonary variables in patients with septic shock, Abraham reported that arterial hypotension was precipitated by a drop of the cardiac index from the high levels classically described in "warm" sepsis to normal ranges (13). These data suggested to the investigators that loss of cardiac compensation for low systemic vascular resistance was the immediate cause of the hypotensive crisis.

Winslow et al. have reported that arterial lactic acid levels are higher in septic patients who died than in those who survived, though the overlap was too great to make this a test of prognostic significance in any individual patient (8). The clinical and laboratory features associated with increased mortality in sepsis are listed in Table 5.

Additional laboratory tests that are reported to be abnormal in patients with sepsis are the levels of cyclo-oxygenase metabolites thromboxane B_2 and 6-keto-prostaglandin $F_{1\alpha}$ (14,15), plasma fibronectin, and angiotensin-converting enzyme. Thromboxane B_2 is a metabolite of thromboxane A_2, a vasoconstrictive and platelet aggregatory lipid. Similarly, 6-keto-$PGF_{1\alpha}$ is a stable metabolite of prostacyclin, a vasodilatory and antiaggregatory metabolite of arachidonic acid metabolism.

Table 5. Clinical and laboratory features that adversely influence survival in sepsis.

Shock
Lactic acidosis
Elevated blood levels of cyclo-oxygenase metabolites
Subtherapeutic levels of antibiotics
Low levels of circulating antibodies to a common core
    lipopolysaccharide antigen of gram-negative bacteria

Although the mean levels of these metabolites were higher in non-surviving than in surviving patients, the separation of values was insufficient to allow this test to be applied prognostically. Angiotensin-converting enzyme (ACE) is a carboxypeptidase that converts angiotensin 1 to angiotensin 2 and is found in highest concentrations in lung capillary endothelial cells. Endothelial cell injury causes release of angiotensin-converting enzyme into the blood, the level of which is reported to be correlated to severity of lung injury (16). Severe sepsis is associated with a decrease in plasma fibronectin, a non-immunologic opsonin that facilitates removal of degradation products by the reticuloendothelial cell system (17). Plasma fibronectin levels are touted as a prognostic indicator in sepsis. Each of these tests is of limited value in an individual patient, since the overlap with control patient populations remains significant.

For nearly 10 years, it has been recognized that high titers of antibody to a core lipopolysaccharide shared by most gram-negative bacteria protects patients against the development of shock and death (18). More recently, levels of circulating antibodies to *Escherichia coli* endotoxin core were shown to correlate well to enhanced survival in patients with *Pseudomonas aeruginosa* septicemia (19). These observations suggested that immunization against this common core antigen may be protective against cardiovascular changes associated with septicemia. Active immunization of sheep using the core glycolipid fraction of a J5 *E. coli* mutant is effective in reducing the pulmonary hypertension and the decrease in cardiac output and alveolar-arterial oxygen gradient that is secondary to gram-negative endotoxemia (20). Passive immunization is also effective in this model, though protection is incomplete. Passive administration of antiserum raised in normal human volunteers against a mutant *E. coli* is reported to reduce mortality and death due to gram-negative bacteremia

(21). These results were reinforced by the observation that administration of plasma rich in antilipopolysaccharide immunoglobulin B provided a survival advantage to gynecologic patients with septic shock (22). Since these two studies were unblinded and suboptimally controlled, however, verification of these results will be critically important.

Kreger and McCabe's study (6) clearly demonstrated that early and appropriate antibiotic therapy is highly effective in reducing mortality secondary to gram-negative bacteremia. In all categories of patients, initial selection of appropriate antibiotic therapy improved outcome. Furthermore, this advantage extended to patients who had already entered into a shock state. These results have been extended by Moore et al., who found that administration of sufficient doses of aminoglycosides to achieve therapeutic levels reduced the mortality rate relative to patients similarly treated but in whom subtherapeutic levels of aminoglycosides were detected (23). These data underscore the importance of delivering to patients judiciously chosen antibiotics in adequate doses as early as sepsis is suspected. New treatments are now being defined and evaluated in animal models and multicenter studies. A graphic example of potential agents for therapeutic use in septic shock is shown in Figure 1.

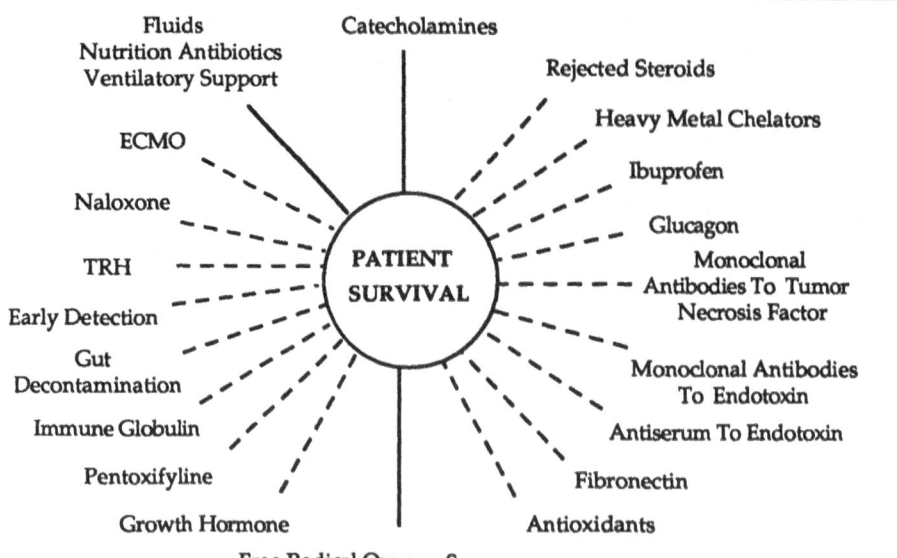

Figure 1. Conventional and proposed treatment of septic shock and multi-organ failure.

REFERENCES

1. McCabe WR: Gram negative bacteremia: Disease-a-month. Chicago, Year Book Medical Publishers, 1973.
2. Sheagren JH: Shock syndromes related to sepsis. Cecil Textbook of Medicine. WB Saunders, Philadelphia, 1986, pp. 1473-77
3. McCabe WR, Treadwell TL, Maria AD: Pathophysiology of bacteremia. Am J Med 75:7-18, 1983
4. National Heart, Lung, and Blood Institute. Extracorporeal support for respiratory insufficiency: Collaborative study. National Heart, Lung, and Blood Institute, Washington, D.C., 1979
5. Goldfarb RD, Tambolini W, Wiener SM, et al: Canine left ventricular performance during LD50 endotoxemia. Am J Physiol 244:H370-7, 1983
6. Kreger BEW, Craven DE, and McCabe WR: Gram-negative bacteremia: IV. Re-evaluation of clinical features and treatment in 612 patients. Am J Med 68:344-55, 1980
7. McCabe WR: Serum complement levels in bacteremia due to gram negative organisms. N Engl J Med 288:21-3, 1973
8. Winslow EJ, Loeb HS, Rahimtoola SH, et al: Hemodynamic studies and results of therapy in 50 patients with bacteremic shock. Am J Med 54:421-32, 1973
9. Hook EW, Horton CA, Schaberg DR: Failure of intensive care unit support to influence mortality from pneumococcal bacteremia. J Am Med Assoc 249:1055-7, 1983
10. Bone RC, Fisher CJ, Clemmer TP, et al: The sepsis syndrome: A valid clinical entity. Crit Care Med 17:389-93, 1989
11. Parker MM, Parillo JE: Hemodynamics and pathogenesis. J Am Med Assoc 250:3324-7, 1983
12. Shubin H, Weil MH: Bacterial shock. J Am Med Assoc 235:421-4, 1976
13. Abraham E, Shoemaker WC, Bland RD, et al: Plasma fibronectin in medical ICU patients. Crit Care Med 11:799-803, 1983
14. Halushka PV, Reines HD, Barrow SE, et al: Elevated 6-keto-prostaglandin F1a in patients in septic shock. Crit Care Med 13:451-453, 1985
15. Reines HD, Cook JA, Halushka PV, et al: Plasma thromboxane concentrations are raised in patients dying with septic shock. Lancet 2:174-5, 1982
16. Fourrier F, Chopin C, Wallaert B, et al: Compared evolution of plasma fibronectin and angio-converting enzyme levels in septic ARDS. Chest 87:191-5, 1985
17. O'Connell MT, Becker DM, Steele BW, et al: Plasma fibronectin in medical ICU patients. Crit Care Med 12:479-82, 1984

18. Zinner SH, McCabe WR: Effects of IgM and IgG antibody in patients with bacteremia due to gram-negative bacilli. J Infect Dis 133:37-45, 1976

19. Pollack M, Huang AI, Prescott RK, et al: Enhanced survival in pseudomonas aeruginosa septicemia associated with high levels of circulating antibody to E. coli endotoxin core. J Clin Invest 72:1874-81, 1984.

20. Girotti, MJ, Menkes E, MacDonald JWD, et al: Effects of immunization on cardiopulmonary alterations of gram-negative endotoxemia. J Appl Physiol 56:582-9, 1984

21. Ziegler EJ, McCutchan JA, Fierer J, et al: Treatment of gram-negative bacteremia and shock with human antiserum to a mutant E. coli. N Engl J Med 307:1225-30, 1982

22. Lachman E, Pitsoe SB, Gaffin SL: Anti-lipopolysaccharide immunotherapy in management of septic shock of obstetric and gynecological origin. Lancet 1:981-3, 1984

23. Moore RD, Smith CR, Lietman PS: The association of aminoglycoside plasma levels with mortality in patients with gram-negative bacteremia. J Infect Dis 149:443-8, 1984

TO PEEP OR NOT TO PEEP ARDS PATIENTS?

V.M. Ranieri, N.T. Eissa, C. Corbeil and J. Milic-Emili

PEEP was introduced in 1967 in the treatment of ARDS (1). Suter et al. (2) introduced the concept of "best PEEP" to describe the optimal level of PEEP at which static compliance was the highest. This level was also associated with maximum oxygen delivery and minimum dead space. In general, the beneficial effects of PEEP are thought to be achieved by recruiting collapsed alveoli and restoring the functional residual capacity (FRC) toward normal (3,4). However, while PEEP is known to increase the end-expiratory lung volume (EELV) in ARDS patients (3,4), with the exception of the studies of Gattinoni's group (5,6) there are no systematic studies in which the recruitment of collapsed lung units due to PEEP has been quantified. Hence, the question remains whether this increase in lung volume simply reflects a displacement of EELV along a fixed static volume-pressure (V-P) curve of the respiratory system with concomitant alveolar overinflation or is associated with an upward shift of the static P-V curve caused by recruitment of previously collapsed lung units. Assessment of static thoracopulmonary V-P curves with the "super-syringe" method has been proposed for diagnosis, staging and management of ARDS patients (7). However, the long time required to perform V-P curves with this method introduces significant errors due to continuing gas exchange. Correction methods have been proposed (8) but are complex and require measurements that are not usually available at the bedside. The "super-syringe" method involves a temporary disconnection of the patients from the ventilator, changing both the previous volume history (9) and the EELV. Indeed, at zero inflation pressure, the EELV after disconnection of the patient from the ventilator should be lower than that obtained during mechanical ventilation and should correspond to the relaxation volume (Vr).

313

T. H. Stanley and R. J. Sperry (eds.), Anesthesia and the Lung 1992, 313–317.
© 1992 Kluwer Academic Publishers.

Recently we studied (10) the effects of PEEP on the static V-P curve in eight septic ARDS patients. In our study the V-P curves were derived from a series of single-breath measurements of static elastic recoil pressure of the respiratory system (Pst,rs) made at different inflation volumes (11) without changing the previous volume history, and without disconnecting the patient from the ventilator. A second order polynomial equation was fitted to the experimental points:

$$\Delta V = a + b\,Pst,rs + c\,Pst,rs^2 \qquad (1)$$

where ΔV is change in volume relative to Vr on zero end expiratory pressure (ZEEP). Alveolar recruitment was calculated as difference in lung volume between PEEP and ZEEP for the same Pst,rs ($=20$ cmH$_2$O) from the V-P curves obtained at the different PEEP levels. Two characteristic morphologies on the V-P curves were identified. In three patients the static inflation V-P curve exhibited a progressive decrease in slope with increasing inflation volume, i.e., it exhibited an upward convexity with a negative value of the constant c (Eq. 1). Application of PEEP to these patients resulted in a volume displacement along the inflation V-P curve obtained on ZEEP. In the other five patients the static V-P curve on ZEEP exhibited an upward concavity, and a positive value of the constant c, i.e., there was a progressive increase in slope with increasing inflation volume, reflecting progressive alveolar recruitment. In these patients PEEP caused an upward shift of the V-P curves. At the highest level of PEEP studied (15 cmH$_2$O), the mean $\pm$SEM recruited alveolar volume amount to 0.23 ± 0.04 L, ranging between 0.16 and 0.36 L. The average percentage ratio of recruited alveolar volume to the change in FRC with PEEP (ΔFRC) was $32.2 \pm 1.5\%$. Volume recruited correlated positively with the coefficient c (Eq. 1), and negatively with end-inspiratory Pst,rs obtained on ZEEP during baseline lung inflation (V$_T$ = 0.7 L).

In ARDS patients, Lemaire's group described an inflection point ("knee") on the static inflation V-P curve of the respiratory system (7) and of the lung (4). According to these authors this inflection point should reflect the critical pressure required to reopen previously closed peripheral airways and/or alveoli. On this basis, Matamis and coworkers (7) proposed that the therapeutic level of PEEP should correspond to the "knee." This notion implies that recruitment is an all-or-none phenomenon, i.e., that there is a single critical pressure at which all closed units reopen. Our results show that in the patients who exhibited alveolar recruitment with PEEP, the inflation V-P curves on ZEEP were characterized by a progressive increase in slope with increasing inflation volume. This suggests that recruitment is a progressive rather than discrete phenomenon. Indeed, the recruited alveolar volume was correlated with the value of the constant c in Eq. 1. This constant is an expression of the rate of change of Cst,rs with increasing lung volume which should reflect recruitment. However, on ZEEP, in three patients the constant c was negative, reflecting a progressive decrease in rate of change of Cst,rs with increasing inflation volume. This was probably due to the fact that in these three patients there was no progressive recruitment with increasing inflation volume and that the functional alveoli were close to their maximal volume.

PEEP was associated with a significant increase in end-inspiratory Pst,rs. At PEEP of 15 cmH_2O, the end-inspiratory values of Pst,rs exceed 40 cmH_2O in most of the patients. At this PEEP level, the patients exhibited a static inflation V-P curve with an upward convexity, indicating alveolar overdistention. The recruited alveolar volume with PEEP of 15 cmH_2O correlated negatively with the end-inspiratory Pst,rs obtained during baseline lung inflation on ZEEP ($V_T = 0.7$ L). This reflects the fact that the patients with high values of end-inspiratory Pst,rs on ZEEP were already in the flat part of the static V-P curve. Higher baseline inflation volumes than 0.7 L should be associated with higher end-inspiratory Pst,rs values with a concomitant recruitment of lung units. In this case, the application of PEEP should elicit a smaller increase in recruited alveolar volume as compared to a lower baseline inflation volume because a high inflation volume should *per se* enhance recruitment due to the concomitant increase in end-inspiratory Pst,rs. In an animal model of ARDS, Corbridge et al. (12) have shown that a small V_T-high PEEP (15 ml/kg and 12 cmH_2O) is a better mode of ventilation than is large V_T-low PEEP (30 ml/kg and 3 cmH_2O) because edema accumulation and shunt are less. In ARDS patients, Kiiski et al. (13) observed that $\dot{D}O_2$ improved after lowering the baseline V_T (10-12 ml/kg) by 25%. Hickling and coworkers (14) reported a reduced ARDS mortality through a reduction of peak airway pressure, low VT and permissive hypercapnia.

We did not find a significant correlation between recruited alveolar volume and change in standard Cst,rs with PEEP. Thus, Cst,rs is not useful to monitor recruitment with PEEP, a conclusion previously reached by Falke (15). Suter and coworkers (2) suggested that "best PEEP" should correspond to the highest value of standard Cst,rs. In their study, however, compliance was not corrected for intrinsic PEEP (PEEPi) (16). According to our results (10), corrected Cst,rs was in most patients highest on ZEEP and hence, using this criterion, "best PEEP" should correspond to ZEEP.

Previous studies (2,3) have shown that the application of PEEP to ARDS patients in general results in an increase in P_aO_2 and $P_{\bar{v}}O_2$ while $\dot{D}O_2$ decreases due to a fall in cardiac output. Our results (10) in eight septic ARDS patients showed that PEEP decreased O_2. Again, according to Suter's criteria (2), "best PEEP" was ZEEP.

In an elegant study of Lemaire's group (17) on patients with acute respiratory failure, PEEP caused a decrease in pulmonary shunting of blood flow and an increase in the nonshunted blood flow. In this study, the fall in cardiac output with PEEP was balanced with dopamine infusion. This supported the hypothesis that PEEP can improve gas exchange by reopening closed alveoli. We agree with this conclusion, when PEEP results in alveolar recruitment. In some patients, however, there is no alveolar recruitment with PEEP (10).

In conclusion, our results suggest that PEEP should not be considered as a standard procedure to be routinely applied to ARDS patients. When PEEP is used, O_2 and static inflation V-P curve should be monitored. Indeed, our study of oxygenation, hemodynamics and respiratory mechanics (10) has shown that in some patients with septic ARDS the optimal physiological pattern was achieved on ZEEP, and hence in these patients "best PEEP" was ZEEP. Other ventilatory strategies such as inverse ratio ventilation, extracorporeal techniques, high frequency ventilation, use of prone posture (18) and mechanical ventilation with low V_T (12-13) should be explored as alternatives.

REFERENCES

1. Ashbaugh DG, Bigelow DB, Petty TL, Levine BE: Acute respiratory disease in adults. Lancet 2:319-23, 1967
2. Suter PM, Fairley HB, Isenberg MD: Optimum end-expiratory airway pressure in patients with acute pulmonary failure. N Engl J Med 292: 284-9, 1975

3. Falke KJ, Pontoppidan H, Kumar A, et al: Ventilation with positive end-expiratory pressure in acute lung disease. J Clin Invest 51:2315-23, 1972

4. Benito S, Lemaire F: Pulmonary pressure-volume relationship in acute respiratory distress syndrome in adults: role of positive end expiratory pressure. J Crit Care 5:27- 34, 1990

5. Gattinoni L, Pesenti A, Avalli L, et al: Pressure-volume curve of total respiratory system in acute respiratory failure. Am Rev Respir Dis 136:730-6, 1987

6. Gattinoni L, Pesenti A, Bombino M, et al: Relationships between lung computed tomographic density, gas exchange, and PEEP in acute respiratory failure. Anesthesiology 69:824-32, 1988

7. Matamis D, Lemaire F, Hart A, et al: Total respiratory pressure-volume curves in the adult respiratory distress syndrome. Chest 86: 58-66, 1984

8. Gattinoni L, Mascheroni D, Basilico E, et al: Volume/pressure curve of total respiratory system in paralyzed patients: artifacts and correction factors. Int Care Med 13: 19-25, 1987

9. Mead J, Collier C: Relation of volume history of lungs to respiratory mechanics in anesthetized dogs. J Appl Physiol 14: 669-78, 1959

10. Ranieri VM, Eissa NT, Corbeil C, et al: Effects of PEEP on alveolar recruitment and gas exchange on ARDS patients. Am Rev Respir Dis (In Press)

11. Levy P, Similowski T, Corbeil C, et al: A method for studying the static volume- pressure curves of the respiratory system during mechanical ventilation. J Crit Care 4:83-9, 1989

12. Corbridge TC, Wood LD, Crawford GP, et al: Adverse effects of large tidal volume and low PEEP in canine acid aspiration. Am Rev Respir Dis 142:311-5, 1990

13. Kiiski R, Takala J, Kari A, Milic-Emili J: Unpublished data.

14. Hickling KG, Henderson SJ, Jackson R: Low mortality associated with low volume pressure limited ventilation with permissive hypercapnia in severe adult respiratory distress syndrome. Crit Care Med 16:372-7, 1990

15. Falke KJ: Do changes in lung compliance allow the determination of "optimal PEEP"? Anaesthetist 29:165-168, 1980

16. Rossi A, Gottfried SB, Zocchi L, et al: Measurement of static compliance of the total respiratory system in patients with acute respiratory failure during mechanical ventilation. Am Rev Respir Dis 131:672-7, 1985

17. Matamis D, Lemaire F, Harf A, et al: Redistribution of pulmonary blood flow induced by positive end-expiratory pressure and dopamine infusion in acute respiratory failure. Am Rev Respir Dis 129:39-44, 1984

18. Stoller JK, Kacmarek RM: Ventilatory strategies in the management of the adult respiratory distress syndrome. Clin Chest Med 4:755-72, 1990

MONITORING CARDIOPULMONARY FUNCTION WITH DUAL OXIMETRY

J. B. Downs

"Assessment" of oxygenation may entail measurement and calculation of a variety of physiologic variables. However, the oxygen tension of arterial blood (P_aO_2) is by far the most common measurement utilized in determining the of "adequacy" of oxygenation. Because of the ease of measurement, P_aO_2, often is used as a guide to oxygen therapy, ventilator adjustment, and other therapeutic interventions. Some clinicians have suggested a mathematical manipulation of P_aO_2, alone or in combination with other variables, to improve diagnostic accuracy and assessment of pulmonary function. The perceived advantage of using the alveolar-arterial O_2 tension difference (AAD), the arterial/alveolar oxygen tension ratio (AAI), the P_aO_2/F_IO_2 ratio (PFI), etc., rather than the P_aO_2 alone, often is far greater than the actual advantage. It is apparent that the ease and efficiency of measurements and calculations have played a greater role in the determination of monitoring practices than accuracy and efficacy. Because of advances in monitoring technology during the last decade, a reassessment of monitoring techniques is indicated.

Ultimately, a primary purpose of the cardiorespiratory system is to deliver an adequate volume of oxygen to the periphery to meet metabolic demand. In the past, measurement techniques for the determination of oxygen delivery (O_2 del) and oxygen consumption ($\dot{V}O_2$ have been cumbersome, time consuming, of questionable accuracy, and difficult to apply in routine clinical situations. Thus, it is not surprising that clinicians have developed only a vague and superficial understanding of oxygen utilization (O_2 util) and its assessment. The flow directed pulmonary artery catheter has brought about significant advances in the monitoring of pulmonary and cardiovascular function. However, until recently, even this

319

T. H. Stanley and R. J. Sperry (eds.), Anesthesia and the Lung 1992, 319–329.
© 1992 Kluwer Academic Publishers.

technology has allowed only intermittent monitoring of some aspects of cardiopulmonary function. Furthermore, guidelines to assist the clinician regarding the efficacy of pulmonary artery catheterization have been vague.

Although the technology for continuous measurement of oxyhemoglobin saturation has been available for more than a decade, widespread interest has been generated only recently. Appropriate use of oximetry requires understanding of the dynamics of oxygen transport and the means by which alteration in cardiopulmonary function may affect arterial and venous oxyhemoglobin saturation. Recent advances in oximetry, both economic and technical, warrant a reconsideration of the appropriateness of current monitoring practices and assessment of newer, and perhaps more accurate, techniques.

For more than two decades, P_aO_2 measurement has formed the basis for pulmonary function monitoring, especially in critically ill patients. For similar period of time, clinicians have debated whether arterial blood oxyhemoglobin saturation (S_aO_2) or P_aO_2 should be monitored. Both measurements have advantages and disadvantages in the accurate assessment of pulmonary function. Similarly, certain clinical circumstances, oxyhemoglobin saturation will allow more accurate monitoring of pulmonary function than will oxygen tension measurement. In a different set of circumstances, the reverse will be true. Arterial hypoxemia may result when some areas of the lung have decreased ventilation ($\dot{V}A$), with relatively higher levels of perfusion ($\dot{Q}$). In addition, as the inspired oxygen concentration (F_IO_2) is decreased, the hypoxemia producing effect of such low $\dot{V}A/\dot{Q}$ areas will be enhanced. Only when an individual breathes pure oxygen will such areas be masked, and subsequent arterial hypoxemia be attributed only to direct, right-to-left intrapulmonary shunting of blood ($\dot{Q}s/\dot{Q}T$). In order to assess the relative importance of areas with low $\dot{V}A/\dot{Q}$, a two-compartment model composed of normal lung and lung with no ventilation, but persistent perfusion, was proposed. In order to calculate physiologic right-to-left intrapulmonary shunting of blood using this two-compartment model ($F_IO_2 < 1.0$), the clinician must have access to mixed venous blood from the pulmonary artery (1,2). Until recently, such access was relatively uncommon. This limitation led clinicians to assume a fixed value for mixed venous blood oxygen content and arterial-venous blood oxygen content difference ($C_{(a-\bar{v})}O_2$). By so doing, any variation in arterial blood oxygen content, saturation, or oxygen tension would be attributed to alteration in pulmonary function. Thus, P_aO_2-based calculations of AAD, AAI, PFI, etc. were proposed to assess the efficiency of pulmonary gas exchange. Unfortunately, a fixed value for the arterial-mixed venous blood oxygen content difference may not be assumed, and any variable based on such and assumption is likely to be grossly inaccurate, especially in critically ill patients (Fig. 1). In fact, any alteration in cardiac output, oxygen consumption, or hemoglobin concentration will have an impact on mixed venous blood oxygen content, and therefore, on arterial oxygen content, saturation, and tension.

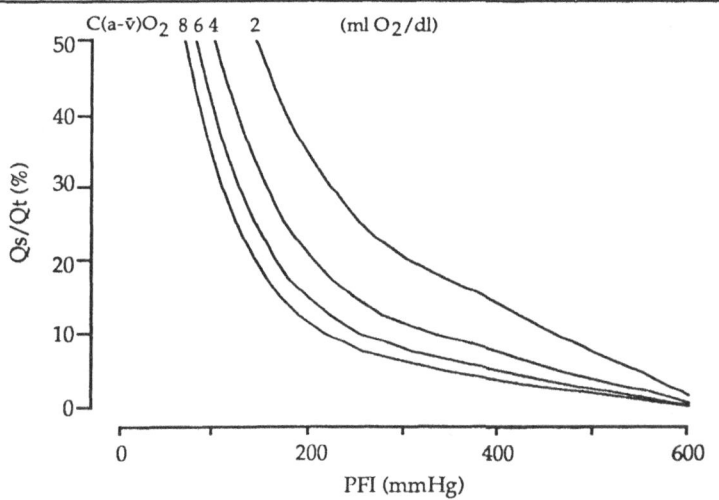

Figure 1. Mathematical relationships between $\dot{Q}_S/\dot{Q}_T$ and PFI, plotted with $C_{(a-\bar{v})}O_2$ levels ranging form 2.0 to 8.0 ml/dl. Average normal values were set for Hgb (15.0 g/dl), P_aCO_2 (40 mmHg), and RQ (0.8). F_IO_2 was assumed to be 0.5.

Analysis of the oxyhemoglobin dissociation curve demonstrates the reason why P_aO_2 alone will not allow accurate assessment of physiologic shunting of blood (Fig. 2). The nonlinear relationship between oxygen tension and oxyhemoglobin saturation has numerous physiologic advantages in terms of oxygen uptake within the lung and oxygen delivery to the periphery. The relatively flat portion of the oxyhemoglobin dissociation curve ensures maximum O_2 loading, even when alveolar O_2 tension is somewhat reduced by $\dot{V}_A/\dot{Q}$ mismatching. At the cellular

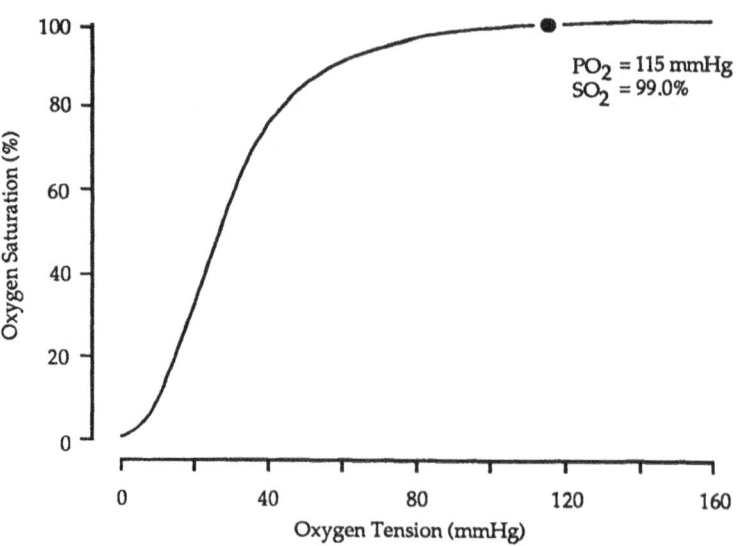

Figure 2. The oxyhemoglobin dissociation curve plotted according to the equation published by Ruiz, et al. (2).

level, the vertical portion of the curve ensures a significant unloading of oxygen with little change in oxygen tension. Even though this nonlinear relationship is advantageous, it causes accurate assessment of pulmonary function to be complex. Small changes in $\dot{V}A/\dot{Q}$ mismatching may cause large changes in P_aO_2 when P_aO_2 is high (i.e., >115 mmHg). However, because of the vertical portion of the oxyhemoglobin dissociation curve, large increases in shunting of blood may be undetected secondary to small changes in P_aO_2 associated with oxyhemoglobin desaturation. For that reason, clinicians have suggested that the F_IO_2 be elevated for P_aO_2 determination, so that arterial oxyhemoglobin saturation approaches 100%. Although the F_IO_2 may be safely elevated for a short period of time on an intermittent basis, routine and continuous monitoring of pulmonary function with elevated F_IO_2 is inaccurate and impractical. When 100% oxygen is used and $(C_{(a-\bar{v})}O_2)$ is normal, P_aO_2 based gas exchange indices reflect pulmonary gas exchange in a linear fashion only up to a $\dot{Q}s/\dot{Q}\tau$ of $\approx 30\%$, and then only when $F_IO_2 = 1.0$ (Fig. 3). If $\dot{Q}s/\dot{Q}\tau$ is higher, the nonlinearity of the oxyhemoglobin dissociation curve will make these indices insensitive to further impairment in gas exchange. Additional inaccuracy is introduced by the increase in $\dot{Q}s/\dot{Q}\tau$ during pure

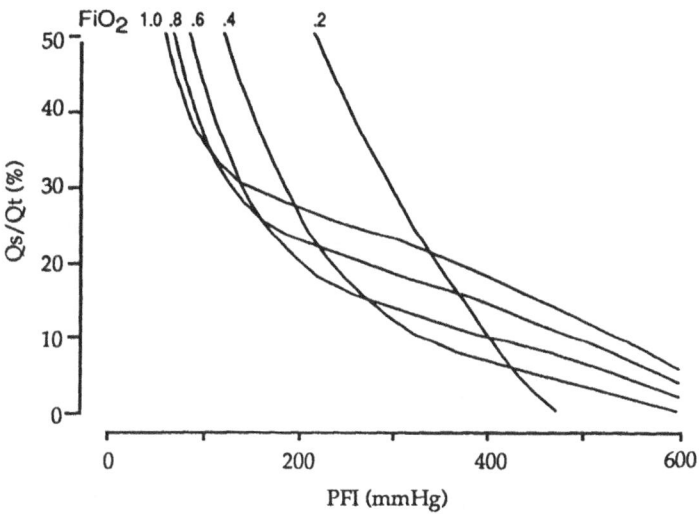

Figure 3. Mathematical relationships between $\dot{Q}_S/\dot{Q}_T$ and PFI, plotted with F_IO_2 levels ranging from 0.21 to 1.0. Average normal values were set for Hgb (15.0 g/dl), P_aCO_2 (40 mmHg), and RQ (0.8). $C_{(a-\bar{v})}O_2$ was assumed to be 4.0 ml/dl.

oxygen breathing (3). Because of the various sources of error, correlation coefficients between $\dot{Q}_S/\dot{Q}_T$ and the oxygen tension based estimates range from 0.45 to 0.75 (4,5). These indices are more accurate when P_aO_2 is high (r = 0.84 - 0.90; P_aO_2 > 115 mmHg; S_aO_2 > 99.0%), but their accuracy is severely reduced (r = 0.10 - 0.54) when P_aO_2 values fall on the descending portion of the oxyhemoglobin dissociation curve (P_aO_2 <115 mmHg, S_aO_2 < 99.0%). Recently, D. Valentine, MD compared the AAD, PFI and AAI to calculated $\dot{Q}_S/\dot{Q}_T$ in patients who received cardiopulmonary bypass. Even when F_IO_2 was elevated to 0.5, the correlation between the O_2 tension based indices and $\dot{Q}_S/\dot{Q}_T$ was clinically unacceptable (Fig. 4) (personal communication).

It long has been our contention that application of low F_IO_2 may have significant benefits (3,6). A low F_IO_2 will avoid oxygen toxicity and absorption atelectasis. In addition, the hypoxemia producing effect of areas of lung with decreased $\dot{V}A/\dot{Q}$ will be more apparent with low F_IO_2. Most importantly, when arterial oxyhemoglobin saturation is less than 100%, accurate assessment of pulmonary function by measurement of arterial oxyhemoglobin saturation becomes possible. Because a linear relationship

324

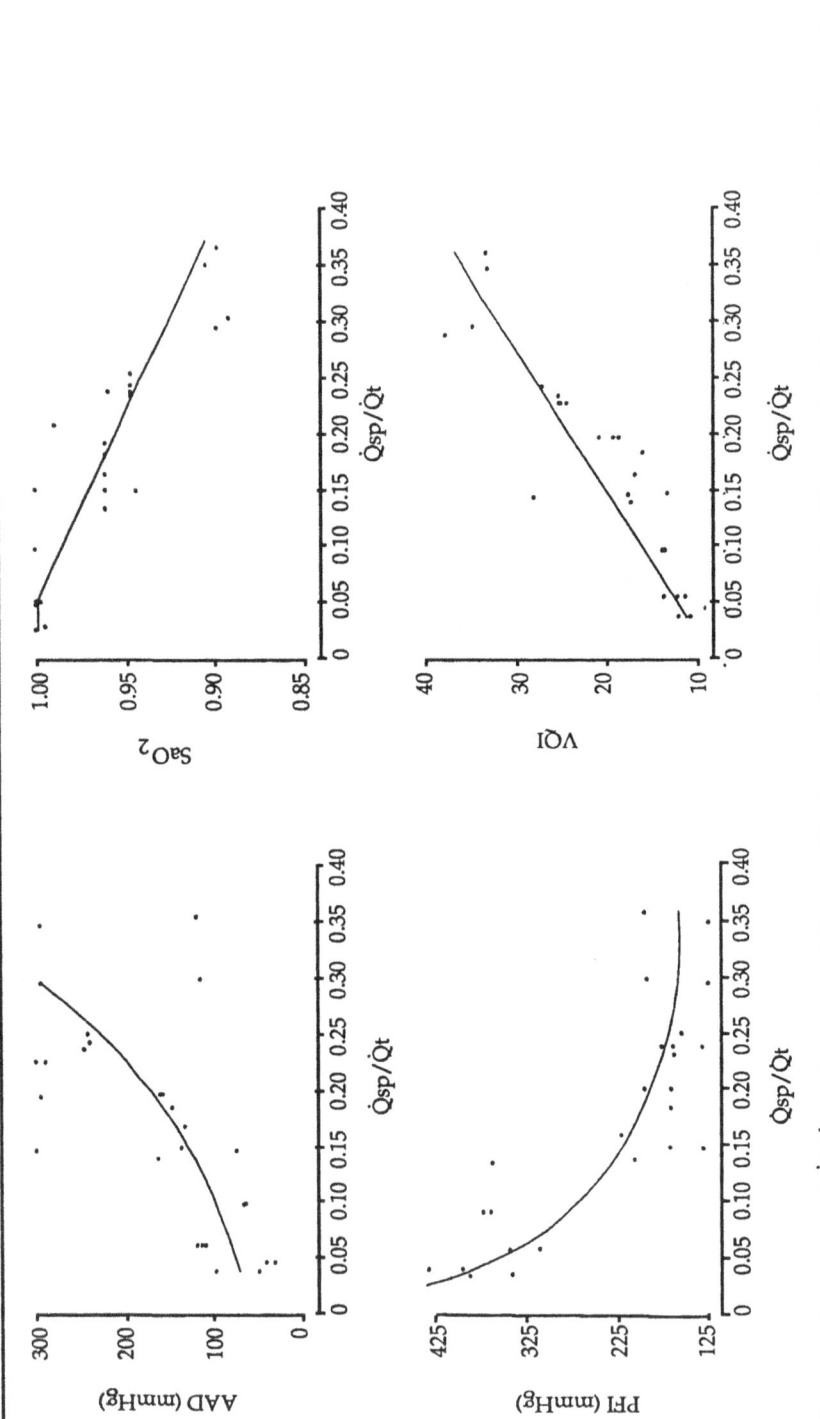

Figure 4. Comparison of Q̇S/Q̇t with AAD, AAI, PFI and VQI (Data provided by Valentine, Hammond and Downs). Data derived from patients following cardiopulmonary bypass breathing 40% oxygen.

exists between S_aO_2 and $\dot{Q}_S/\dot{Q}_T$, estimation of pulmonary function is _easier_ for the clinician when using S_aO_2, than when using O_2 tension based indices. In contrast to intermittent sampling of blood for measurement of P_aO_2, continuous measurement of arterial oxyhemoglobin saturation is clinically practical. Thus, continuous assessment of pulmonary function may occur when arterial oxyhemoglobin saturation measurement is employed. By combining measurement of arterial oxyhemoglobin saturation with mixed venous oxyhemoglobin saturation, accurate estimation of physiologic shunting of blood is possible. Right-to-left intrapulmonary shunt can be approximated by the ventilation perfusion index (VQI) derived as follows:

$$\frac{\dot{Q}_S}{\dot{Q}_T} = \frac{S\acute{c}O_2 - S_aO_2}{S\acute{c}O_2 - S\bar{v}O_2} \approx VQI$$

Here, SO_2 is the oxyhemoglobin saturation of arterial (a) mixed venous ($\bar{v}$) and pulmonary end-capillary ($\acute{c}$) blood. Thus, measurement of arterial and venous oxyhemoglobin saturation will permit continuous assessment of pulmonary function without alteration of clinically applicable F_IO_2. Calculation of VQI provides a linear estimate of $\dot{Q}_S/\dot{Q}_T$ because the effect of the oxyhemoglobin dissociation curve is absent. Since changes in mixed venous oxygenation are taken into account, alterations in peripheral oxygen delivery and consumption have little effect on the estimate (Fig. 5). We found a correlation coefficient of 0.92 between $\dot{Q}_S/\dot{Q}_T$ and its oxyhemoglobin saturation based estimate, VQI (5). Valentine found the same correlation (r=.92) when he compared the VQI to shunting by measuring with the multiple inert gas elimination technique described Drs. Wagner, West and Saltzman (Fig. 4) (personal communication). Thus, VQI is a clinically useful and accurate calculation. The accuracy of this index is maintained as long as arterial oxyhemoglobin saturation has value other than 100%.

Alteration of respiratory therapy may occur frequently in critical care settings. Usually, major changes in therapy are assessed no more frequently than hourly. However, changes in continuous positive airway pressure (CPAP) have been shown to result in equilibration of functional residual capacity in less than one minute. Equilibration of arterial oxygen tension occurs in a similar time frame (7). Change in F_IO_2 results in rapid

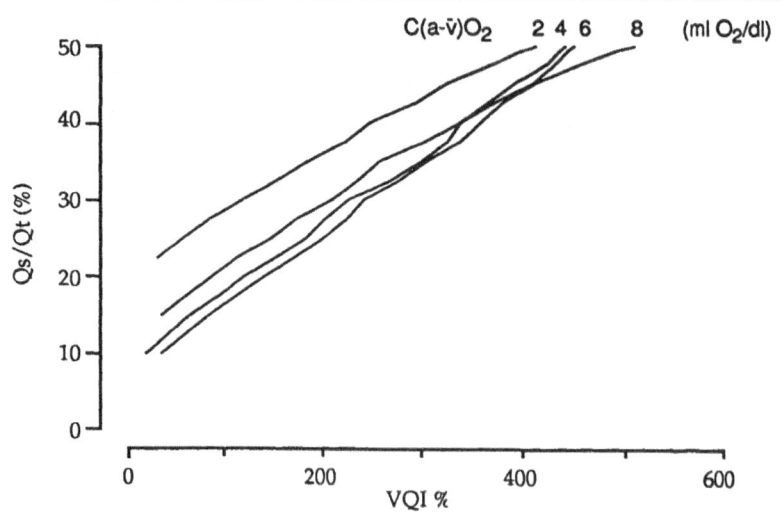

Figure 5. Mathematical relationships between $\dot{Q}S/\dot{Q}T$ and VQI, plotted with $C_{(a-\bar{v})}O_2$ levels ranging from 2.0 to 8.0 ml/dl. Average normal values were set for Hgb (15.0 g/dl), P_aCO_2 (40 mmHg), and RQ (0.8). F_IO_2 was assumed to be 0.5.

alteration in P_aO_2. Therefore, it is evident that major alterations in respiratory therapy should be evaluated within minutes, rather than the current practice of waiting one or two hours following change. Continuous measurement of arterial and mixed venous oxyhemoglobin saturation using combined pulse and pulmonary artery oximetry (dual oximetry) permits such assessment. In addition, clinically unsuspected changes in the patient's pulmonary function will be detected more rapidly with continuous measurement techniques than with intermittent sampling of arterial and venous blood. Alterations in therapy then will be triggered directly by the primary change in lung function rather than by secondary hemodynamic change that normally would initiate blood sampling. Data from arterial and mixed venous saturation monitors easily can be transformed to estimate gas exchange in a real-time fashion using on-line calculation of VQI. This procedure obviates the delay associated with data interpretation at the monitor-observer interface (Fig. 6).

Invasive monitoring of cardiac function has become commonplace in most critical care units. Usually, clinically appropriate assessment of cardiac function includes measurement of cardiac filling pressure and stroke volume. However, "adequacy" of cardiac performance, in terms of

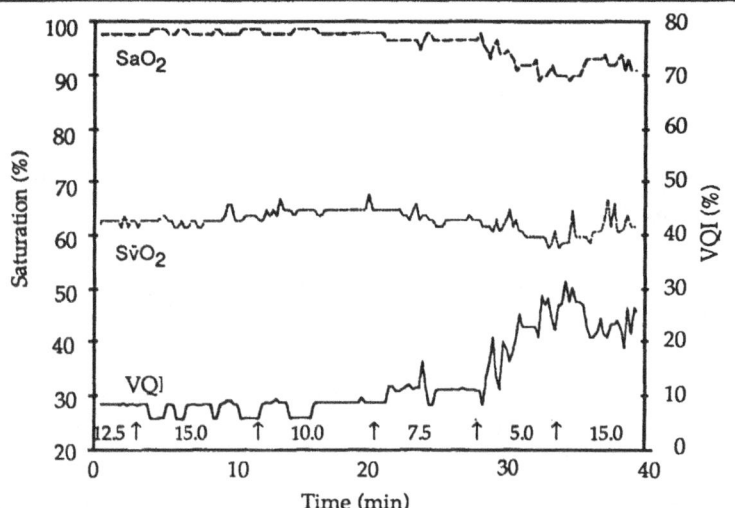

Figure 6. Changes in S_aO_2, SO_2, and VQI at varying levels of CPAP in a patient with acute pulmonary insufficiency.

oxygen delivery, has only recently been widely appreciated. For example, a cardiac output of 10 L/min would be more than adequate in most clinical settings. However, an anemic patient with increased oxygen consumption might require an even higher cardiac output to meet peripheral oxygen demand. Ideally, the clinician should have some means of assessing oxygen delivery relative to oxygen demand. Oxygen delivery depends not only on cardiac output, but on arterial oxygen content, as well. Arterial blood oxygen content is determined by hemoglobin concentration and oxyhemoglobin saturation, and is relatively independent of the dissolved oxygen. Oxygen consumption of an organ system depends on metabolic demand. However, blood flow to the organ system, distribution of blood flow within the system, distance from the capillary to the cell, and the oxygen tension gradient between the capillary and the cell also play critical roles. The diffusion gradient may depend on the oxyhemoglobin saturation and the relative position of the oxyhemoglobin dissociation curve.

The relationship between oxygen delivery and oxygen consumption for any organ system will determine the "adequacy" of oxygenation. Although it is possible to assess oxygen utilization of some organ systems, for most such assessment is clinically difficult. It is possible to assess global oxygen utilization by measurement of systemic oxygen delivery and total body oxygen consumption.

$$O_2 \text{ utilization } = \frac{O_2}{O_2 \text{ del}}$$

Further expansion of this equation results in a readily applicable oxygen extraction index (O_2EI):

$$O_2 \text{ utilization } = \frac{CO \times Ca\text{-}\bar{v}O_2}{CO \times CaO_2} = \frac{Ca\text{-}\bar{v}O_2}{CaO_2} = 1 - \frac{C\bar{v}O_2}{CaO_2}$$

$$= 1 - \frac{Hgb \times 1.34 \times S\bar{v}O_2 + P\bar{v}O_2 \times .0031}{Hgb \times 1.34 \times S_aO_2 + P_aO_2 + P_aO_2 \times .0031} \approx 1 - \frac{S\bar{v}O_2}{S_aO_2}$$

Thus, mixed venous oxygen saturation accurately represents total body oxygen utilization (8). Several investigators have shown that mixed venous oxygen saturation more accurately predicts the ratio between oxygen consumption and oxygen delivery than does cardiac output, arterial oxygen tension, arterial oxygen delivery, oxygen consumption, or any other variable suggested for assessment of "adequacy" of oxygenation (1). Use of SO_2 to estimate oxygen utilization assumes complete saturation of arterial blood oxyhemoglobin. When dual oximetry is used, such an assumption no longer is necessary, and the accuracy of the estimate will improve accordingly. Thus, we suggest use of the oxygen extraction index (O_2EI).

$$O_2EI = 1 - \frac{S_a\bar{v}O_2}{S_aO_2}$$

There is sound physiologic basis for continuous monitoring of arterial and mixed venous oxyhemoglobin saturation. Dual oximetry will provide simultaneous, real-time estimates of two critically important body functions, pulmonary gas exchange and peripheral tissue oxygen utilization (9). There is little doubt that application of these techniques will improve the efficacy of therapy with vasoactive and cardiotonic drugs, oxygen, mechanical ventilation, and CPAP. It is likely that time and cost savings will result and that morbidity and mortality may decrease.

GENERAL REFERENCES

1. Mitchell LA, Downs JB, Dannemiller FJ: Extrapulmonary influences on A-aDO$_2$ following cardiopulmonary bypass. Anesthesiology 43:583-86, 1975
2. Ruiz BC, Tucker WK, Kirby RR: A program for calculating intrapulmonary shunt, blood-gas, and acid-base values with a programmable calculator. Anesthesiology 42:88-95, 1975
3. Douglas ME, Downs JB, Dannemiller FJ, et al: Change in pulmonary venous admixture with varying inspired oxygen. Anesth Analg 55:688-95, 1976
4. Covelli HD, Nessan VJ, Tuttle WK: Oxygen derived variables in acute respiratory failure. Crit Care Med 11:646-49, 1983
5. Räsänen J, Downs JB, Malec DJ, et al: Oxygen tensions and oxyhemoglobin saturations in the assessment of pulmonary gas exchange. Crit Care Med 15:1058- 61, 1987
6. Register SD, Downs JB, Stock MC, et al: Is 50% oxygen harmful? Crit Care Med 15:598-601, 1987
7. Rose DM, Downs JB, Heenan TJ: Temporal responses of functional residual capacity and oxygen tension to changes in positive end-expiratory pressure. Crit Care Med 9:79-82, 1981
8. Nelson LD: Continuous venous oximetry in surgical patients. Ann Surg 203:349-52, 1983
9. Räsänen J, Downs JB, Malec DJ, et al: Real-time continuous estimation of gas exchange by dual oximetry. Intensive Care Med 14:118-22, 1988

DEVELOPMENTS IN
CRITICAL CARE MEDICINE AND ANESTHESIOLOGY

DEVELOPMENTS IN
CRITICAL CARE MEDICINE AND ANESTHESIOLOGY

KLUWER ACADEMIC PUBLISHERS – DORDRECHT / BOSTON / LONDON

The manufacturer's authorised representative in the EU is Springer
Nature Customer Service Centre GmbH, Europaplatz 3, 69115 Heidelberg,
Germany. If you have any concerns regarding our products, please
contact ProductSafety@springernature.com

Printed and bound by CPI Group (UK) Ltd, Croydon, CR0 4YY

23/04/2026

02095629-0003